W9-BSA-201

The Cardiac Renin-Angiotensin System

edited by

Klaus Lindpaintner, M.D.

*Brigham and Women's Hospital
and Children's Hospital;
Harvard Medical School
Boston, Massachusetts*

and

Detlev Ganten, M.D., Ph.D.

*Max-Delbrück Center for Molecular Medicine (MDC)
Berlin-Buch, Germany*

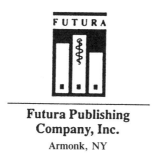

**Futura Publishing
Company, Inc.**
Armonk, NY

Library of Congress Cataloging-in-Publication Data

The Cardiac renin-angiotensin system / edited by Klaus
    Lindpaintner and Detlev Ganten.
        p.   cm.
    Includes bibliographical references and index.
    ISBN 0-87993-571-5
    1. Heart—Molecular aspects. 2. Renin. 3. Angiotensin.
    4. Heart—Pathophysiology. I. Lindpaintner, Klaus. II. Ganten, D.
    (Detlev), 1941–
    [DNLM: 1. Renin-Angiotensin System—physiology. 2.
    Myocardium—enzymology. 3. Myocardial Diseases—
    physiopathology. WG 280 C26664 1994]
    QP114.M65C37 1994
    612.1'73—dc20
    DNLM/DLC
    for Library of Congress   93-39407
                                                                    CIP

Copyright 1994
Futura Publishing Company, Inc.

Published by
Futura Publishing Company, Inc.
135 Bedford Road
Armonk, New York 10504

LC #: 93-39407
ISBN #: 0-87993-571-5

Printed in the United States of America.

This book is printed on acid-free paper.

Contributors

R. Wayne Alexander, M.D., Ph.D.
R. Bruce Logue Professor of Medicine, Division of Cardiology, Emory University, Atlanta, Georgia

Andrew M. Allen, Ph.D.
NHMRC Australian C.J. Martin Research Fellow, Howard Florey Institute of Experimental Physiology and Medicine, University of Melbourne, Victoria, Australia

Michael Bader, Ph.D.
German Institute for High Blood Pressure Research and Department of Pharmacology, University of Heidelberg, Heidelberg, Germany

Kenneth M. Baker, M.D.
Staff scientist, Weis Center for Research, Geisinger Clinic, Danville, Pennsylvania

George W. Booz, Ph.D.
Associate Scientist, Weis Center for Research, Geisinger Clinic, Danville, Pennsylvania

Christian G. Brilla, M.D., Ph.D.
Associate Professor of Medicine, Division of Cardiology, Philipps University of Marburg, Marburg, Germany

F. Merlin Bumpus, Ph.D. (deceased)
Emeritus Staff, Department of Cardiovascular Biology, Research Institute, Cleveland Clinic Foundation, Cleveland, Ohio

Scott E. Campbell, Ph.D.
Assistant Professor of Medicine, Division of Cardiology, Department of Internal Medicine, University of Missouri-Columbia, Columbia, Missouri

Pieter A. de Graeff, M.D., Ph.D.
Assistant Professor, Department of Pharmacology/Clinical Pharmacology, University of Groningen, Groningen, The Netherlands

Rainer Dietz, M.D.
Universitätsklinikum Rudolf Virchow, Franz-Volhard-Klinik, Max-Delbrück Centrum für Molekulare Medizin, Berlin-Buch, Germany

David E. Dostal, Ph.D.
Associate Scientist, Weis Center for Research, Geisinger Clinic, Danville, Pennsylvania

Victor Dzau, M.D.
William G. Irwin Professor of Medicine and Chief, Division of Cardiovascular Medicine, Stanford University School of Medicine, Stanford, California

Maria S. Fernandez-Alfonso, Ph.D.
German Institute for High Blood Pressure Research and Department of Pharmacology, University of Heidelberg, Heidelberg, Germany

Detlev Ganten, M.D., Ph.D.
Scientific Director, Max-Delbrück Center for Molecular Medicine, Berlin-Buch, Germany

Peter Gohlke, Ph.D.
German Institute for High Blood Pressure Research and Department of Pharmacology, University of Heidelberg, Heidelberg, Germany

Kathy K. Griendling, Ph.D.
Assistant Professor of Medicine, Division of Cardiology, Emory University, Atlanta, Georgia

Traudel Hellmann, D.MSc.
German Institute for High Blood Pressure Research and Department of Pharmacology, University of Heidelberg, Heidelberg, Germany

Alan Hirsch, M.D.
Assistant Professor of Medicine and Director, Vascular Medicine Program, University of Minnesota Medical School, Minneapolis, Minnesota

Ahsan Husain, Ph.D.
Associate Staff, Department of Cardiovascular Biology, Research Institute, Cleveland Clinic Foundation, Cleveland, Ohio

Manwen Jin, D. MSc.
Department of Pharmacology, University of Wuhan, Wuhan, People's Republic of China, and German Institute for High Blood Pressure Research, Heidelberg, Germany

Reinhold Kreutz, M.D.
Division of Cardiology, Children's Hospital, Boston, Massachusetts

Akio Kinoshita, M.D.
Assistant, Department of Medicine, Fukuoka University, Fukuoka, Japan

Gervasio Lamas, M.D.
Chief of Cardiology, Mount Sinai Medical Center, Miami Beach, Florida

Young-Ae Lee, M.D.
Department of Cardiology, Children's Hospital, Harvard Medical School, Boston, Massachusetts

Klaus Lindpaintner, M.D., F.A.C.P.
Assistant Professor of Medicine, Harvard Medical School; Division of Cardiovascular Medicine, Brigham and Women's Hospital, Boston, Massachusetts; and Department of Cardiology, Children's Hospital

Wolfgang Linz, V.M.D.
Department of Pharmacology, Hoechst AG, Frankfurt/Main, Germany

Beverly H. Lorell, M.D.
Associate Professor of Medicine, The Charles A. Dana Research Institute and the Department of Cardiology, Beth Israel Hospital and Harvard Medical School, Boston, Massachusetts

Yi-kun Lou, B.M.
Graduate student (Ph.D. program), Department of Physiology, University of Sydney, Sydney, Australia

Xixian Liu, M.D.
German Institute for High Blood Pressure Research and Department of Pharmacology, University of Heidelberg, Heidelberg, Germany

Frederick A.O. Mendelsohn, M.D., Ph.D., F.R.A.C.P.
Professor of Medicine, University of Melbourne, Austin and Repatriation General Hospitals, Victoria, Australia

Brian J. Morris, D.Sc.
Reader in Physiology, Molecular Biology and Hypertension Laboratory, Department of Physiology, University of Sydney, Sydney, Australia

Michael R. Muellerleile, M.D.
Cardiology Fellow, University of Minnesota Medical School, Minneapolis, Minnesota

Masahiro Nagano, M.D.
Assistant Professor of Medicine, Department of Geriatric Medicine, Osaka University Medical School, Yamadaoka, Japan

Nikolaj Niedermaier, M.D.
Department of Medicine, University of Heidelberg Hospitals and Clinics, Heidelberg, Germany

Toshio Ogihara, M.D.
Professor of Medicine, Department of Geriatric Medicine, Oshaka University Medical School, Yamadaoka, Japan

Karl Josef Osterziel, M.D.
Universitätsklinikum Rudolf Virchow, Franz-Volhard-Klinik, Max-Delbrück Centrum für Molekulare Medizin, Berlin-Buch, Germany

Martin Paul, M.D.
German Institute for High Blood Pressure Research and the Department of Pharmacology, University of Heidelberg, Heidelberg, Germany

Marc A. Pfeffer, M.D., Ph.D.
Associate Professor of Medicine, Harvard Medical School, Cardiovascular Division, Brigham and Women's Hospital, Boston, Massachusetts

Richard N. Re, M.D.
Vice-President and Director of Research, Alton Ochsner Medical Foundation, Division of Research, New Orleans, Louisiana

Juan M. Saavedra, M.D.
Chief, Section on Pharmacology, Laboratory of Clinical Science, National Institute of Mental Health, National Institutes of Health, Bethesda, Maryland

Bernwald A. Schölkens, M.D.
Professor of Pharmacology, Hoechst AG, Frankfurt/Main, Germany

Heribert Schunkert, M.D.
Instructor in Medicine, Department of Internal Medicine II, University of Regensburg, Regensberg, Germany

Kazuto Shigematsu, M.D., Ph.D.
Associate Professor, Department of Pathology, Nagasaki University Medical School, Nagasaki, Japan

Yao Sun, M.D.
Department of Medicine, Division of Cardiology, University of Missouri, Columbia, Missouri

Shen-Shu Sung, Ph.D.
Assistant Staff, Department of Cardiovascular Biology, Research Institute, Cleveland Clinic Foundation, Cleveland, Ohio

Thomas Unger, M.D.
Professor of Pharmacology, German Institute for High Blood Pressure Research, University of Heidelberg, Heidelberg, Germany

Hidenori Urata, Ph.D.
Fellow, Max-Delbrück Center for Molecular Medicine, Berlin-Buch, Germany

Wiek H. van Gilst, Ph.D.
Assistant Professor, Department of Pharmacology/Clinical Pharmacology, University of Groningen, Groningen, The Netherlands

Mohan Viswanathan, Ph.D.
Visiting Scientist, Section of Pharmacology, Laboratory of Clinical Science, National Institute of Mental Health, National Institutes of Health, Bethesda, Maryland

Jürgen Wagner, M.D.
German Institute for High Blood Pressure Research and Department of Pharmacology, University of Heidelberg, Heidelberg, Germany

Karl T. Weber, M.D.
Chairman, Department of Internal Medicine, and Director, Division of Cardiology, University of Missouri-Columbia, Columbia, Missouri

Harry Wesseling, M.D., Ph.D.
Professor of Clinical Pharmacology, Department of Pharmacology/Clinical Pharmacology, University of Groningen, Groningen, The Netherlands

Gabriele Wiemer, Ph.D.
Professor of Pharmacology, Hoechst AG, Frankfurt/Main, Germany

Hiroshi Yamada, M.D.
Department of Pediatrics, Osaka City University Medical School, Osaka, Japan

Jialong Zhuo, Ph.D.
NHMRC Australian Postdoctoral Research Fellow, University of Melbourne, Department of Medicine, Austin and Repatriation General Hospitals, Victoria, Australia

To Lyn, Julia, Eva, and Ursula,

*who have contributed in so many ways
to this work.*

K.L.
D.G.

Preface

The past decade has witnessed the accumulation of a body of knowledge about a hitherto unrecognized facet of the renin-angiotensin system: the heart, too, among a number of organs, harbors its own renin-angiotensin system. Owing to the potential implications that local synthesis and the action of angiotensin peptides in the heart may have, much interest and the work of many laboratories worldwide have focused on the elucidation of the nature and role of this system. As a result, we have arrived at a still sketchy but, in its principal outlines, well-founded conceptual understanding of this system. The process by which the present understanding came about is, in itself, remarkable and exemplary for the fruits that the interaction of basic research and clinical investigation may bear: rarely in the history of biomedical research has there been as intensive a give-and-take between clinicians and basic scientists that resulted so quickly in the implementation and understanding of novel therapeutic modalities. Important advances in the clinical management of entities such as congestive heart failure and postmyocardial infarction ventricular remodeling, ushered in by the use of angiotensin-converting enzyme inhibitors, prompted the research community to search with increased enthusiasm for underlying mechanisms. Their work has not only provided us with solid evidence for the existence of the cardiac renin-angiotensin system but is unraveling complex regulatory interactions between hemodynamic parameters and the expression of components of this system in normal and diseased states. The progress made in the elaboration of this system was heavily dependent on the use of recombinant DNA technology; in this respect, again, the work on the cardiac renin-angiotensin system was exemplary in the early application of these techniques and stands as a paradigm for recent developments and advances in molecular cardiology.

Although much remains to be learned about the nature and role of the cardiac renin-angiotensin system, enough information has been accumulated to take stock and assemble a volume that, although by necessity incomplete owing to the rapid pace of research activities in the field, will provide an easily accessible review of the current state of knowledge about this system. We have been privileged to orchestrate this effort and are deeply indebted to all the contributing authors whose generosity and cooperation have made this book possible. We hope that it will not only serve as a reference base but that it will foster new ideas and innovative investigational approaches. These, in turn, will further enhance our understanding of this system and may eventually contribute to novel therapeutic strategies to combat human illness, thus fulfilling biomedical research's noblest and ultimate goal.

Klaus Lindpaintner, M.D.
Detlev Ganten, M.D., Ph.D.

Foreword

The ongoing story of the renin-angiotensin system (RAS) is one of the most important and fascinating in modern biology and medicine. In 1898, Tigerstedt and Bergmann isolated a pressor substance from the kidney, and in 1934 Goldblatt demonstrated that constriction of one renal artery caused release of this substance, now known to be renin, from the kidney. These observations led to the appreciation of the role of the RAS in renal vascular hypertension and later, when the important role of angiotensin II in the control of mineralocorticoid metabolism and thirst became clarified, it became evident that the renal RAS (more properly, the renin-angiotensin-aldosterone system) had a central role in circulatory homeostasis and control—a role comparable in importance to that of the sympathoadrenal system. By 1970, the renal RAS had emerged as an important endocrine system, complete with feedback inhibition loops.

In the last two decades the situation has become more complex and interesting. First, it has been shown that many extrarenal tissues contain renin. Indeed, *all* of the components of the RAS system—including renin, angiotensinogen, angiotensin converting enzyme (ACE), angiotensin II, and its receptors—are found in numerous organs. Simultaneously, it was discovered that ACE inhibitors are effective not only in hypertensive patients with elevated circulating renin levels, but also in those patients with normal and even low renin levels. The convergence of these two streams of observations led to the hypothesis that the tissue RASs might be as, or more, important than the circulating RAS. Subsequent work has shown that tissue RASs operate in paracrine, autocrine, and intracrine modes.

Considerably more information is available on the RAS in the cardiovascular system than in any other extrarenal system. This information is summarized lucidly and comprehensively in this volume, superbly planned and edited by Lindpaintner and Ganten, two distinguished investigators who themselves have contributed so much to this important field. The cardiac RAS is involved in a broad array of critical functions—control of cardiac contraction, relaxation, heart rate, the electrical properties of the cardiac conduction system, coronary vascular tone, cardiac metabolism, the expression of protooncogenes that enhance myocyte protein synthesis and thereby hypertrophy, and in the proliferation of fibroblasts and of coronary vascular smooth muscle. Angiotensin II also plays an important role in the release of sympathetic neurotransmitters and of the potent vasoconstrictor endothelin. Angiotensin II receptors are abundant in areas of the brain involved in the control of cardiac function via the autonomic nervous system as well as in peripheral sympathetic ganglia. Activation of these receptors appears to influence cardiovascular function both directly and indirectly.

Although not strictly a component of the cardiac RAS, the kinin-kallikrein system is appropriately reviewed since it influences the mechanism of action of ACE inhibitors. There is a discussion of chymase, a serine protease, which is not blocked by ACE inhibitors, and whose activity in the formation of angiotensin II in the human ventricle is greater than that of ACE.

This book reviews the accumulating evidence that interference with the cardiac RAS by means of ACE inhibition can ameliorate the deleterious effects of activation of the system. The interesting clinical observations that blockade of the RAS improves survival in postmyocardial infarct patients who are neither hypertensive nor in heart failure and that it reduces the incidence of recurrent myocardial infarction and the need for coronary revascularization provide strong, albeit indirect, evidence for the importance of the cardiac RAS in ischemic heart disease.

This volume also casts a sharp eye on the future and outlines areas that are now ripe for intensive investigation. These include the study of different classes of angiotensin II receptors (including those situated on nuclear chromatin), a clearer definition of the manner in which angiotensin II affects gene transcription and expression, the potential use of antisense oligonucleotides directed against angiotensinogen mRNA to interfere with the synthesis of angiotensin, and the application of transgenic animals in elucidation of the role of the cardiac RAS.

An understanding of the role of the cardiac RAS is of growing importance to a variety of cardiovascular scientists—molecular biologists, biochemists, physiologists, and pharmacologists—as well as to clinical investigators and trainees. All will be richly rewarded by the extensive, up-to-date, and critically reviewed information in this valuable book.

Eugene Braunwald, M.D.
Hersey Professor of the Theory
and Practice of Medicine
Brigham and Women's Hospital
Harvard Medical School
Boston, Massachusetts

Contents

Preface: Klaus Lindpaintner, M.D., and Detlev Ganten
M.D., Ph.D. ix
Foreword: Eugene Braunwald, M.D. xi
Abbreviations xvi

1. **The Cardiac Renin-Angiotensin System:**
    An Overview
    David E. Dostal, George W. Booz,
    and Kenneth M. Baker 1

2. **Cardiac Renin, Gene Expression, and Regulation**
    Brian J. Morris and Yi-kun Lou 21

3. **Cardiac Angiotensinogen: Its Local Activation to**
    Angiotensin Peptides and Its Regulation
    Young-Ae Lee, Manwen Jin, Traudel Hellmann,
    Nikolaj Niedermaier, Detlev Ganten, and
    Klaus Lindpaintner 47

4. **Localization and Properties of the Angiotensin-**
    Converting Enzyme and Angiotensin Receptors in
    the Heart
    Jialong Zhuo, Andrew M. Allen, Hiroshi Yamada,
    Yao Sun, and Frederick A.O. Mendelsohn 63

5. **Cloning of the Angiotensin AT_1 Receptor and Its**
    Expression in Cardiac Tissue
    Kathy K. Griendling and R. Wayne Alexander 89

6. **Regulation of Cardiac Second Messengers by**
    Angiotensins
    George W. Booz, David E. Dostal,
    and Kenneth E. Baker 101

7. **Characterization and Localization of Angiotensin**
    Receptors in Central and Autonomic Nervous
    Systems Regulating Heart Function
    Juan M. Saavedra, Mohan Viswanathan,
    and Kazuo Shigematsu 125

8. **The Renin-Angiotensin System As a Growth Regulator in Cardiovascular and Non-Cardiovascular Tissues**
   Richard N. Re 141

9. **Myocardial Fibrosis: Structural Basis for Pathological Remodeling and the Role of the Renin-Angiotensin-Aldosterone System**
   Scott E. Campbell, Christian G. Brilla,
   and Karl T. Weber 153

10. **Role of the Cardiac Renin-Angiotensin System in Left-Ventricular Hypertrophy**
    Masahiro Nagano and Toshio Ogihara 167

11. **Induction of the Cardiac Angiotensin-Converting Enzyme in Pressure-Overload Hypertrophy: Implications for Diastolic Function**
    Beverly H. Lorell and Heribert Schunkert 183

12. **The Cardiac Renin-Angiotensin System in Different Ischemic Syndromes of the Heart**
    Pieter A. de Graeff, Wiek H. van Gilst,
    and Harry Wesseling 201

13. **The Contribution of Tissue Renin-Angiotensin Systems to Disease Progression in Experimental Heart Failure**
    Alan T. Hirsch, Michael R. Muellerleile,
    and Victor J. Dzau 233

14. **The Contribution of Bradykinin to the Cardiovascular Actions of ACE Inhibitors**
    Wolfgang Linz, Gabriele Wiemer, Peter Gohlke,
    Thomas Unger, and Bernward A. Schölkens 253

15. **Transgenic Rats Expressing Components of the Renin-Angiotensin System: Focus on Cardiovascular Regulation**
    Martin Paul, Jürgen Wagner, Reinhold Kreutz,
    Maria S. Fernandez-Alfonso, Yixian Liu,
    Michael Bader, and Detlev Gantlen 289

16. **Human Heart Chymase**
    Ahsan Husain, Akio Kinoshita, Shen-Shu Sung,
    Hidenori Urata, and F. Merlin Bumpus 309

17. **The Cardiac Renin-Angiotensin System and Human Coronary Physiology and Pathology**
Karl-Josef Osterziel and Rainer Dietz 333

18. **Ventricular Remodeling Following Myocardial Infarction: Experimental and Clinical Benefits of ACE Inhibition**
Marc A. Pfeffer and Gervasio A. Lamas 345

Index 359

Color Appendix A1

Some Abbreviations Used in This Book

A I: angiotensin I
A II: angiotensin II
A III: angiotensin III
ACE: angiotensin-converting enzyme
AMP: adenosine monophosphate
ATP: adenosine triphosphate

bFGF: basic fibroblast growth factor

cGMP: cyclic guanosine monophosphate
CHF: congestive heart failure

EDRF: endothelium-derived relaxing factor
EGF: epidermal growth factor

IP_3: inositol triphosphate

JGA: juxtaglomerular apparatus

LVEDP: left-ventricular end-diastolic pressure
LVH: left-ventricular hypertrophy
LVP: left-ventricular pressure

mRNA: messenger ribonucleic acid

PCR: polymerase chain reaction
PKC: protein kinase C
PLC: phospholipase C

RAAS: renin-angiotensin aldosterone system
RAS: renin-angiotensin system

SHR: spontaneously hypertensive rat

VSMC: vascular smooth muscle cells

WKY: Wistar Kyoto rat

The Cardiac Renin-Angiotensin System: An Overview

David E. Dostal, George W. Booz, and Kenneth M. Baker

Introduction

The renin-angiotensin system (RAS) has been recognized as an important hormonal regulator of cardiovascular homeostasis.[1,2] The principle mediator of the physiological actions of the RAS is the octapeptide, angiotensin II (A II). Angiotensinogen, the precursor of A II, is produced in the liver and hydrolyzed in the plasma by the aspartyl protease renin, producing a decapeptide, angiotensin I (A I). The angiotensin-converting enzyme (ACE), localized primarily on the surface of the vascular endothelium, cleaves the two carboxyl-terminal amino acids of A I to form A II. Over the past two decades, it has become apparent that A II mediates several important functions in the myocardium, such as modulation of coronary vascular tone, increased inotropy and chronotropy,[1] and stimulation of myocardia] growth.[3] Angiotensin II can affect cardiac function both indirectly and directly. Indirect effects of A II include stimulation of the sympathetic nervous system,[4–6] inhibition of vagal tone,[7] decreased renal excretion of sodium, and maintenance of vascular tone.[8] Direct actions of A II include activation of voltage-sensitive calcium channels,[9,10] stimulation of phospholipase C resulting in phosphoinosi-

Lindpaintner K and Ganten D (editors): *The Cardiac-Renin Angiotensin System,* © Futura Publishing Co., Inc., Armonk, NY, 1994.

tide metabolism,[11,12] production of diacylglycerol, and activation of protein kinase C (unpublished data).

As is the case in many other organs and tissues, the effects on the heart involving the RAS have been viewed in the context of a classical hormonal system in which circulating A II mediates the biological effects. In the last decade, several local RASs have been described in various tissues including adrenal,[13] blood vessel,[14,15] brain,[16] and kidney,[17] which have provided evidence for paracrine and autocrine pathways for the actions of A II. This review will provide experimental evidence for the presence of cardiac renin-angiotensin components within cardiac cells and discuss the possible functional relevance of the cardiac RAS.

Components of the Cardiac Renin-Angiotensin System

The identification of an independent cardiac RAS requires the demonstration of tissue synthesis of the components necessary for the generation of A II. Several lines of evidence obtained from biochemical and molecular biology studies suggest the presence of a functional RAS within the heart. The localization of RAS components in various regions of the heart and individual cell types is presented below.

Evidence for Cardiac Renin Production

Initial evidence for intracardiac renin was demonstrated in the dog heart in which nephrectomy had no effects on renin activity and sodium depletion resulted in enhanced enzyme activity.[18] Renin activity measured in the homogenates of mouse and rat hearts is identical to kidney renin activity with regard to pH optimum, reaction velocities, and other physical characteristics.[19,20] Since these biochemical results could be explained by sequestration of renin from the circulation, the most convincing evidence for cardiac-derived renin has been obtained from molecular biology studies. Renin mRNA has been detected in the heart by Northern hybridization analysis, S_1 nuclease protection assay, and in situ hybridization.[20-24] In the adult rat heart, the level of renin transcripts has been reported to be approximately 2% of that in the kidney.[23] Stimulated increases in renin mRNA levels by sodium depletion in the heart and kidney, but not in the submandibular gland and the testes, suggests that intracardiac renin gene expression is regulated.[19] The concept of tissue-specific regulation is further supported by evidence that stimulation of β-adrenoreceptors increased cardiac and renal renin mRNA but not in submandibular, testicular, or adrenal tissue.[19] Renin activity in the heart, like renin gene expression, has been shown to be influenced by various manipulations. Sodium depletion,[19] β-adrenoreceptor agonists,[25] nifedipine,[26] and the vasodilator hydralazine[27] have been shown to increase renin activity in the heart. Renin activity has also been documented in isolated rat cardiomyocytes and is inhibitable by a renin-specific antibody.[20] Cardiomyocytes isolated from rats treated with hydralazine also show an increase in renin activity, but no changes in renin activity were observed in cardiomyocytes from rats treated with nifedipine, alpha methyldopa, or ACE inhibitors.[20,27] The difference in renin activity in the whole heart compared to isolated cardiomyocytes following in vivo administration of nifedipine may reflect differential regulation of renin in nonmyocytes. The concept of renin production by nonmyocytes is supported by a recent study that demonstrated the presence of renin mRNA and renin protein in cultures of ventricular myocytes and fibroblasts obtained from neonatal rat hearts.[22] In these cultures, immunoreactive renin was evident in the perinuclear regions of the cultured cardiomyocytes and fibroblasts, suggesting constitutive production of the protein.[22]

Evidence for Cardiac Angiotensinogen Production

Angiotensinogen mRNA has been detected by Northern hybridization analysis, S_1 nuclease protection assay, and in situ hybridization in the adult rat and mouse heart.[21–23,28–30] The levels of angiotensinogen transcripts in the whole heart have been estimated to be 1% to 5% of those in the liver.[23] Angiotensinogen mRNA in the adult rat heart is in highest abundance in the right chambers of the heart, with greater amounts in the atria than in the ventricles.[29] This is in contrast to the neonatal rat heart in which the amounts of angiotensinogen mRNA in the ventricles are markedly greater than in the atria.[22] Recently, angiotensinogen protein and mRNA have been localized to cultured cardiomyocytes and fibroblasts isolated from the ventricles of neonatal rats.[22] The perinuclear and diffuse cytoplasmic localization of immunoreactive angiotensinogen staining suggests that the protein is constitutively released rather than stored in a secretory compartment.[22] Pharmacological, experimental, and developmental stimuli have been used to study the regulation of the angiotensinogen gene. Glucocorticoid, estrogen, and thyroid hormone administration produce marked increases in angiotensinogen mRNA levels in the heart analogous to responses observed in the liver.[29,31] Nephrectomy stimulates angiotensinogen gene expression in the liver, but does not influence levels of cardiac angiotensinogen mRNA, suggesting that regulation of the cardiac RAS is independent of the endocrine system. The upregulation of angiotensinogen mRNA in the hypertrophied left ventricle, but not in other tissues, following coarctation of the aorta,[28,32] suggests that increased stress on the ventricular wall may be a potent stimulus for inducing angiotensinogen gene expression. Angiotensinogen mRNA is markedly elevated in the ventricles of the neonatal rat heart,[22] which indicates that developmental stimuli regulate the angiotensinogen gene.

Evidence for the Cardiac Angiotensin-Converting Enzyme

The gene for the angiotensin-converting enzyme (ACE) in humans, rabbits, and mice has been cloned, and the amino acid sequence has been derived from the nucleotide sequence.[33–35] The angiotensin-converting enzyme acts not only on A I but is identical to kininase II, one of the bradykinin-degrading enzymes,[36] and therefore also acts on neuropeptide substrates such as enkephalin, the gonadotropin-releasing hormone, neurotensin, and substance P.[37,38] Radioligand binding, autoradiographic labeling, and enzymatic assays have been used to detect ACE in the four chambers of the heart with higher levels in the atria than in the ventricles.[26,39,40–42] The concentration of ACE in adult rat heart membranes has been reported to be approximately 1% of that of membrane homogenates from the lung.[40,43] Radioligand binding of ACE in membrane fractions of the rat heart demonstrated that the atria had a significantly lower affinity for the labeled antagonist than did the ventricles.[41] This suggests that two forms of cardiac ACE may exist in the rat heart. On the basis of differences such as substrate specificity,[44] monovalent cation requirements, and isoeletric point,[45] it has been suggested that ACE isolated from the human heart is different from that present in other tissues. Patterns of ACE labeling using autoradiography in the normal rat heart show a high density of ACE associated with cardiac valves and the adventitial and endothelial layers of major arteries.[41] The presence of ACE in coronary vessels has been corroborated by biochemical studies, which demonstrate conversion of A I to A II by the coronary vasculature.[46,47] The endocardium has small amounts of ACE, whereas sinoatrial and atrioventricular nodes lack ACE.[41] The association of ACE with vascular smooth muscle,[48] adult rat cardiomyocytes,[40] cultured ventricular myocytes, and fibroblasts from neonatal rat hearts[49] suggests that conversion of A I to A II may take place within coronary vessels and the myocardium. The regulation of ACE activity and gene expression in cardiac tissue is poorly understood. Recently, a substance that inhibits ACE[50] has been identified in the rat heart. However, it remains to be determined whether this endogenous substance is an important regulator of ACE activity in vivo. In vivo administration of calcium antagonists and diuretics increases ACE activity in the ventricles of the rat heart.[15] Experimentally induced pressure-overload hypertrophy[51,52] and ischemic congestive heart failure[53] also increase ACE activity and ACE mRNA. The increase in ACE mRNA in the left ventricles of rats with left ventricular hypertrophy suggests that ACE expression is associated directly with the hypertrophic response.[52]

Recent evidence suggests that conversion of A I to A II in the human heart may occur by a pathway that does not require ACE.[54] A chymotrypsinlike proteinase (chymase) has been characterized[54,55] and cloned[56] in the human heart. This heart chymase demonstrates a high degree of catalytic efficiency and substrate specificity for the formation of A II from A I, which is unaffected by ACE inhibitors but is inhibited by a soybean-trypsin inhibitor.[54] Further investigation, however, is required to determine the contribution of this enzyme to A II production in the heart under physiological and pathological conditions.

Cardiac Angiotensin Receptors

The functioning of a cardiac RAS requires the presence of appropriate angiotensin receptors coupled to signal transduction pathways. Cardiac receptors have been demonstrated in sarcolemmal membrane preparations from avian,[12,57–59] bovine,[60,61] guinea pig,[62] rat,[28] and human[63] myocardium. In the human heart, A II receptors have been localized in the coronary vessels, the myocardium, and the sympathetic nerves.[63] High affinity sites with kds ranging from 0.6 to 4.5 nm have been described in neonatal rat cardiomyocytes and left ventricular myocardial membranes, respectively.[64,65] A receptor density of 45,000 sites/cell has been estimated for neonatal rat cardiomyocytes.[65] In a recent autoradiographic study, A II binding sites were localized in atrial and ventricular myocardium and associated with the medial layer of larger vessels.[66] In this study, dense binding was associated with the intracardiac ganglia and the parasympathetic nerves, and moderate density binding was associated with the conduction system including the sinoatrial node, the atrioventricular node, and the atrioventricular bundle.[66] There is a decrease in cardiac receptor sites in the first ten days of the neonatal rat heart, with few A II receptors present in the adult rat myocardium.[63,65] The presence of a relatively high number of A II receptors in neonatal tissue compared to adult tissue suggests a specialized role for A II receptors, perhaps related to the growth process.

Recently, a high-affinity binding protein for A II has been described in the cytosol of cardiomyocytes.[67] Even though the function of this protein is unknown, it may serve to transport A II derived from internalization or intracellular synthesis to target sites within the cell. One possible target is the nucleus. A high-affinity ^{125}I-A II binding site has been characterized in neonatal rat cardiomyocyte nuclei (GW Booz, unpublished data) and liver nuclear membranes, which has properties distinct from plasma membrane and cytosolic binding sites.[68] The binding of A II to a nuclear receptor could be directly involved in protein/DNA interactions or could generate nuclear second messengers leading to transcriptional regulation of the genes involved in growth.

Cardiac Synthesis of Angiotensin II

There are several lines of evidence suggesting that local synthesis of angiotensins occurs within the myocardium. Concentrations of A I and A II, sufficiently high to have biological effects, have been demonstrated in the atria and ventricles of the hearts of rhesus monkeys.[69] The concentrations of angiotensin per gram of wet tissue ranged between 30 and 150 fmol for A I and between 100 and 500 fmol for A II.[69] The highest concentrations of both peptides have been reported in the right atrium followed by the right ventricle, the left atrium, the interventricular septum, and the left ventricle.[69] It is conceivable that angiotensins detected in tissue could result from local synthesis or from sequestration of peptide or precursors from the circulatory system. A variety of approaches have been used to differentiate angiotensin peptides sequestered by cardiac tissue from the circulation versus those derived from local synthesis. One approach has been the use of nephrectomized animals that have low or undetectable plasma levels of angiotensins. The levels of A I have been shown to be increased in the atria and ventricles of rats following nephrectomy,[70] which suggests that the cardiac RAS may function separately from the circulating system. Treatment of nephrectomized rabbits with the ACE inhibitor captopril decreased A II in the atria but had no effect on A II concentrations in the ventricles, suggesting that regulation of A II synthesis may differ in the atria and ventricles.[71]

Accumulating evidence suggests that various cell types within the heart have components of the RAS. The localization of the converting enzyme on the luminal surface of the coronary arteries [41] suggests that endothelial cells may play a role in the conversion of A I to A II. This concept is supported by the observation that isolated perfused rat hearts convert A I (in perfusate) to A II.[52,69,72] It has been demonstrated that vascular smooth muscle has immunoreactive renin[73] and angiotensinogen mRNA,[74] suggesting that the coronary vessels may produce angiotensins. There is also substantial evidence to suggest that angiotensins are synthesized by ventricular myocytes and fibroblasts. Renin activity has been reported in adult rat ventricular myocytes.[20] The complete RAS cascade has been reported in cultured neonatal rat ventricular myocytes and fibroblasts.[22,49] The presence of nanomolar concentrations of A I and A II in media from cultured cardiomyocytes and fibroblasts suggests that sufficient levels of peptide may be produced by these cells to be physiologically relevant.[49]

Even though localization of intracellular renin, angiotensinogen, and ACE in cardiomyocytes and fibroblasts may reflect synthesis and cellular processing of these components, it is conceivable that, following processing in the Golgi apparatus, RAS components may be copackaged in intracellular vesicles where they could interact to form A II. This concept is supported by the observation that A I and A II have inununoreactive staining patterns that are similar to those of renin, angiotensinogen, and ACE.[22,49] Alternatively, endocytosis of RAS components can be envisaged. Intracellularly generated A II may be exported and have paracrine or autocrine functions or remain within the cell and exert intracellular effects. The latter possibility is supported by evidence that internalized A II localizes in mitochondria and nuclei.[75] Nuclear envelope binding sites have been reported for liver nuclei[68] and for neonatal rat cardiomyocytes (GW Booz, unpublished data). In rat liver preparations, A II binds to nuclear chromatin, resulting in decreased stabilization of chromatin treated with micrococcal nuclease or deoxyribonuclease I.[76,77] These findings suggest that A II internalized from outside of or synthesized within the cell may regulate gene transcription by interacting with receptors on the nuclear envelope and/or directly by interacting with nuclear elements.

Putative Functions of the Cardiac Renin-Angiotensin System

Information concerning possible physiological roles of the cardiac RAS is primarily based on in vitro models in which cardiac preparations have been treated with exogenous A II. To date, there is no direct evidence that links activity of the cardiac RAS to normal cardiac function. On the basis of physiological and pharmacological evidence obtained from in vitro systems, it is possible that local production of A II could regulate or modulate the following cardiac functions: coronary blood flow,[46,78] the cardiosympathetic nervous system,[79,80] positive inotropic[9,81,82] and chronotropic actions,[11,83] and cardiac growth.[28,58,84–87]

Effects on Coronary Blood Flow

The physiological significance of locally generated A II is suggested indirectly by the cardioprotective effect of converting enzyme inhibitors in regional myocardial ischemia.[88–90] Angiotensin II has a pronounced vasoconstrictor effect on coronary arteries, even at concentrations that do not affect systemic pressure and cardiac work.[91] Several lines of evidence, based on the use of ACE inhibitors in pathological conditions, suggest that locally produced peptide affects the cardiac vasculature. In the dog heart, ACE inhibition reduces the size of myocardial infarction.[88] Angiotensin I and A II reduce coronary blood flow in the isolated rat, guinea pig, and rabbit heart, and pretreatment with the ACE inhibitor blocks the effects of A I.[92] In isolated perfused rat hearts, administration of an ACE inhibitor significantly reduces the frequency of occurrence and the duration of postischemic arrhythmias while concomitantly preserving myocardial energy-rich phosphates and glycogen with limited lactate accumulation.[93,94] This finding indicates that persistent changes occur with ACE inhibition that are localized in cardiac tissue and are independent of changes in preload or afterload in this experimental model. The presence of dense ACE labeling in coronary vessels,[41] together with the above observations, suggests that the A II, which is involved in these effects, could be derived from the coronary vasculature. Even though these studies provide good evidence for the local production of A II within the heart, kinins, which accumulate after ACE inhibition, may also have an important role. This possibility is suggested by the marked effect that bradykinin has on increasing coronary blood flow.[95] With the recent development of specific renin blockers and nonpeptide angiotensin receptor antagonists, it may be easier to evaluate the effects of locally produced A II on the coronary vasculature since these agents would not be expected to affect bradykinin metabolism.

Effects on Contractility

Angiotensin II can affect contraction of cardiac tissue directly or indirectly through interactions with the sympathetic nervous system.[4] It has been well documented that the facilitation of sympathetic nervous effects on the heart by A II contributes to the inotropic actions of the peptide.[1,2,4] This action of A II is due to an increase in the amount of the neurotransmitter that is released from the presynaptic sympathetic nerve terminals[4] and to a decreased uptake of the neurotransmitter by nerve terminals.[79] Isolated perfused rabbit hearts, which have been pretreated with ramipril (an ACE inhibitor), had significantly reduced contractility and heart rates upon sympathetic nerve stimulation compared to untreated animals.[5] These results suggest that a local RAS may be important for potentiation of mechanical activity through the nervous system since the observed effects were presumably due to an inhibition of tissue synthesis of A II in the absence of exogenous angiotensins. In the normal and cardiomyopathic hamster heart, in which there is no saturable A I binding, the inotropic effects produced by A I are blocked by an A II receptor antagonist but not by an ACE inhibitor, suggesting that another enzyme may convert A I to A II in this system.[81] This suggests that during ACE inhibition, elevated tissue levels of A I could be converted to A II by heart chymase,[54] resulting in beneficial inotropic effects in the failing heart.

Effects on the Heart Rate

The stimulatory effect of A II on the contractile frequency of spontaneous beating in neonatal rat cardiomyocytes[65,66] is blocked by specific receptor antagonists,[65] suggesting that A II may have a direct chronotropic effect. Angiotensin II may have a greater physiological role in the regulation heart rate in the neonate, where there is a greater number of cardiac A II receptors compared to the adult.[65] Locally produced A II may also mediate chronotropic effects through sinoatrial and atrioventricular nodes since this specialized conduction tissue has a large number of angiotensin-binding sites.[63]

Regulation of Myocardial Growth

The effectiveness of ACE inhibitors in preventing and reversing myocardial growth in experimental animal models and the prevention of hypertrophy in patients has been documented.[28,96-98] However, it has been difficult to differentiate between the indirect effects of ACE inhibitors on hemodynamics and bradykinin metabolism from those associated with reduced cardiac levels of A II. The direct involvement of A II in mediating cardiac growth has been demonstrated by studies in which low doses of the ACE inhibitor, which did not affect blood pressure[99] or afterload,[28] were demonstrated to prevent or cause regression of cardiac hypertrophy in aortic-banded rats. A recent study in which rats were infused with A II, also provides evidence of a direct role for A II in mediating cardiac growth. In this study, after seven days of infusion with subpressor doses of A II, significant left- ventricular hypertrophy developed.[100] The experimentally induced cardiac hypertrophy was completely blocked by the nonpeptide AT_1 receptor antagonist Losartan (DuP 753). Blockade of the RAS with enalapril or with an AT_1 receptor antagonist also greatly attenuated myocardial growth in the newborn pig, indicating an important role for A II in the developing and neonatal heart.[85,86] It is unlikely that an increase in production of bradykinin following ACE inhibition is responsible for preventing remodeling of the ventricle since this peptide has been reported to be a mitogen in cultured human fibroblasts[101] and therefore would be expected to augment the nonmyocyte proliferative response in the heart.[102,103] The importance of an intracardiac RAS in mediating hypertrophic growth is suggested by the observation that ACE activity and mRNA levels for ACE[40,52,53] and angiotensinogen[28] are increased in the hypertrophic myocardium. In addition, treatment with ACE inhibitors normalizes ACE content[40] and prevents the cardiac hypertrophy.[28,40] The increased fractional conversion of A I to A II observed in perfused, hypertrophied adult rat hearts is also significantly decreased by ACE inhibitors.[52] Evidence based on clinical and experimental use of ACE inhibitors has led to speculation concerning the possible roles of the cardiac RAS in various pathological states, such as congestive heart failure, ischemic heart disease, and cardiac hypertrophy. It has been documented that ACE inhibition improves symptoms associated with congestive heart failure and reduces mortality in patients with this pathological condition.[97,98,104] Even though the beneficial effects of ACE inhibitors may in part be related to prevention of A II production in coronary vessels, cardiomyocytes, and cardiac fibroblasts, the secondary effects of these agents may also contribute. Angiotensin-converting enzyme inhibitors may not only affect cardiac function by inhibiting circulating or tissue angiotensin production, but these agents also prevent bradykinin metabolism as well as inhibit norepinephrine release from sympathetic nerve terminals. In addition, some ACE inhibitors may have unique properties because of chemical structure, such as the presence of a sulphydryl group, which may account for possible differences observed when these agents are used in the treatment of various cardiac diseases.[89,105] Differentiation of the role of the cardiac RAS from other hormonal pathways may become apparent by inhibiting the cardiac RAS with specific renin blockers or angiotensin receptor antagonists.

Several in vitro studies have demonstrated that A II is a growth factor in 3T3 fibroblasts,[106] neuroblastoma cells,[107] vascular smooth muscle cells,[108] and cardiomyocytes.[57,58] The cellular hypertrophy induced by A II in cultured embryonic chick cardiomyocytes was associated with an increased rate of protein synthesis and was prevented by an angiotensin receptor antagonist.[57] The effects of A II were not related to changes in contractility since the protein synthetic response was also observed in depolarized, nonbeating cells.[58] Angiotensin- converting enzyme inhibitors have been reported to inhibit the increased collagen production and DNA synthesis in nonmyocytes (primarily fibroblasts), which occur after experimental myocardial infarction in the rat.[109] These findings indicate that the intracardiac actions of A II are not restricted to cardiomyocytes but involve cardiac fibroblasts as well. This concept is further supported by observations that show that A II increases DNA and protein synthesis in cultured neonatal rat ventricular fibroblasts (unpublished observations).

The mechanisms by which intracardiac A II promotes hypertrophic growth in cardiomyocytes and proliferative growth in cardiac fibroblasts are still poorly understood. In cardiomyocytes and vascular smooth muscle, A II has been shown to activate protein kinase C (PKC) and growth-related genes such as *c-fos*.[110] Nanomolar concentrations of the protein kinase C inhibitor, staurosporine, have been found to prevent A II-induced hypertrophy of embryonic chick and neonatal rat cardiomyocytes, suggesting an involvement of PKC in the growth process (unpublished data). Activation of PKC might result in gene transcription by a variety of mechanisms, which include phosphorylation of nuclear lamins[111] and activation of sarcolemmal Na^+/H^+ exchange resulting in intracellular alkalinization.[112] Induction of proto-oncogenes, such as *c-fos*, may also be an important control step in the stimulation of protein synthesis since introduction of antisense oligonucleotides to *c-fos* inhibits this process.[113] The growth effects of A II could also be mediated by intracellular A II. In support of this concept, the localization of ^{3}H-A II has been reported in the perinuclear regions of vascular smooth muscle and cardiomyocytes following intraventricular injection.[75] Angiotensin II may also stimulate growth by affecting the production of other growth factors which activate transcriptional pathways necessary for growth. Angiotensin II stimulates the release of the platelet-derived growth factor A-chain[114] and transforming growth factor beta-1[115] from vascular smooth muscle cells. Thus, angiotensin singularly or in concert with other growth-promoting factors may regulate cardiomyocyte hypertrophy and proliferation of nonmyocytes (i.e., smooth muscle cells and fibroblasts).

Conclusion

The evidence reviewed supports the concept of a cardiac RAS as having an important role as a paracrine and/or autocrine effector in the heart. The physiological relevance of this system is illustrated by the identification of the biological components within cells and tissues of the heart and the putative links to cardiac function. The potential significance of the cardiac RAS is indicated by the potent beneficial effect of ACE inhibitors in the treatment of congestive heart failure and in regional myocardial ischemia. A considerable amount of investigative work will be required for the assessment of the physiological and pathophysiological importance of the cardiac RAS. This includes further identification and localization of cell types responsible for producing components of the RAS; regulation of the synthesis, storage, and secretory pathways for the individual components; integration of the cardiac RAS with other effector pathways in the heart; and determination of the functional actions of the cardiac RAS. It can be anticipated that several new physiological and pathophysiological facets of the cardiac RAS will be discovered as these questions are answered.

Acknowledgements

The authors thank Dr. H. A. Singer for his critical review of the manuscript and Ms. Kathleen McGann for preparing the manuscript in its final form. Research from the authors' laboratories was supported by the National Institutes of Health (K.M.B. HL44883, and HL44379), the American Heart Association (K.M.B. 900607), the Pennsylvania Affiliate of the American Heart Association (K.M.B. and DED), by the Geisinger Clinic, and by the Mars Foundation. Dr. G. W. Booz is a recipient of a postdoctoral National Research Service Award (HL08477). Dr. K. M. Baker is an Established Investigator of the American Heart Association.

Summary

The renin-angiotensin system (RAS) is recognized as an important hormonal regulator of cardiovascular homeostasis. In the past decade, an accumulation of experimental evidence suggests that the RAS is not solely an endocrine system but is present within several peripheral tissues, including the heart. Recent biochemical, molecular biological, and functional evidence suggests the presence and regulated synthesis of renin-angiotensin components in the heart where angiotensin II (A II) may have an important role as a paracrine and/ or autocrine effector. The physiological relevance of the cardiac RAS is illustrated by the identification of the biological components within cells and tissues of the heart and the putative links to cardiac function. The potential significance of this system is indicated by the beneficial effects of angiotensin-converting enzyme inhibitors in the treatment of congestive heart failure and in regional myocardial ischemia. Locally derived A II may modulate coronary blood flow, inotropy, and chronotropy, whereas, under pathological conditions, the cardiac RAS may influence ventricular growth and myocardial metabolism, may induce ventricular arrhythmias during ischemia and reperfusion-induced myocardial injury, and may contribute to postinfarction ventricular remodeling. Future studies directed toward cellular and subcellular localization of the various components of the RAS will provide vital information concerning the interaction of the components as a locally functioning, integrated unit.

References

1. Peach MJ. Renin-angiotensin systems: biochemistry and mechanisms of action.Physiol Rev 1977; 57:313–370.
2. Peach MJ. Pharmacology of angiotensin II. In: Fisher JW, ed. Kidney

Hormone, vol. 3. London, England: Academic Press Inc., 1986: 273–308.

3. Dostal DE, Baker KM, Peach MJ. Growth promoting effects of angiotensin II in the cardiovascular system. In: Maggi M, Greenen V., eds. Horizons in Endocrinology, vol. 2. New York: Raven Press, 1991; 76: 265–272.

4. Blumberg AL, Ackerly JA, Peach MJ. Differentiation of neurogenic and myocardial angiotensin II receptors in isolated rabbit atria. Circ Res 1976; 36:719–726.

5. Xiang JZ, Schoelkens BA, Ganten D, Unger T. Effects of sympathetic nerve stimulation are attenuated by the converting enzyme inhibitor HOE-498 in isolated rabbit hearts. Clin Exper Hypertens 1984; 6: 1853–1857.

6. Xiang JZ, Linz W, Becker H, Ganten D, Lang RE, Schoelkens B, et al. Effects of converting enzyme inhibitors: ramipril and enalapril on peptide action and sympathetic neurotransmission in the isolated heart. Eur J Pharmacol 1984; 113:215–223.

7. Lee WB, Ismay MJ, Lumbers ER. Mechanisms by which angiotensin affects the heart rate of the conscious sheep. Circ Res 1980; 47: 286–292.

8. Baker KM. Cardiac actions of angiotensin. J Vasc Med Biol 1991; 3(1): 30–37.

9. Freer R, Pappano A, Peach M, Bing K, McLean M, Vogel S, et al. Mechanisms for the positive inotropic effect of angiotensin II on isolated cardiac muscle. Circ Res 1976; 39:178–183.

10. Kass, RS, Blair ML. Effects of angiotensin II on membrane current in cardiac Purkinje fibers. J Mol Cell Cardiol 1981; 13:797–809.

11. Allen IS, Cohen NM, Dhallan RS, Gaa ST, Lederer WJ, Rogers TB. Angiotensin II increases spontaneous contractile frequency and stimulates calcium current in cultured neonatal rat heart myocytes: insights into the underlying biochemical mechanisms. Circ Res 1988; 62: 524–534.

12. Baker KM, Aceto JF. Characterization of avian angiotensin II cardiac receptors: coupling to mechanical activity and phosphoinositide metabolism. J Mol Cell Cardiol 1989; 21:375–382.

13. Aguilera G, Schirar A, Baukal A, Catt KJ. Circulating angiotensin II and adrenal receptors after nephrectomy. Nature (London) 1981; 289: 507–509.

14. Dzau VJ. Vascular renin-angiotensin system in hypertension. New insights into the mechanism of action of angiotensin converting enzyme inhibitors. Amer J. Med 1988; 84 (suppl 4A):4–8.

15. Rosenthal JH, Pfeifle B, Michailov ML, Pschorr J, Jacob ICM, Dahleim H. Investigations of components of the renin-angiotensin system in rat vascular tissue. Hypertension 1984; 6:383–390.

16. Unger T, Badoer E, Ganten D, Lang RE, Rettig R. Brain angiotensin: pathways and pharmacology. Circulation 1988; 77(suppl I):I-140–I-154.

17. Naruse K, Inagami T, Celio MR, Workman RJ, Takii Y. Immunohistochemical evidence that angiotensins I and II are formed by intracellular mechanism in juxtaglomerula cells. Hypertension 1982; 4(suppl II):II-70–II-74.

18. Hayduk K, Boucher R, Genest J. Renin activity and content in various tissues in dogs under different pathophysiological states. Proc Soc Exp Biol Med 1070; 134:252–255.

19. Dzau VJ, Brody T, Ellison KE, Pratt RE, Ingelfinger JR. Tissue-specific regulation of renin expression in the mouse. Hypertension 1987; 9 (suppl III):III-36–-III-41.

20. Dzau VJ, Re RN. Evidence for the existence of renin in the heart. Circulation 1987; 73 (suppl I):I-134–I-136.

21. Chernin MI, Candia AF, Stark LL, Aceto JF, Baker KM. Fetal expression of renin angiotensin and atriopeptin genes in chick heart. Clin Exp Hypertens 1990; A12:617–629.

22. Dostal DE, Rothblum KC, Chernin MI, Cooper GR, Baker KM. Intracardiac detection of angiotensinogen and renin: evidence for a localized renin-angiotensin system in neonatal rat heart. Am J Physiol (Cell Physiol) 1992; 263 (4Pt1):C838–C850.

23. Dzau VJ, Ellison KE, Brody T, Ingelfinger JR, Pratt R. A comparative study of the distribution of renin and angiotensinogen messenger ribonucleic acids in rat and mouse tissues. Endocrinology 1987; 120: 2334–2338.

24. Suzuki F, Hellmann W, Paul M, Ludwig G. Renin gene expression in rat tissues: a new quantitative assay method for rat renin mRNA using synthetic cRNA. Clin Exp Hypertens 1988; A10:345–359.

25. Dzau VJ, Ellison KE, Ouelette AJ. Expression and regulation of renin in the mouse heart. Clin Res 1984; 33:181A.

26. Rosenthal J, von Lutterotti N, Thunreiter M, Gomba S, Rothemund J, Reiter W, et al. Suppression of renin-angiotensin system in the heart of spontaneously hypertensive rats. J Hypertens 1987; 5:S23–S31.

27. Dzau VJ. Cardiac renin-angiotensin system: molecular and functional aspects. Amer J Med 1988; 84:22–27.

28. Baker KM, Cherin MI, Wixon SK, Aceto JF. Renin angiotensin system involvement in pressure-overload cardiac hypertropy in rats. Am J Physiol 1990; 259:H324–H332.

29. Campbell DJ, Habner JF. Angiotensinogen gene is expressed and differentially regulated in multiple tissues of the rat. J Clin Invest 1986; 78:31–39.

30. Kunapuli SP, Kumar A. Molecular cloning of human angiotensinogen cDNA and evidence for the presence of its mRNA in rat heart. Circ Res 1987; 60:786–790.

31. Lindpaintner K, Jin M, Niedermaier N, Wilhelm MJ, Ganten D. Cardiac angiotensinogen and its local activation in the isolated perfused beating heart. Circ Res 1990; 67:564–573.

32. Drexler H, Lindpaintner K, Lu W, Schieffer B, Ganten D. Transient increase in a rat model of myocardial infaction and failure. Circulation 1989; 8O:II-459.

33. Bernstein KE, Martins BM, Bernstein EA, Linton J, Striker L, Striker G. The isolation of angiotensin converting enzyme cDNA. J Biol Chem 1988; 263:11021–11024.

34. Roy SN, Kusari J, Soffer RL, Lai CY, Sen GC. Isolation of cDNA clones of rabbit angiotensin converting enzyme: identification of two distinct mRNAS for the pulmonary and testicular isozymes. Biochem Biophys Res Commun 1988; 155:678–684.

35. Soubrier F, Alenc-Gelas F, Hubert C, Allelgrini J, John M, Tregear G, et al. Two putative active centers in human angiotensin I-converting enzyme revealed by molecular cloning. Proc Natl Acad Sci USA 1988; 85:9386–9390.
36. Yang HYT, Erdos EG, Levin Y. A dipepidyl carboxypeptidase that converts angiotensin I and inactivates bradykinin. Biochimica et Biophysica Acta 1970; 214:374–376.
37. Erdos EG, Skidgel RA. The unusual substrate and the distribution of human angiotensin I converting enzyme. Hypertension 1986; 8 (suppl I):I34–I37.
38. Ganten D, Lang RE, Archelos J, Unger T. Peptidergic systems: effects on blood vessels. J Cardiovasc Pharmacol 1984; 6:S598–S607.
39. Fabris B, Jackson B, Cubela R, Mendelsohn FAO, Johnston CI. Angiotensin converting enzyme in the rat heart: studies of its inhibition in vitro and ex vivo. Clin Exp Pharmacol Physiol 1989; 16:309–313.
40. Johnston CI, Mooser V, Sun Y, Fabris B. Changes in cardiac angiotensin converting enzyme after myocardial infarction and hypertrophy in rats. Clin Exper Pharmacol Physiol 1991; 18:107–110.
41. Yamada H, Fabris B, Allen AM, Jackson B, Johnston CI, Mendelsohn FAO. Localization of angiotensin converting enzyme in rat heart. Circ Res 1991; 68:141–149.
42. Pinto JE, Viglione P, Vaavedra JM. Autoradiographic localization and quantification of rat heart angiotensin converting enzyme. Am J Hypertens 1991; 4:321–326.
43. Welsch C, Grima M, Griesen EM, Helwig JJ, Barthelmebs M, Coquard C, et al. Assay of tissue angiotensin converting enzyme. J Cardiovasc Pharmacol 1987; 14 (suppl 4):S26–S31.
44. Sakharov IY, Dukhanina EA, Molokoedov AS, Danilov SM, Ochvinnikov MV, Bespalova ZD, et al. Atriopeptin 2 is hydrolysed by cardiac but not by pulmonary isozyme of angiotensin-converting enzyme. Biochem Biophys Res Commun 1988; 151:109–113.
45. Sakharov IY, Danilov SM, Dukhanina EA. Affinity chromatography and some properties of the angiotensin-converting enzyme from human heart. Biochem Biophys Acta 1987; 923: 143–149.
46. Cornish KG, Joyner WL, Gilmore JP. Evidence for conversion of angiotensin II by the coronary microcirculation. Blood Vessels 1979; 16: 241–246.
47. Jackson B, Mendelsohn FAO, Jonston CI. Angiotensin-converting enzyme inhibition: prospects for the future. J Cardiovasc Pharm 18 (suppl 7):S4–S8.
48. Hial V, Gimbrone MA, Peyton MP, Wilcox CM, Pisano JJ. Angiotensin metabolism by cultured human vascular endothelial and smooth muscle cells. Microvasc Res 1979; 17:314–329.
49. Dostal DE, Rothblum KC, Conrad KM, Cooper GR, Baker KM. Detection of angiotensin I and II in cultured rat cardiac myocytes and fibroblasts: evidence for local production. Am J Physiol (Cell Physiol) 1992; 263(4Pt1):C851–C863.
50. Ikemoto F, Song GB, Tominaga M, Yamamoto K. Endogenous inhibitor of angiotensin converting enzyme in the rat heart. Biochem Biophys Res Commun 1989; 159:1093–1099.
51. Lorell BH, Schunkert H, Grice WN, Tang SS, Apstein CS, Dzau VJ.

Alteration in cardiac converting enzyme activity in pressure overload hypertrophy (abstract). Circulation 1989; 80:II-297.

52. Shunkert H, Dzau VJ, Tang SS, Hirsh AT, Apstein CS, Lorell BH. Increased rat cardiac angiotensin converting enzyme activity and mRNA expression in pressure overload left ventricular hypertrophy: effects on coronary resistance, contractility, and relaxation. J Clin Invest 1990; 86:1913–1920.

53. Fabris B, Jackson B, Kohzuki M, Perich R, Johnston CI. Increased cardiac converting enzyme in rats with chronic heart failure. Clin Exper Pharmacol Physiol 1990; 17:309–314.

54. Urata H, Kinoshita A, Misono FM, Bumpus FM, Husain A. Identification of a highly specific chymase as the major angiotensin II-forming enzyme in the human heart. J Biol Chem 1990; 265:22348–22357.

55. Kinoshita A, Urata H, Bumpus FM, Husain A. Multiple determinants for the high substrate specificity of an angiotensin II-forming chymase from the human heart. J Biol Chem 1991; 266:19192–19197.

56. Urata H, Kinoshita A, Perez DM, Misono KS, Bumpus FM, Graham RM, et al. Cloning of the gene and cDNA for human heart chymase. J Biol Chem 1991; 266:17173–17179.

57. Aceto JF, Baker KM. [Sar[1]] Angiotensin II receptor-mediated stimulation of protein synthesis in chick heart cells. Am J Physiol 1990; 258: H806–H813.

58. Baker KM, Aceto JF. Angiotensin II stimulation of protein synthesis and cell growth in chick heart cells. Am J Physiol 1990; 259: H610–H618.

59. Baker KM, Singer HA, Aceto JF. Angiotensin II receptor-mediated stimulation of cytosolic free calcium and inositol phosphates in chick myocytes. J Pharmacol Exp Ther 1989; 251:578–585.

60. Mukherjee A, Kulkarni PV, Haghani Z, Sutko JL. Identification and characterization of angiotensin II receptors in cardiac sarcolemma. Biochemn Biophys Res Commun 1982; 105:575–581.

61. Rogers TB. High affinity angiotensin receptors in myocardial sarcolemmal membranes. J Biol Chem 1984; 259:8106–8114.

62. Baker KM, Singer HA. Identification and characterization of the guinea pig angiotensin II ventricular and atrial receptors: coupling to inositol phosphate production. Circ Res 1988; 62:896–904.

63. Urata H, Healy B, Stewart RW, Bumpus FM, Husain A. Angiotensin receptors in normal and failing human hearts. J Clin Endocrinol Metab 1989; 69:54–66.

64. Baker KM, Campanile C, Trachte G, Peach MJ. Identification and characterization of the rabbit angiotensin II myocardial receptor. Circ Res 1984; 54(3):286–293.

65. Rogers TB, Gaa ST, Allen IS. Identification and characterization of functional angiotensin II receptors on cultured heart myocytes. J Pharmacol Exp Ther 1986; 236:438–444.

66. Allen AM, Yamada H, Mendelsohn FAO. In vitro autoradiographic localization of binding to angiotensin receptors in the rat heart. Int J Cardiol 1990; 28:25–33.

67. Sen I, Rajasekaran AK. Angiotensin II-binding protein in adult and neonatal rat heart. J Mol Cell Cardiol 1991; 23:563–572.

68. Booz GW, Conrad KM, Hess AL, Singer HA, Baker KM. Angiotensin

II binding sites on hepatocyte nuclei. Endocrinology 1992; 130: 3641–3649.
69. Lindpaintner K, Wilhelm MJ, Jin M, Unger T, Lang RE, Schoelkens BA, et al. Tissue renin-angiotensin systems: focus on the heart. J Hypertens 1987; 5(suppl 2):S33–S38.
70. Wilhelm AJ, Lindpaintner K, Jin MW, Unger T, Lang RE, Ganten D. Evidence for local regulatory properties of an intrinsic cardiac renin-angiotensin system (abstract). Circulation 1987; 76:340.
71. Unger T, Ganten D, Lang RE. Tissue converting enzyme and cardiovascular actions of converting enzyme inhibitors. J Cardiovas Pharmacol 1986; 8:S75–S81.
72. Lindpaintner K, Jin M, Wilhelm MJ, Suzuki F, Linz B, Schoelkens BA, et al. Intracardiac generation of angiotensin and its physiologic role. Circulation 1988; 77(suppl I): 1–18.
73. Re R, Fallon JT, Dzau VJ, Quay SC, Haber E. Renin synthesis by canine aortic smooth muscle cells in culture. Life Sci 1982; 30:99–106.
74. Naftilan AJ, Zuo WM, Ingelfinger J, Ryan TJ, Pratt RE, Dzau VJ. Localization and differential regulation of angiotensinogen mRNA expression in the vessel wall. J Clin Invest 1991; 87:1300–1311.
75. Robertson AL, Khairallah PA. Angiotensin: rapid localization in nuclei of smooth and cardiac muscle. Science 1971; 172:1138–1139.
76. Re RN, LaBiche RA, Bryan SE. Nuclear-hormone mediated changes in chromatin solubility. Biochem Biophys Res Commun 1983; 110: 61–68.
77. Re RN, Vizard DL, Brown J, Bryan S. Angiotensin II receptors in chromatin fragments generated by micrococcal nuclease. Biochem Biophys Res Commun 1984; 119:220–227.
78. Ertl B, Alexander RW, Kloner RA. Interaction between coronary occulusion and the renin-angiotensin system in the dog. Basic Res Cardiol 1983; 78:518–533.
79. Khairallah PA. Action of angiotensin on adrenergic nerve endings. Fed Proc 1972; 31:1351–1357.
80. Knape JTA, van Zwieten PA. Positive chronotropic activity of angiotensin II in the pithed normotensive rat is primarily due to activation of cardiac B_1-adrenoreceptors. Naunyn Schmiedeberg's Arch Pharmacol 1988; 338:185–190.
81. Hirakata H, Fouad-Tarazi FM, Bumpus FM, Khosla M, Healy B, Husain A, et al. Angiotensin and the failing heart. Enhanced positive inotropic response to angiotensin I in cardiomyopathic hamster heart in the presence of captopril. Circ Res 1990; 66:891–899.
82. Kobayashi M, Furukawa Y, Chiba S. Positive chronotropic and inotropic effects of angiotensin II in the dog heart. Eur J Pharmacol 1978; 50:17–25.
83. Nakashima A, Angus JA, Johnston CI. Chronotropic effects of angiotensin I, angiotensin II, bradykinin, and vasopressin in guinea pig atria. Eur J Pharmacol 1982; 81:479–485.
84. Baker KM, Booz GW, Dostal DE. Cardiac actions of angiotensin II: role of an intracardiac renin-angiotensin system. Ann Rev Physiol 1992; 54:227–241.
85. Beinlich CJ, Baker KM, White GJ, Morgan ME. Control of growth in the neonatal pig heart. Am J Physiol 1991; 261:3–7.

86. Beinlich CJ, White GJ, Baker KM, Morgan HE. Angiotensin II and left ventricular growth in newborn pig heart. J Mol Cell Cardiol 1991; 23(9):1031–1038.
87. Moravec CS, Schluchter MD, Paranandi L, Czerska B, Stewart RW, Rosenkranz E, et al. Inotropic effects of angiotensin II on human cardiac muscle in vitro. Circulation 1990; 82:1973–1984.
88. Ertl G, Kloner RA, Alexander RW, Braunwald E. Limitation of experimental infarct size by an angiotensin converting enzyme inhibitor. Circulation 1982; 65:40–48.
89. Grover GJ, Sleph PG, Dzwonczyk S, Wang P, Fung W, Tobias D, et al. Effects of different angiotensin-converting enzyme (ACE) inhibitors on ischemic isolated rat hearts: relationship between cardiac ACE inhibition and cardioprotection. J Pharmacol Exper Ther 1991; 257: 919–929.
90. Liang C, Gavras H, Black J, Sherman L, Hood W. Renin angiotensin system inhibition in acute myocardial infarction in dogs: effect on systemic hemodynamics, myocardial blood flow, segmental myocardial function, and infarct size. Circulation 1982; 66:1249–1259.
91. Fowler NO, Holmes JC. Coronary and myocardial actions of angiotensin. Circ Res 1964; 14:191–201.
92. Xiang J, Linz W, Becker H, Ganten RE, Lang RE, Schoelkens B, et al. Effects of converting enzyme inhibitors: ramipril and enalapril on peptide action and sympathetic neurotransmission in the isolated heart. Eur J Pharmacol 1985; 113:215–223.
93. Linz W, Schoelkens BA, Han YF. Beneficial effects of converting enzyme inhibitor, ramipril, in ischemic rat hearts. J Cardiovas Pharmacol 1986; 8(suppl 10):S91–S99.
94. Schoelkens BA, Linz W, Lindpaintner K, Ganten D. Angiotensin deteriorates but bradykinin improves cardiac function following ischaemia in isolated rat hearts. J Hypertens (London) 1987; 5(suppl 5):S7–S9.
95. Schoelkens BA, Linz W, Koenig W. Effects of the angiotensin converting enzyme inhibitor, ramipril, in isolated ischemic rat heart abolished by a bradykinin antagonist. J Hypertens 1988; 6:S25–S28.
96. Brilla CG, Janicki JS, Weber KT. Cardioprotective effects of lisinopril in rats with genetic hypertension and left ventricular hypertrophy. Circulation 1991; 83:1771–1779.
97. Chatterjee K, Parmley VW, Cohen JN, Levine TB, Awan NA, Mason DT, et al. A cooperative muticenter study of captopril in congestive heart failure: hemodynamic effects and long term response. Am Heart J 1985; 110:439–447.
98. CONSENSUS Trial Study Group. Effects of enalapril on mortality in severe congestive heart failure: results of the Cooperative North Scandinavian Enalapril Survival Study (CONSENSUS). N Engl J Med 1987; 316:1429–1435.
99. Linz W, Schoelkens BA, Wonten D. Converting enzyme inhibitor specifically prevents development and induces the regression of cardiac hypertrophy in rats. Clin Exp Hypertens 1989; 11:1325–1350.
100. Dostal DE, Baker KM. Angiotensin II stimulation of left ventricular hypertrophy in adult rat heart: mediation by the AT_1 receptor. Am J Hypertens 1992; 5(number 5, part I):276–280.
101. Owen NE, Villereal ML. Lys-bradykinin stimulates Na^+ influx and DNA synthesis in cultured human fibroblasts. Cell 1983; 32:979–985.

102. Brilla G, Pick R, Tan LB, Janicki JS, Weber KT. Remodeling of the rat right and left ventricles in experimental hypertension. Circ Res 1990; 67:1355–1364.
103. Zak R. Cell proliferation during cardiac growth. Amer J Cardiol 1973; 31:211–219.
104. SOLVD Investigators. Effect of enalapril on survival in patients with reduced left ventricular ejection fraction and congestive heart failure. New Engl J Med 1991; 325:293–302.
105. Packer M, Lee WH, Yushak M, Medina N. Comparison of captopril and enalapril in patients with severe chronic heart failure. N Eng J Med 1986; 315:847–853.
106. Schelling P, Ganten D, Speck G, Fisher H. Effects of angiotensin II and angiotensin II antagonist saralasin on cell growth and renin in 3T3 and SV3T3 cells. J Cell Physiol 1979; 98:503–513.
107. Chen L, Re RN, Prakash 0, Mondale D. Angiotensin-converting enzyme inhibition reduces neuroblastoma cell growth rate. Proc Soc Exper Biol Med 1991; 196:280–283.
108. Geisterfer AA, Peach MJ, Owens GK. Angiotensin II induces hypertrophy not hyperplasia of cultured rat aortic smooth muscle cells. Circ Res 1988; 62:749–756.
109. van Krimpen C, Smits JF, Cleutjens JP, Debets JJ, Schoemaker RG, Struyker-Boudier HA, et al. DNA synthesis in the non-infarcted cardiac interstitium after left coronary artery ligation in the rat: effects of captopril. J Mol Cell Cardiol 1991; 23:1245–1253.
110. Taubman MB, Berk BC, Izumo S, Tsuda T, Alexander RW, Nadal-Ginard B. Angiotensin II induces c-fos mRNA in aortic smooth muscle: role of Ca^{2+} mobilization and protein kinase C activation. J Biol Chem 1989; 264:526–530.
111. Tsuda T, Alexander RW. Angiotensin II stimulates phosphorylation of nuclear lamins via a protein kinase C-dependent mechanism in cultured vascular smooth muscle cells. J Biol Chem 1990; 265:1165–1170.
112. Moolenaar WH. Effects of growth factors on intracellular pH regulation. Annu Rev Physiol 1986; 48:363–376.
113. Rainer RS, Eldridge CS, Gilliland GK, Naftilan AJ. Antisense oligonucleotide to c-fos blocks the angiotensin II-induced stimulation of protein synthesis in rat aortic smooth muscle cells. Hypertension 1990; 16:326.
114. Naftilan AJ, Pratt RE, Dzau VJ. Induction of platelet-derived growth factor A-chain and c-myc gene expressions by angiotensin II in cultured rat vascular smooth muscle cells. J Clin Invest 1989; 83: 1419–1424.
115. Stouffer GA, Owens GK. Angiotensin II-induced mitogenesis of spontaneously hypertensive rat-derived cultured smooth muscle cells is dependent on autocrine production of transforming factor-β. Circ Res 1992; 70:820–828.

2

Cardiac Renin, Gene Expression, and Regulation

Brian J. Morris and Yi-kun Lou

Introduction

The question of whether renin is synthesized in cardiac tissue has, until recently, been controversial. At the outset, however, it should be noted that local synthesis of renin in the heart is nevertheless a different issue than the existence of a cardiac renin-angiotensin system (RAS) since renin enzyme activity in the heart could arise as a consequence of uptake from plasma rather than from intracardiac synthesis. Thus, the questions that have to be answered are (1) Is renin synthesized by cells in the heart? (2) Is renin taken up from the bloodstream? and (3) Do both of these processes occur? If renin is present, then there is a likely capacity for A II formation in the heart, assuming that cardiac renin comes into contact and reacts with angiotensinogen, and that the A I formed is subsequently converted to A II by dipeptidyl carboxypeptidase 1 (the angiotensin I-converting enzyme (ACE)), or heart chymase, or both. The present chapter provides an overview of the conflicting evidence that has prevailed until recently for and against cardiac-renin synthesis and then goes on to show how new results from the use of the highly sensitive polymerase chain reaction (PCR) technique now appear to have resolved this issue, at least in relation to the heart of the rat.

Cardiac Renin

Reninlike Enzymatic Activity in the Heart

Interestingly, the first attempt to determine whether the heart (of the hog) contained renin resulted in a negative finding, even

Lindpaintner K and Ganten D (editors): *The Cardiac-Renin Angiotensin System,* © Futura Publishing Co., Inc., Armonk, NY, 1994.

though renin activity could be detected readily in the artery and vein and, at lower levels, in several other tissues.[1] Reninlike activity in the mammalian heart (left-ventricular wall of the dog) was first described by Genest's group.[2,3] Others then went on to support these findings in other species.[4-7] In the Wistar Kyoto (WKY) rat, the mean reninlike activities reported for different regions of the heart ranged from 189 ng A I·h^{-1}. ml^{-1} (right ventricle) to 266 ng (septum) A I·h^{-1}·g tissue^{-1},[7] and in the mouse, cardiac reninlike activity was estimated as 11 ng A I·h^{-1}. mg protein^{-1}.[6] Is such cardiac reninlike activity true renin, however? In the marmoset heart, reninlike activity was found to be 5.5 ng A I·h^{-1}. mg protein^{-1} (compared with 1,150 ng A I·h^{-1}. mg protein^{-1} in the kidney) when assayed at pH 6.0, which is near the pH optimum of renin, but was only 0.052 at the more physiological pH of 7.4.[8] Although true renin activity, when measured at pH 7.4, is less than that which one can measure near the optimum pH, it is nevertheless much more than a mere 1% of the activity at pH 6.0. On this basis, the data therefore tend to suggest that much of the reninlike activity that had been measured at pH 6.0 was not due to renin but to other proteases. Notably, in studies of apparent reninlike activity in other tissues, the related aspartyl protease cathepsin D has been found to possess A I-generating activity at acidic pHs but is inactive at pH 7.4.[9-12] Wood et al. also tested the effect of a primate renin inhibitor, which was said to be ten thousandfold less active against cathepsin D, and found that although it was ineffective in inhibiting cardiac reninlike activity if given i.v., when added to reaction vessels in vitro at a concentration of 5×10^{-6} mol·l^{-1}, at pH 6.0, it suppressed the reninlike activity by 87%. The renin inhibitor was also tested at pH 7.4, at which pH the reninlike activity was more likely to be true renin and was effective: the concentration needed for 50% inhibition being 8×10^{-10} mol·l^{-1}.[8] Despite the specificity of the inhibitor at the concentrations used, the inhibition observed at pH 6.0 could, at least in part, still have been a reflection of the inhibition of the related aspartyl protease rather than renin itself because the former would be present in concentrations far exceeding that of any renin. Nevertheless, on the whole, the results do suggest that at least a small fraction of the reninlike activity in the heart was quite likely to have been renin.

Immunochemical Evidence for Cardiac Renin

A different approach to the identification and, in some experiments, the localization of renin in the heart has involved immunochemical techniques. The antirenin antibody has been reported to neutralize renin in mouse heart tissue,[6] and antibodies directed against renin showed localization in veins and coronary vessels of the normal rat heart, being present in smooth muscle cells of the tunica media.[13] No antibody reaction was found in endothelial cells of the blood vessels nor in atrial or ventricular myocytes. In contrast, in the case of the neonatal Sprague-Dawley rat, Dostal et al. found that both primary cultures of neonatal ventricular cardiomyocytes and single-passage cardiac fibroblasts gave immunofluorescent staining with renin antibodies[14] and suggested a role during development.

Uptake of Circulating Renin by the Heart

What then is the origin of cardiac renin? Early work showed that cardiac renin did not disappear, and in fact was unchanged, after nephrectomy,[2] and this was taken as evidence for a cardiac origin of the reninlike activity in the heart. It is, however, by no means certain that the reninlike activity being measured was renin itself, as opposed to nonspecific protease activity, as discussed above. Also, the time after nephrectomy might not have been sufficient for the clearance and metabolism of any renin that might have been taken up from the bloodstream by the heart. In blood vessels, by comparison, nephrectomy experiments have shown that the renin disappears with time and is derived entirely through uptake from the bloodstream.[15-17] Indeed, good evidence now exists to suggest that vascular renin (of renal origin) accounts for much of the A I generated in peripheral vascular beds.[18-21] The possibility that at least a certain portion of renin in the heart is derived from the circulation is suggested by the findings of a prorenin gradient of 35% to 58% across the coronary vascular bed,[22] although these findings remain to be confirmed.

Regulation of Levels of Reninlike Activity in the Heart

Reninlike activity in the heart is enhanced by sodium depletion,[2,23,24] β-adrenoceptor agonists,[25] the calcium antagonist nifedipine,[7] and the vasodilator hydralazine[26] and is decreased by castration.[23] It is not entirely clear from these experiments, however, whether such changes are a result of effects on the secretion of renin from the kidney that change the level of circulating renin, which is then taken up by the heart in greater or lesser amounts, or to more direct effects on the production of renin by the heart itself, or to a mixture of both. Similarly, it is not clear whether the finding that the ventricle and septum of the spontaneously hypertensive rat (SHR) contained ~60% as much reninlike activity as in the WKY rat [7] reflects a strain difference, a pathophysiological response to the hypertension, or a difference in uptake reflecting a difference in circulating concentrations of renin. In the atrium, interestingly, reninlike activity was similar in the SHR and WKY strains in this study.

Renin in Cultured Cardiac Cells

Myocytes isolated from the left ventricle of rats and placed into culture have also been found to contain reninlike activity.[27–29] This activity may reflect the situation in vivo or may be a result of de novo production of renin in the artificial environment of cell culture, where the cells are removed from possible repressive influences such as hemodynamic factors and neural input to the heart, as well as hormonal and chemical factors. The concentration detected, 4 pg A I·h^{-1}·µg DNA^{-1}, was very low, being less than the concentration in plasma. The fact that the reninlike activity was inhibited by 80% with the antibody directed against renin nevertheless supports the identity of this activity as genuine renin. Similarly, reninlike activity has been detected in cultured myocytes from the mouse heart and was inhibited by antimouse renin.[30] Nifedipine caused a decrease in reninlike activity in the cultured rat cardiac myocytes,[23] that is, had an effect opposite to that observed in the whole animal. The fact, moreover, that the reninlike activity was capable of regulation can be taken as evidence in favor of it being true renin; cathepsin D, for example, would not be expected to respond to these kinds of influences.

Conclusion in Relation to Renin in the Heart

From these various findings it would appear that small quantities of renin could be present in cardiac tissue, but these experiments do not make it clear whether the source of such cardiac renin is uptake from the circulation or endogenous synthesis. The next section will address the issue of whether or not the heart manufactures renin.

Cardiac Renin mRNA

Evidence from Hybridization Probing for Renin RNA

The decision as to whether the heart synthesizes renin has depended on the valid detection of genuine renin gene transcripts in cardiac tissue. The earliest methods of detection of renin mRNA, by dot-blot hybridization, were only sensitive enough to detect transcripts in the kidney, where renin is present in the less than 0.01% of the kidney cell population that constitutes the juxtaglomerular cells.[31,32] Subsequently, Northern blotting, which uses large amounts of RNA obtained by pooling tissues from several animals [23,33–35] and the more sensitive solution hybridization/ribonuclease protection approach,[33,35,36–38] have been used to detect what was concluded to be renin mRNA in cardiac tissues of rats and mice. The findings were based on the appearance of bands of radioactive exposure on autoradiographs, obtained following hybridization probing of blots from electrophoretic gels; such bands were in a position corresponding to that expected for renin mRNA (1.6 kb for Northerns and, for ribonuclease protection, a position corresponding to the size of the double-stranded fragment protected by the particular renin DNA fragment used for the probe). This appeared to suggest the presence of small concentrations of renin mRNA in cardiac tissues of the rat and mouse, at least for some researchers.[6,13,26] The relative concentration of renin mRNA in the CD-1 mouse heart determined by Northern blotting by Dzau et al. was 5% to 10% of that in the kidney, and for the rat heart it was 2% of the renal value.[34] Sensitivity was said to be improved by the use of renin cRNA, instead of cDNA, as the probe. By developing a quantitative solution hybridization assay, Paul et al. reported values of 0.07 pg/μg total RNA for male CD-1 mice but state that in NMRI mice renin mRNA was at or below the limit of detection.[36] Similarly, in the DBA mouse, Field et al. have been unable to detect renin mRNA in the heart.[39] It has thus been concluded that there are strain differences in renin gene expression in the mouse heart. The values obtained for CD-1 mice are, however, similar to those found for the male rat heart by Suzuki et al. of 0.11 pg/μg total RNA for the ventricle and 0. 04 pg/μg total RNA for the atrium.[35] The value obtained by Suzuki et al. for the kidney was only 0.43 pg/μg total RNA and for the adrenal was 0.01 pg/μg total RNA. The fact that no signal was obtained for the spleen, which is rich in cathepsin D, was used to support their assertion of specificity. The sixfold higher concentration of renin mRNA they obtained in the kidney versus the heart is, moreover, markedly different from the seven hundredfold higher renin concentration they obtained for the kidney over the heart. It is difficult to reconcile this difference unless one postulates, for example, that there is preferential cardiac production of prorenin rather than renin. There is, however, no evidence for this, and as mentioned above, one paper has reported extraction rather than generation of prorenin across the coronary vascular bed.[22] Any prorenin produced could, however, remain intracellular. Are results then obtained by hybridization probing of the heart valid, or do they reflect nonspecific hybridization? One way to be certain would be to obtain sequence information by, for example, using a cDNA library prepared from the heart and analyzing clones that hybridize to renin cDNA or oligonucleotide probes. This has not been done to date.

Regulation Studies Involving Hybridization Probing

Sodium depletion of 40-day-old male Swiss mice by a low sodium diet and i.p. furosemide for 2 weeks has been reported to result in an apparent 4.5 times higher concentration of cardiac renin mRNA on Northern blots than found for mice fed a high sodium diet.[23] Interestingly, treatment of 8-week-old NMRI female mice with testosterone had no effect on cardiac renin mRNA, although cardiac reninlike activity was said to be increased 1.6 times after 2 hours and 1.9 times after 3 weeks, but not at 1 week and 2 weeks;[40] this suggested that the changes observed were from effects that increased renin by an extracardiac action (presumably on the kidney), with the resulting renin in plasma being taken up by the heart to account for the rise. Another treatment besides sodium depletion that has been found to increase cardiac renin mRNA is furosemide: when given i.p. for 1 week, furosemide increased cardiac renin mRNA 2.4 times in adult male WKY rats.[41] In 5-week-old WKY rats, however, renin mRNA was undetectable in the heart, whereas a faint protected band was seen in SHR of this age, but by 12 weeks a faint band of similar intensity could be seen for both WKY and SHR.[42] Production of two-kidney, one-clip hypertension in female WKY rats resulted in a progressive increase in the protected band for the heart, which was more intense at 20 weeks than at 4 weeks postclipping.[43]

Negative Findings by Northern Blotting and Ribonuclease Protection

Although the results cited above have led to a general impression by many that the heart does indeed contain renin mRNA, suggesting that at least some of the renin in the heart is from expression of the renin gene in this tissue, it is noteworthy that a number of investigators have been unable to detect renin mRNA by these techniques.[13,39,44,45] Tada et al., for example, did not obtain a protected band of 202 bp for the exon 9 probe in a ribonuclease protection assay with 20 μg poly(A)$^+$ RNA from the Sprague-Dawley rat heart.[44] Their technique of purifying total mRNA before ribonuclease protection assay, rather than using total RNA as in the studies above, is superior, although it also introduces the potential for degradation because of the greater number of steps and the time involved in sample preparation. Nevertheless, renin mRNA was detected in a range of other tissues in relative concentrations that are consistent with the general findings by others. Could then the results of others reflect nonspecific effects such as hybridization to homologous cathepsin D or other sequences, assay conditions, species and strain differences, diet, age, or other factor(s)? Interestingly, even after sodium depletion or captopril treatment, no protected fragment was seen in the study by Tada et al., and they point out how their results differ from those of Dzau et al. who found an increase in signal for renin mRNA after such treatments.[23,34]

Localization of Renin mRNA in the Heart

In situ hybridization has been used in an attempt to detect, as well as to localize, renin mRNA in the hearts of neonatal and adult rats.[46] In neonatal rats the signal for the renin mRNA probe was found to be distributed evenly among the four cardiac chambers, whereas in the adult rat, although the signals were still detectable in each chamber, the highest signals were found in the right atrium.

Transgenic Studies

Introduction of the duplicated *Ren-2*^{d} gene of DBA/2 mice into a one-renin gene mouse strain led to its expression in kidney, adrenal, and a number of other tissues, but not in the heart.[47] Mice made transgenic for the human renin gene, however, have been reported to express human renin mRNA in the heart. This was seen for studies that involved microinjection of the gene plus 3 kb of upstream DNA and 1.2 kb of downstream DNA by Fukamizu et al., but the signal was faint and only evident after 72 hours' exposure for an assay involving 50 μg total RNA.[48] In a later study by Sigmund et al., who introduced the gene plus 0.9 kb of upstream DNA and 0.4 kb of downstream DNA, the signal seen was at the lower limit of detection of the ribonuclease protection method used, which could distinguish human from mouse transcripts by taking advantage of sequence differences between each one, and then in only one of four transgenic lines.[49] Sigmund and coworkers point out, however, the possibility that their results could have been artifactual, resulting from chromosomal position effects on transgene expression in individual transgenic lines, or may not have reflected the tissue-specificity or level of expression in particular human tissues. In a subsequent review, they state that human renin mRNA was not demonstrated in the heart of transgenic mice.[50]

Polymerase Chain Reaction for Renin mRNA Detection

Over the last few years, the highly sensitive polymerase chain reaction (PCR) technique has been brought to bear in addressing the question of low-level renin gene transcription in extrarenal tissues. This involves isolation of total RNA from a tissue, copying it into cDNA using reverse transcriptase[51] or Taq polymerase,[52] and then using PCR to amplify a particular region within the renin cDNA produced. Figure 1 outlines the scheme currently employed in the authors' laboratory for renin mRNA PCR. The PCR process involves a reaction mixture containing the cDNA and synthetic oligonucleotide primers of approximately 20 nucleotides in length that are complementary to and will therefore hybridize to defined sequences on opposite strands of the double-stranded cDNA (Figure 2), Taq polymerase, each of the four deoxynucleotide triphosphates, $MgCl_2$, Tris buffer, and other ingredients. The reaction tubes are placed in a DNA thermal cycler set at three particular temperatures and times for undergoing the successive cycles of strand-dissociation at 92° to 95°C, primer annealing at 52° to 62°C, and extension at 70° to 72°C. Extension of the primers involves the DNA strand-copying action of Taq polymerase, which is a heat-stable enzyme, and leads to a doubling, with each cycle, of that portion of the cDNA bounded by the primer sequences. After 25 to 30 cycles, an increase in the particular fragment within the renin cDNA of the order of a millionfold is obtained. This can be visualized on an ethidium bromide-stained polyacrylamide or agarose electrophoretic gel. For greater sensitivity and confirmation of specificity, the DNA can be then transferred to a membrane and probed with a labeled oligonucleotide corresponding to a suitable region of the amplified DNA fragment.

RENIN mRNA PCR PROTOCOL

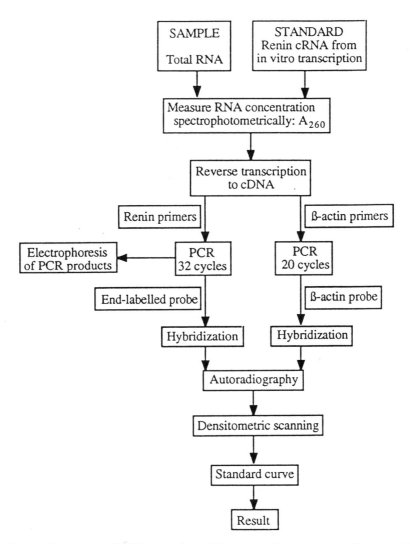

Fig. 1. Flowchart of PCR method used by the authors for quantification of renin mRNA in rat tissues. PCR of β-actin mRNA monitors intersample variability.

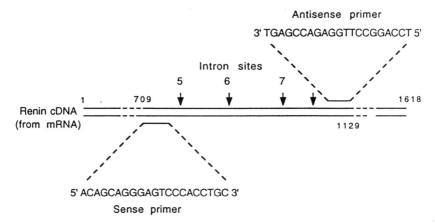

Fig. 2. The PCR strategy adopted by the authors for amplification of a segment of the cDNA copy obtained from reverse transcription of renin mRNA (which is 1,618 bp long, excluding the poly(A) tail). Shown are the oligonucleotides used as primers and the number of the nucleotide residue to which the 5' end of the oligonucleotide hybridizes. Also shown are the locations of several of the nine introns in the corresponding renin genomic sequence. By choosing a region that spans such intron sites, one can readily distinguish between PCR products derived from renin mRNA and PCR products derived from renin genomic DNA since the latter will be longer.

Another approach is to use labeled primers to generate a radioactive PCR product, which can then be detected by autoradiography of the gels themselves, without the need to perform DNA transfer onto a membrane. After autoradiography, a band corresponding in position to that on the stained gel will be obtained, but it is generally more intense and therefore more easily discerned. Since preparations of total RNA obtained from tissues can sometimes be contaminated with genomic DNA, it is important to ensure that the PCR products produced are derived from renin cDNA copies of renin mRNA and not renin genomic DNA, which of course is present in all nucleated cells. The strategy employed is to select primer sequences, which each correspond to different exons. Since exons are separated by often long stretches of intronic DNA, a PCR product arising from the renin gene can be readily discerned as a much longer fragment of predefined length and so may be distinguished readily from products emanating from renin mRNA.

Cardiac Renin mRNA Detected by PCR

In the first report involving PCR for renin mRNA detection, which involved one primer corresponding to a sequence in exon 7 and the other corresponding to a region of exon 9, and PCR of cDNA obtained from 5 μg total RNA, Ekker et al. were unable to detect renin mRNA in cardiac and vascular tissues of two-gene DBA/2 mice after 30 amplification cycles,[51] even though a PCR product of expected size was found for the kidney and a number of other extrarenal tissues. No data were presented for the rat heart, although, using corresponding primers specific for rat renin sequences, they were able to detect a renin mRNA PCR product in other extrarenal tissues, such as brain, liver, testis, and hypothalamus, and at very low levels in the spleen, lung, prostate, and thymus of the Wistar rat. In contrast, starting with 1 μg total RNA, Dostal et al. were able, after 30 PCR cycles, to detect a signal of a size corresponding to the PCR product for renin mRNA in the adult Sprague-Dawley rat heart.[14] Okura et al. were the first to employ PCR in the development of an assay for quantification of renin mRNA in tissues of 16-week-old male WKY rats.[53] Their approach involved primers in exons 8 and 9 that would result in a 189 bp renin mRNA/cDNA-derived PCR product and, as an internal standard, serially diluted renin cDNA obtained from cRNA of in vitro transcripts from a genomic fragment spanning the same region. Thus, PCR products from the tissue renin mRNA were 189 bp and those from standards were 853 bp. These were in separate tubes. After 25 cycles, using labeled primers, subsequent autoradiography revealed a faint band for the heart and artery, where cDNA for these particular samples was made from 250 pg of total mRNA. The concentration of renin mRNA in the heart was reported as 0.15 pg/μg total RNA, which compares with values of 56 pg/μg they obtained for the kidney, 0.16 pg/μg for the adrenal, and 0.11 pg/μg for the aorta. The values were generally higher than concentrations of 0.43, 0.11, 0.04, and 0.01 pg/μg reported by Suzuki et al. for the kidney, cardiac ventricle and atrium, and adrenal, respectively,[35] but the value of Okura et al. for rat cardiac tissue was of the same order as a value of 0.07 pg/μg found by Paul et al. for the CD-1 mouse heart.[36]

In contrast to these results, Iwai and Inagami were unable to detect renin mRNA in the ventricle or the aorta of adult rats of the Sprague-Dawley, WKY, or SHR strains or in cultured vascular smooth muscle cells, starting with 10 μg total RNA and a quantitative PCR involving 30 to 35 cycles; but they found values of 0.01, 0.01, and 0.02 to 0.03 pg/μg total RNA in the brains of the respective strains and 0.008 and 0.03 pg/μg total RNA for the adrenal of Dahl salt-sensitive and salt-resistant rats, respectively, after 4 weeks of a low salt diet.[54] No values were reported for the kidney. Known quantities of a shortened renin mRNA fragment transcribed from a deletion mutant were included in each reaction so that cDNA derived from this fragment and renin mRNA could be coamplified in a PCR that included $[\alpha^{32}P]$-dCTP to give radioactive products. The signal intensity for the internal standard (263 bp) was then compared with that for native renin mRNA (372 bp) for quantification of the latter. The values thus appear to be lower than those obtained by Okura et al. in those tissues where renin mRNA was detected. It is difficult to explain the discrepancy between these different reports, although one omission from the paper by Okura et al. is any mention of controls for contamination, where false positives resulting from PCR-product carryover in the laboratory environment can be a major problem in this highly sensitive technique and requires rigid precautions to prevent it from happening.[55] Moreover, the finding by Okura et al. of similar concentrations for the heart as for the adrenal differs from results using earlier techniques, where levels in the heart, when present, were always lower than in the adrenal.[7,38]

As in the study by Iwai and Inagami, a study by Holycross et al. was unable to detect renin mRNA by PCR in aortas of adult male Sprague-Dawley rats, even after 3 days of treatment with 0.2 mg/ml enalapril p.o., although no tests for the heart appear to have been carried out.[56] Interestingly, the primers used were also able to hybridize to and amplify a fragment of cathepsin D and cathepsin E mRNA-derived cDNA, although the product differed in size for cathepsin D (303 bp) but not cathepsin E (282 bp), which was the same as the 282 bp renin PCR product, and each was distinguished

Table 1
PCR Primers Used for Renin mRNA Detection in Rat Tissues and Their Location with Respect to the Nucleotide Sequence of 1.6 kb Rat Renin mRNA

Reference	Sense Primer	Antisense Primer	Size of PCR Product
Ekker et al.[51]	940–959	1,181–1,200	261 bp
Lou et al.[52]	768–788	1,079–1,099	331 bp
Okura et al.[53]	1,053–1,072	1,221–1,241	189 bp
Iwai & Inagami[54]	747–776	1,118–1,089	372 bp
Holycross et al.[56]	334–361	594–615	282 bp
Wang et al.[57]	876–896	1,041–1,061	186 bp
Lou et al.[58]	709–730	1,080–1,099	390 bp
Lou & Morris (unpubl.)*	709–730	1,109–1,129	421 bp

* As used in the quantitative method described in this chapter.

by hybridization probing. In another quantitative renin mRNA PCR study, involving adult female Sprague-Dawley rats, much lower values of approximately 0.001 pg/μg total RNA were obtained for the kidney, with considerable interassay variability.[57] The hearts were not tested. Table 1 shows the region amplified in the various reports of renin mRNA PCR. A summary of the data obtained in the various attempts by different groups to quantify renin mRNA in the heart and other tissues by PCR, dot-blot hybridization, and ribonuclease protection/solution hybridization techniques is provided in Table 2. In considering this data, it is worthwhile performing a calculation to estimate, to an order of magnitude, the concentration of renin mRNA in the kidney, where renin is present in cells that occupy approximately 0.01% or less of the tissue mass. On the basis of an estimated total RNA concentration of 3 mg/g tissue and a total mRNA of 2% of total RNA, the concentration of renin mRNA can

Table 2

Values for Renin mRNA Concentration in the Heart and Other Tissues from Various Studies Using Different Techniques

Reference	Method	Species	Renin mRNA (pg/μg total RNA)			
			Heart	Kidney	Adrenal	Brain
Mesterovic et al.[31]	Dot-blot	SW mouse	—	2–5	—	—
Catanzaro et al.[32]	Dot-blot	SW mouse	—	1–2	—	—
Morris et al.[85]						
Paul et al.[36]	RP/SH	NMRI mouse	<0.01	5	—	0
	RP/SH	CD-1 mouse	0.07	5	—	0.03
Suzuki et al.[35]	RP/SH	WKY rat	0.04–0.1	0.4	0.01	0.06
Okura et al.[53]	PCR	WKY rat	0.15	56	0.16	—
Iwai & Inagami[54]	PCR	Dahl S	0	—	0.01–0.03	0.01
	PCR	WKY, BN, Lewis	0	—	—	0.01
	PCR	SHR	0	—	—	0.03
Lou & Morris (unpubl.)	PCR	SD rat	0.01	3	—	—

Abbreviations: RP, ribonuclease protection; SH, solution hybridization; SW, Swiss-Webster; BN, Brown-Norway; SD, Sprague-Dawley be calculated to be of the order of 1 pg/μg total RNA if one assumes that renin mRNA is half of the total mRNA in the juxtaglomerular cell. Values that deviate markedly from this value might therefore be judged to be incorrect, and the values reported for other tissues, such as heart tissue, in that particular study might then need to be reconsidered. Even if the kidney value appears approximately correct, this does not, however, offer assurance that values for other tissues are also correct since the latter could still include nonspecific influences on the value obtained, or, in the case of PCR, degradation of mRNA prior to cDNA synthesis or PCR-product carryover contamination.

Regulation of Renin mRNA Shown by PCR

Recently, Lou et al., using PCR for 35 cycles, followed by hybridization probing of PCR products, have found that although renin mRNA is only just able to be detected in the atria, but not in the ventricles, of sodium-replete, adult, female, 7-week-old, 150 g Wistar rats, when the rats are treated for 1 week with enalapril (1 mg/ml in drinking water) and a low sodium diet, an enormous increase in the amount of PCR product occurred.[58] This suggested that the renin gene is quiescent in cardiac tissue under sodium-replete conditions, but that under similar conditions known to act as potent stimuli to renin expression in the kidney,[32] renin gene expression in the heart can be switched on. Interestingly, another extrarenal tissue, the adrenal, also responds to sodium depletion—with a doubling of renin mRNA.[59] The ability of the renin gene to respond to such stimuli was, moreover, first determined for the kidney.[32]

Regulation of Cardiac Renin mRNA by Quantitative PCR

A quantitative PCR has since been devised by us, as outlined in Figures 1 and 2. In this procedure, which was based on a method devised for platelet-derived growth factor (PDGF) mRNA,[60] total mRNA was isolated, and a dilution series for samples and standards underwent PCR in separate tubes. For the standard, renin cRNA was transcribed from a rat renin cDNA in an expression plasmid. In addition, the PCR of cDNA reverse transcribed from β-actin was used as an internal monitor of intersample variability. After electrophoresis of the post-PCR mixture on a 3% agarose gel to confirm that any PCR product present was of the size expected from renin

Renin mRNA PCR – Heart

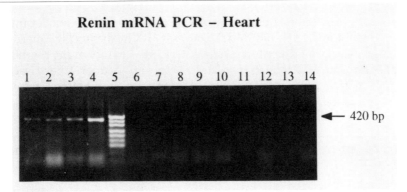

Fig. 3. Ethidium-bromide-stained 3% agarose electrophoretic gel on which the post-PCR mixture was run. Lanes 1–4: 3μl of products from 1 μg kidney total RNA—lane 1: NaCl-replete control rat; lane 2: enalapril-treated; lane 3: low NaCl diet; lane 4: enalapril + low NaCl. Lane 5: DNA size marker (pUC19 cut with *Hpa*II). Lane 6: negative control (submandibular gland total RNA). Lanes 7–14: 10 μl of products from 10 μg of heart total RNA—lane 7: atrium of NaCl-replete control rat; lane 8: atrium of enalapril-treated rat; lane 9: atrium of low NaCl rat; lane 10: atrium of enalapril + low NaCl rat; lane 11: ventricle of NaCl-replete control; lane 12: ventricle of enalapril-treated rat; lane 13: ventricle of low NaCl rat; lane 14: ventricle of enalapril + low NaCl rat.

mRNA, 420 bp (Figure 3), the post-PCR mixture was then subjected to slot-blot hybridization using an oligonucleotide probe (5'-CTG CAG TTG ATC ATG CAA GCC CTG GGA GTC AA-3') corresponding to nucleotides 931–962 of the full-length renin cDNA and directed at a target sequence within the renin PCR product (nucleotides 709 to 1,129). The intensity of bands on the autoradiograph obtained (Figure 4) was determined using a scanning laser densitometer, and values for standards were used to construct a standard curve (Figure 5). From this, the quantity of renin mRNA in samples was determined. For atrial tissue, this was 0.010 ± 0.001 pg/μg total RNA. The concentration in the ventricle was lower. The values obtained compare favorably with those in several other studies, and in the case of the kidney were similar to those reported for the renal tissue of the mouse in our early dot-blot experiments (Table 2). Using this method, we have found that the concentration of renin mRNA in atrial tissue can be markedly stimulated by the A I-converting enzyme inhibitor, enalapril (5 mg/kg per day in drinking water), and by sodium depletion, with the most marked stimulation obtained with a combination of both enalapril and a low sodium diet (Figure 6). The combination of a low sodium diet and an ACE inhibitor has

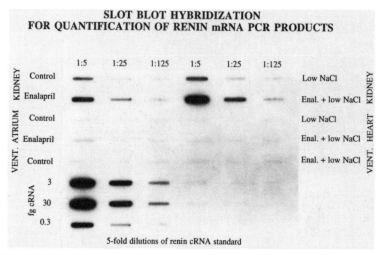

Fig. 4. Autoradiograph obtained after slot-blot hybridization of post-PCR DNA samples on Zeta probe nylon membrane with ^{32}P-end-labeled renin oligonucleotide probe. Renin cRNA standard was mixed with 10 μg of total RNA from a tissue that does not express the renin gene—the rat submandibular gland (SMG)—as the carrier, prior to reverse transcription. The last two slots at the right-hand side of the bottom row were from PCR of SMG total RNA (negative control).

similarly been found to be more effective than either alone in stimulating renin mRNA in the kidney.[23,32,61–65] We have also used our PCR method to quantify changes in renin mRNA concentration in the kidney, as well as in other tissues. It therefore appears that a phenomenon similar to that occurring in the kidney with such stimuli also operates for renin gene expression in the heart.

Recruitment

It is not known whether the changes seen in renin mRNA concentration are due to increased expression of the renin gene in cells already expressing renin mRNA at a lower level, or whether it involves recruitment for renin synthesis of cells that were previously dormant in relation to renin gene expression. In this regard, it is noteworthy that recruitment of quiescent cells for renin synthesis under stimulated conditions occurs in the classic site of renin synthesis in the kidney—the juxtaglomerular apparatus (JGA). After sodium depletion,[66] adrenalectomy,[67,68] renal artery constriction,[69] a

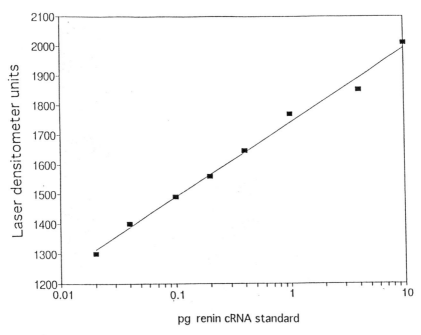

Fig. 5. A standard curve used for determination of renin mRNA concentration. Intensity of bands on autoradiograph such as in Figure 4 were determined with a laser densitometer and plotted against the corresponding quantity of the renin cRNA standard used for reverse transcription and PCR.

high protein diet,[70] or ACE-inhibitor treatment,[64,71–73] not only do more JGAs contain renin and renin mRNA, but renin and renin mRNA each appear de novo in previously negative cells extending farther up the afferent arteriolar tree.

Switching Off of Renin Gene Expression with Maturation

A similar situation applies in reverse during development: in newborn WKY rats and SHRs, renal renin has been reported to be two and five times higher than in adults of each strain, respectively; renin mRNA was eight times higher; and renin immunoreactivity was distributed throughout the entire length of the afferent arterioles and interlobular arteries, whereas by adulthood the pattern had contracted to the well-known juxtaglomerular location.[65] Similar developmental changes have been reported earlier in the mouse,[74]

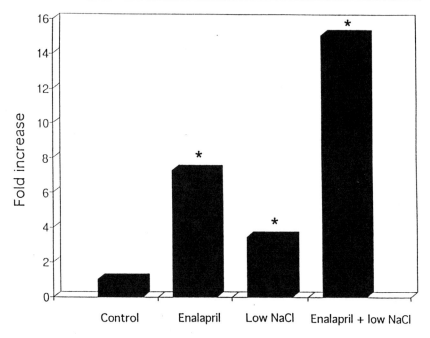

Fig. 6. Response in cardiac renin mRNA, quantified by PCR, after treatment of groups of six Sprague-Dawley rats for one week with enalapril (6 mg/kg per day in drinking water), or a low sodium diet, or both. In each case S.E.(not shown) was <10% of the value for the mean. A t-test comparing each treatment with the control showed that the change was highly significant ($^*p<0.001$).

pig,[75] and human.[76] Interestingly, PCR has shown recently that in the kidney, proximal tubule cells do not contain renin mRNA in untreated rats, but that after enalapril treatment, renin expression can be detected.[77] This, coupled with the finding of angiotensinogen in the kidney, suggests the operation of a local intrarenal RAS.[78]

Renin mRNA PCR of the Neonatal Heart and Localization

In the heart, Dostal et al. have found a considerably greater signal intensity after a renin mRNA PCR involving 1 μg total RNA from the cardiac tissue of neonatal Sprague-Dawley rats than was apparent in adult animals.[14] In situ hybridization indicated that, in contrast to the situation in adult rats, the left ventricle of neonatal rats had more renin mRNA than the atrium, and it was proposed that this might be due to the rapid ventricular growth at this early stage of development. In embryonic chicks at day 18, renin mRNA has similarly been detected in all 4 cardiac chambers but was found only in the atria 10 days after birth.[79]

Role of Renin Expression in the Heart

Thus, cardiac renin expression would appear to be highly regulatable and therefore of potential physiological and pathophysiological importance. The quantity of angiotensinogen mRNA and protein (reviewed in the next chapter) far exceeds that of renin mRNA and protein. This implies that renin might be rate limiting in the operation of a putative intracardiac RAS. The increase in renin mRNA that can occur under certain circumstances is suggestive of increased transcription of the renin gene, although the contribution of decreased degradation has not yet been examined. There is, however, no information on the nature of the protein synthesized, and experiments that have been carried out for other tissues[80] would resolve this issue. Prorenin would, nevertheless, be the anticipated translation product. Prorenin is generally regarded as inactive, although evidence is beginning to accumulate that suggests the possibility that prorenin, under certain circumstances, might have intrinsic enzymatic activity without being converted to renin.[81,82] This could apply in the specialized environment of a particular intracellular compartment or local extracellular milieu, but there is no hard evidence yet for prorenin activity in vivo, certainly not in the heart. The extent to which prorenin might be converted to renin in cardiac cells in vivo is not known. It is also uncertain whether or not renin or prorenin that might be produced in the heart is secreted. It is possible that there might be intracellular activity, either exclusively or in addition to local extracellular activity. An intracellular form of renin/prorenin could arise, for example, from the use of alternate promoter(s) that lead to synthesis of a renin precursor having a different, more hydrophilic N-terminal leader sequence which could prevent the molecule from entering the secretory compartment.[83] Evidence to date shows, however, that even though this may occur for some extrarenal tissues, only the proximal (major) promoter is used in the heart of DBA/2 mice.[84]

Acknowledgements

The authors' research is supported by a grant from the National Heart Foundation of Australia.

Summary

This chapter examines the evidence for renin enzymatic activity, renin immunoreactivity, and renin mRNA in cardiac tissue. The data does not appear to be convincing, at least for measurements made under basal conditions, and leads to the conclusion that renin and gene expression is, at best, extremely low and not consistently seen across the various species and strains tested. Possible reasons for the discrepancies between the results of different studies are discussed. Emerging evidence, however, from the use of sensitive polymerase chain reaction (PCR) technology points to the presence of renin mRNA in the heart but at very low concentrations (10 fg/µg total RNA). Most notably, this work has recently demonstrated that the renin gene in cardiac tissue can undergo marked stimulation under certain conditions, such as sodium depletion and converting-enzyme inhibitor treatment. These new findings strengthen suggestions about a role for renin, possibly as the rate-limiting enzyme, in an intracardiac RAS in particular physiological situations and, potentially, in pathophysiological cardiovascular states as well.

References

1. Gould AB, Skeggs LT, Kahn JR. The presence of renin activity in blood vessel walls. J Exp Med 1964; 119:389–399.
2. Hayduk K, Boucher R, Genest J. Renin activity and content in various tissues in dogs under different pathophysiological states. Proc Soc Exp Biol Med 1970; 134:252–255.
3. Ganten D, Ganten U, Granger P, Boucher R, Genest J. Renin in heart muscle and arterial tissue (abstract). Verh Dtsch Ges Kreislaufforsch 1972; 38:268.
4. Yunge L, Ballak M, Beuzeron M, Lacasse J, Cantin M. Ultrastructural cytochemistry of atrial and ventricular cardiocytes of the bullfrog *(Rana catesbeiana)*: relationship of specific granules with reninlike activity of the myocardium. Can J Pharmacol 1980; 58:1436–1476.
5. Needleman P, Marshall GR, Sobel BE. Hormone interactions in the isolated rabbit heart. Circ Res 1975; 37:802–808.
6. Dzau VJ, Re RN. Evidence for the existence of renin in the heart.Circulation 1987; 75(suppl. I):I-134–I-136.
7. Rosenthal J, von Lutterotti N, Thurnreiter M, Gomba S, Rothemund

J, Reiter W, et al. Suppression of renin-angiotensin system in the heart of spontaneously hypertensive rats. J Hypertens 1987; 5(suppl. 2): S23–S31.

8. Wood JM, Baum H-P, Carleton J, Dzau VJ. Inhibition of renin-like activity in marmoset tissue by the renin inhibitor CGP 29 287. J Hypertens 1987; 5(suppl. 2):S67–S69.

9. Day RP, Reid IA. Renin activity in dog brain: enzymological similarity to cathepsin D. Endocrinology 1976; 99:93–100.

10. Dorer RE, Lentz KE, Kahn JR, Levine M, Skeggs LT. A comparison of the substrate specificities of cathepsin D and pseudorenin. J Biol Chem 1978; 253:3140–3142.

11. Hackenthal E, Hackenthal R, Hilgenfeldt U. Isorenin, pseudorenin, cathepsin D, and renin: a comparative enzymatic study of angiotensin-forming enzymes. Biochim Biophys Acta 1978; 522:574–578.

12. Morris BJ, Reid IA. A "renin-like" enzymatic action of cathepsin D and the similarity in subcellular distributions of "renin-like" activity and cathepsin D in the midbrain of dogs. Endocrinology 1978; 103: 1289–1296.

13. Mebazzaa A, Chevalier B, Mercadier JJ, Echter E, Rappaport L, Swynghedauw B. A review of the renin-angiotensin system in the normal heart. J Cardiovasc Pharmacol 1989; 14(suppl. 4):S16–S20.

14. Dostal DE, Rothblum KN, Chernin MI, Cooper GR, Baker KM. Intracardiac detection of angiotensinogen and renin: a localized renin-angiotensin system in neonatal rat heart. Am J Physiol 1992; 263:C838–C850.

15. Fordis CM, Megorden JS, Ropchak TG, Keiser HR. Absence of reninlike activity in rat aorta and microvessels. Hypertension 1983; 5:635–641.

16. Loudon M, Bing RF, Thurston H, Swales JD. Arterial wall uptake of renal renin and blood pressure control. J Hypertens 1983; 5:629–634.

17. Swales JD, Abramovici A, Beck F, Bing RF, Loudon M, Thurston H. Arterial wall renin. J Hypertens 1983; 1(suppl.1):17–22.

18. Admiral PJJ, Derkx FHM, Danser AHJ, Pieterman H, Schalekamp MADH. Metabolism and production of angiotensin I in different vascular beds. Hypertension 1990; 15:44–55.

19. Campbell DJ. The site of renin production. J Hypertens 1985; 3: 199–207.

20. Campbell DJ. Circulating and tissue angiotensin systems. J Clin Invest 1987; 79:1–6.

21. Mizuno K, Tani M, Niimura S, Hashimoto S, Satoh A, Shimamoto K, et al. Direct evidence for local generation and release of angiotensin II in human vascular tissue. Biochem Biophys Res Commun 1989; 165: 457–463.

22. Skinner SL, Thatcher RL, Whitworth JA, Horowitz JD. Extraction of plasma prorenin by human heart. Lancet 1986; i:995–997.

23. Dzau VJ, Brody T, Ellison KE, Pratt RE, Ingelfinger JR. Tissue-specific regulation of renin expression in the mouse. Hypertension 1987; 9(suppl. III):III-36–III-41.

24. Dzau VJ, Ingelfinger JR, Pratt RE. Regulation of tissue renin and angiotensinogen gene expressions. J Cardiovasc Pharmacol 1986; 8:45–52.

25. Dzau VJ, Ellison KE, Ouelette AJ. Expression and regulation of renin in the mouse heart (abstract). Clin Res 1984; 33:181A.

26. Dzau VJ. Cardiac renin-angiotensin system: Molecular and functional aspects. Am J Med 1988; 84:22–27.

27. Re R, Fallon JT, Dzau VJ, Quay SC, Haber E. Renin synthesis by canine aortic smooth muscle cells in culture. Life Sci 1982; 30:99–106.
28. Re R. The myocardial intracellular renin-angiotensin system. Am J Cardiol 1987; 59:56A–58A.
29. Re R, Ravigatt U. New approaches to the study of the cellular biology of the cardiovascular system. Circulation 1988; 77(suppl I):I-14–I-17.
30. Dzau VJ, Ellison KE, Ouelette AJ. Expression and regulation of renin in the mouse heart (abstract). Clin Res 1984; 33:181A.
31. Mesterovic N, Catanzaro DF, Morris BJ. Detection of renin mRNA in mouse kidney and submandibular gland by hybridization with renin cDNA. Endocrinology 1983; 113:1179–1181.
32. Catanzaro DF, Mesterovic N, Morris BJ. Studies of the regulation of mouse renin genes by measurement of renin messenger ribonucleic acid. Endocrinology 1985; 117:872–878.
33. Ganten D, Ludwig G, Hennhoefer C. Genetic control of renin in the tisues of different strains of mice (abstract). Nuayn Schmeideberg's Archiv Pharmacol 1986; 332:R59.
34. Dzau VJ, Ellison KE, Brody T, Ingelfinger J, Pratt RE. A comparative study of the distributions of renin and angiotensinogen messenger ribonucleic acids in rat and mouse tissues. Endocrinology 1987; 120: 2334–2338.
35. Suzuki F, Ludwig G, Hellmann W, Paul M, Lindpaintner K, Murakami K, et al. Renin gene expression in rat tissues: a new quantitative assay method for rat renin mRNA using synthetic cRNA. Clin Exp Hypertens 1988; A10:345–359.
36. Paul M, Wagner D, Metzger R, Ganten D, Lang RE, Suzuki F, et al. Quantification of renin mRNA in various mouse tissues by a novel solution hybridization assay. J Hypertens 1988; 6:247–252.
37. Samani NJ, Morgan K, Brammar WJ, Swales JD. Detection of renin messenger RNA in rat tissues: increased sensitivity using an RNAse protection technique. J Hypertens 1987; 5(suppl. 2):S19–S21.
38. Samani NJ, Swales JD, Brammar WJ. Expression of the renin gene in extra-renal tissues of the rat. Biochem J 1988; 253:907–910.
39. Field LJ, McGowan RA, Dickinson DP, Gross KW. Tissue and gene specificity of mouse renin expression. Hypertension 1984; 6: 597–603.
40. Metzger R, Wagner D, Takahashi S, Suzuki F, Lindpainter K, Ganten D. Tissue renin-angiotensin systems. Aspects of molecular biology and pharmacology. Clin Exp Hypertens 1988; A10:1227–1238.
41. Suzuki F, Lindpaintner K, Keuneke C, Hellmann W, Takahashi S, Nakamura Y, et al. Tissue-specific regulation of gene expression for renin and angiotensinogen. Clin Exp Hypertens 1988; A10: 1317–1319.
42. Samani NJ, Swales JD, Brammar WJ. A widespread abnormality of renin gene expression in the spontaneously hypertensive rat: modulation in some tissues with the development of hypertension. Clin Sci 1989; 77:629–636.
43. Samani NJ, Brammar WJ, Swales JD. Renal and extra-renal levels of renin mRNA in experimental hypertension. Clin Sci 1991; 80:339–344.
44. Tada M, Fukamizu A, Seo MS, Takahashi S, Murakami K. Renin expression in the kidney and brain is reciprocally controlled by captopril. Biochem Biophys Res Commun 1989; 159:1065–1071.
45. Aldred GP, Fu P, Crawford RJ, Fernley RT. The sequence and tissue expression of ovine renin. J Mol Endocrinol 1992; 8:3–11.

46. Baker KM, Chernin MI, Cooper GR. Localization of heart angiotensinogen and renin mRNA by hybridization histochemistry (abstract). Physiologist 1990; 33:A-96.
47. Mullins JJ, Sigmund CD, Kane-Haas C, Gross KW. Expression of the DBA/2J *Ren-2* gene in the adrenal gland of transgenic mice. EMBO J 1989; 8:4065–4072.
48. Fukamizu A, Seo MS, Hatae T, Hokoyma M, Nomura T, Katsuki M, et al. Tissue-specific expression of the human renin gene in transgenic mice. Biochem Biophys Res Commun 1989; 165:826–832.
49. Sigmund CD, Jones CA, Kane CM, Wu C, Lang JA, Gross KW. Regulated tissue- and cell-specific expression of the human renin gene in transgenic mice. Circ Res 1992; 70:1070–1079.
50. Sigmund CD, Fabian JR, Gross KW. Expression and regulation of the renin gene. Trends Cardiovasc Med 1992; 2:237–245.
51. Ekker M, Tronik D, Rougeon F. Extra-renal transcription of the renin genes in multiple tissues of mice and rats. Proc Natl Acad Sci USA 1989; 86:5155–5158.
52. Lou Y-k, Smith DL, Robinson BG, Morris BJ. Renin gene expression in various tissues determined by single-step polymerase chain reaction. Clin Exp Pharmacol Physiol 1991; 18:357–362.
53. Okura T, Kitami Y, Iwata T, Hiwada K. Quantitative measurement of extra-renal mRNA by polymerase chain reaction. Biochem Biophys Res Commun 1991; 179:25–31.
54. Iwai N, Inagami T. Quantitative analysis of renin gene expression in extrarenal tissues by polymerase chain reaction method. J Hypertens 1992; 10:717–724.
55. Kwok S, Higuchi R. Avoiding false positives with PCR. Nature 1989; 339:237–238.
56. Holycross BJ, Saye J, Harrison JK, Peach MJ. Polymerase chain reaction analysis of renin in rat aortic smooth muscle. Hypertension 1992; 19:697–701.
57. Wang Y, Yamaguchi T, Franco-Saenz R, Mulrow PJ. Regulation of renin gene expression in rat adrenal zona glomerulosa cells. Hypertension 1992; 20:776–781.
58. Lou Y-k, Robinson BG, Morris BJ. Renin messenger RNA, detected by polymerase chain reaction, can be switched on in rat atrium. J Hypertens 1993; 11:237–243.
59. Brecher AS, Shier DN, Dene H, Wang SM, Rapp JP, Franco-Saenz R, et al. Regulation of adrenal renin messenger ribonucleic acid by dietary sodium chloride. Endocrinology 1989; 124:2907– 2913.
60. Ballagi-Pordány A, Ballagi-Pordány A, Funa K. Quantitative determination of mRNA phenotypes by the polymerase chain reaction. Analyt Biochem 1991; 196:89–94.
61. Nakamura N, Soubrier F, Menard J, Panthier J-J, Rougeon F, Corvol P. Nonproportional changes in plasma renin concentration, renal renin content, and rat renin messenger RNA. Hypertension 1985; 7:855–859.
62. Iwao H, Fukui K, Kim S, Nakayama K, Ohkubo H, Nakanishi S, et al. Effect of changes in sodium balance on renin, angiotensinogen and atrial natriuretic factor messenger RNA levels in rats. J Hypertens 1988; 6(suppl. 4):S297–S299.
63. Miller CCJ, Samani NJ, Carter AT, Brooks JI, Brammar WJ. Modula-

tion of mouse renin gene expression by dietary sodium chloride intake in one-gene, two-gene and transgenic animals. J Hypertens 1989; 7: 861–863.

64. Berka JLA, Alcorn D, Coghlan JP, Fernley RT, Morgan TO, Ryan GB, et al. Granular juxtaglomerular cells and prorenin synthesis in mice treated with enalapril. J Hypertens 1990; 8:229–238.

65. Gomez R, Lynch KR, Chevalier RL, Wilfong N, Everett A, Carey RM, et al. Renin and angiotensinogen gene expression in maturing rat kidney. Am J Physiol 1988; 254:F582–F587.

66. Taugner R, Hackenthal E, Nobling R, Harlacher M, Reb G. The distribution of renin in the different segments of the renal arterial tree: immunocytochemical investigation in the mouse kidney. Histochemistry 1981; 73:75–88.

67. Szabo J, Devenyi I. Ultrastructural data on different types of hyperplasia and hyperfunction of the juxtaglomerular apparatus. Acta Morphol Hung 1972; 20:39–48.

68. De Senarclens CF, Pricam CE, Banichahi FD, Vallotton MB. Renin synthesis, storage and release in the rat: a morphological and biochemical study. Kidney Int 1977; 11:161–169.

69. Taugner R, Marin-Grez M, Keilbach R, Hackenthal E, Nobling R. Immunoreactive renin and angiotensin II in the afferent glomerular arterioles of rats with hypertension due to unilateral renal artery constriction. Histochemistry 1982; 76:61–69.

70. Tufro-McReddie A, Arrizurieta EE, Brocca S, Gomez RA. Dietary protein modulates intrarenal distribution of renin and its mRNA during development. Am J Physiol 1992; 263:F427–F435.

71. Taugner R, Hackenthal E, Helmchen U, Ganten D, Kugler P, Marin-Grez M, et al. The intra-renal renin-angiotensin system: an immunocytochemical study on the localization of renin, angiotensinogen, converting enzyme and the angiotensins in the kidney of mouse and rat. Klin Woschenschr 1982; 60:1218–1222.

72. Zaki FG, Keim GR, Takii Y, Inagami T. Hyperplasia of juxtaglomerular cells and renin localization in kidneys of normotensive animals given captopril: electron microscopic and immunohistochemical studies. Ann Clin Lab Sci 1982; 12:200–215.

73. Gomez RA, Chevalier RL, Everett AD, Elwood JP, Peach MJ, Lynch KR, et al. Recruitment of renin gene-expressing cells in adult rat kidneys. Am J Physiol 1990; 259:F660–F665.

74. Minuth M, Hackenthal E, Poulsen K, Rix E, Taugner R. Renin immunocytochemistry of the differentiating juxtaglomerular apparatus. Anat Embryol 1981; 162:173–181.

75. Egerer G, Taugner R, Tiedmann K. Renin immunohistochemistry in the mesonephros and metanephros of the pig embryo. Histochemistry 1984; 81:385–390.

76. Celio M, Groscurth P, Inagami T. Ontogeny of renin immunoreactive cells in the human kidney. Anat Embryol 1985; 173: 149–155.

77. Moe OW, Ujiie K, Star RA, Miller RT, Widell J, Alpern RJ, et al. Renin expression in renal proximal tubule. J Clin Invest 1993; 91:774–779.

78. Morris BJ, Johnston CI. Renin substrate in granules from rat kidney cortex. Biochem J 1976; 154:625–637.

79. Chernin MI, Candia AF, Stark LL, Aceto JF, Baker KM. Fetal expres-

sion of renin, angiotensinogen, and atriopeptin genes in chick heart. Clin Exp Hypertens 1990; 12:617–629.

80. Catanzaro DF, Mullins JJ, Morris BJ. The biosynthetic pathway of renin. J Biol Chem 1983; 258:7364–7368.

81. Lenz T, Sealey JE. Tissue renin systems as a possible factor in hypertension. In: Laragh JH, Brenner BM, eds. Hypertension: Pathophysiology, Diagnosis, and Management. New York: Raven Press, 1990:1319–1328.

82. Derkx FHM, Deinum J, Lipovski M, Verhaar M, Fischli W, Schalekamp MADH. Nonproteolytic "activation" of prorenin by active site-directed renin inhibitors as demonstrated by renin-specific monoclonal antibody. J Biol Chem 1992; 267:22837–22842.

83. Morris BJ. New possibilities for intracellular renin and inactive renin now that the structure of the human renin gene has been elucidated (editorial review). Clin Sci 1986; 71:345–355.

84. Paul M, Burt DW, Kreiger JE, Nakamura N, Dzau VJ. Tissue specificity of renin promoter activity and regulation in the mouse. Am J Physiol 1992; 262:644–650.

85. Morris BJ, Catanzaro DF, Hardman J, Mesterovic N, Tellam J, Hort Y, et al. Human renin gene sequence, gene regulation and prorenin processing. J Hypertens 1984; 2(suppl. 3):231–233.

3

Cardiac Angiotensinogen: Its Local Activation to Angiotensin Peptides and Its Regulation

Young-Ae Lee, Manwen Jin, Traudel Hellmann, Nikolaj Niedermaier, Detlev Ganten, and Klaus Lindpaintner

Introduction

Although the renin-angiotensin system (RAS) was originally understood as a classical endocrine system, where soluble effector molecules originate from a secretory gland and reach their target organs via the bloodstream, we now recognize that the RAS produces its effects on different levels of organization. There is now definitive evidence for the expression of all components of what would classically be required for the definition of the RAS (renin, angiotensinogen, the angiotensin-converting enzyme, and the specific angiotensin receptor) in a variety of organs or tissues, and their presumed mode of action is paracrine, autocrine, or, perhaps, even intracrine. Proof of the existence of these local "tissue renin-angiotensin systems" relied heavily on the demonstration of local synthesis of the components of the catalytic cascade in individual tissues, as well as on their local interaction, resulting in the activation of precursor molecules to biologically active peptides. It is the purpose of this chapter to review the evidence, from our own work and from that

Lindpaintner K and Ganten D (editors): *The Cardiac-Renin Angiotensin System,* © Futura Publishing Co., Inc., Armonk, NY, 1994.

molecules to biologically active peptides. It is the purpose of this chapter to review the evidence, from our own work and from that of other laboratories, that supports the local intracardiac synthesis, the potential for activation, and regulatory modulation of angiotensinogen, the 55 kd glycoprotein of the α_2-globulin class that represents the precursor of biologically active angiotensin peptides.

Intracardiac Synthesis of Angiotensinogen

Early efforts to demonstrate the existence of a cardiac RAS focused on measurements of the protein and peptide components of the system in homogenized tissues. Initial measurements of angiotensin peptides in the ventricles, atria, and septum of hearts of rhesus monkeys revealed that concentrations per gram of wet tissue weight ranged between 100 fmol and 500 fmol for A II and between 30 fmol and 150 fmol for A I.[1] For both peptides, concentrations were highest in the right atrium, followed by the right ventricle, the left atrium, the interventricular septum, and the left ventricle. In a subsequent experiment, we presented additional evidence for the cardiac origin of these peptides by documenting that converting- enzyme inhibition lowers cardiac A II in nephrectomized rabbits. Although the measured concentrations, akin to values found in plasma, are certainly indicative of the potential for biological effects of the peptides in cardiac tissues, and although the inhibition by the converting-enzyme inhibitor treatment is consistent with local synthesis of the peptides, the experiment by no means provided proof for such local generation. Adsorption and extraction from the circulating pool and sequestration of peptides into the myocardium could not be excluded by these experimental results. A somewhat more convincing indication, at least for the intracardiac conversion of the precursor decapeptide to the biologically active octapeptide, if not for the intracardiac synthesis of angiotensinogen itself, came from a series of experiments using isolated, perfused rabbit hearts in which the sympathetic cardiac nerves were preserved intact. Electrical stimulation of these nerves resulted in the expected marked increase in heart rate, cardiac contractility, and coronary resistance. When this experiment was repeated in the presence of a converting-enzyme inhibitor in the crystalloid perfusate, all these responses were significantly attenuated and were consistent with the predicted loss of the facilitating effect of A II on sympathetic neurotransmission.[2] Although the preparation eliminated the possibility that this effect may have been due to a decrease in systemic A II, the possibility that the substrate for intracardiac A II was sequestrated from the circulating angiotensinogen pool could again not be excluded.

The dilemma of not being able to distinguish intracardially synthesized angiotensinogen from extracardially synthesized angiotensinogen was quickly resolved with the availability of sequence information and specific molecular probes for rat angiotensinogen in the early 1980s.[3] Our initial work on demonstrating angiotensinogen gene expression in the heart was done in both rats and mice by Northern blot hybridization,[4] followed by the development of a specific and rapid liquid hybridization assay that allowed processing of large sample numbers in an efficient manner.[5] For greater sensitivity, as well as specificity, we later adapted an RNAse protection assay to perform these analyses.[6] All analyses were based on the use of radiolabeled antisense cRNA molecules prepared from cloned angiotensinogen fragments by using the 5'-located RNA polymerase promoter site. In keeping with results obtained on the protein and peptide levels, we found that cardiac expression of angiotensinogen was highest in the right atrium, followed by the left atrium and, with considerably lower concentrations of mRNA, by the right and left ventricles.[7,8] These results from our laboratory correspond with those of a number of other groups.[9-13] In a comparative study, cardiac angiotensinogen mRNA levels were measured as 5% and 1% of those found in the livers of rats and mice, respectively.[10]

Source of Intracardiac Angiotensinogen

Since it stands to reason that the circulating angiotensinogen pool contributes to the overall intracardiac stores of angiotensinogen, and since most experiments addressing the functional integration of the elements of the cardiac RAS were to be performed in explanted, perfused hearts, it was important to demonstrate that intracardiac synthesis does, in fact, contribute measurable amounts of angiotensinogen and to assess the relative contribution from the two sources with regard to their magnitude and their kinetics.

The experiments were performed by measuring the spontaneous release of angiotensinogen from isolated, perfused rat hearts. Fractions of the coronary sinus effluent were collected and subsequently assayed for angiotensinogen concentrations by in vitro generation of A I after incubation at 37°C for 1 hour in the presence of purified hog renin. The data obtained show two distinct phases of release:

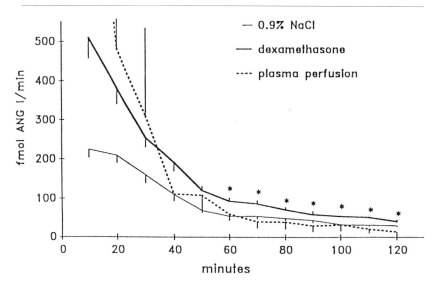

Fig. 1. Angiotensinogen release from isolated, perfused hearts under base-line conditions after a 10-minute perfusion with angiotensinogen-rich plasma and after pretreatment of experimental animals with dexamethasone 7mg/kg i.p. Asterisks denote statistically significant differences between baseline and dexamethasone-stimulated angiotensinogen release during the late phase of angiotensinogen release ($p < 0.05$) (from Lindpaintner K, et al.[7]).

during an early phase, large, but rapidly declining, amounts of angiotensinogen appeared in the effluent, whereas a second, more prolonged period was characterized by the release of lower, but relatively constant, amounts. We interpret the initial phase as the washout of plasma-derived angiotensinogen still present in the heart. Calculated cumulative data suggest that this pool has a fairly constant size. The second, delayed phase of angiotensinogen release at a relatively low, but stable, rate may thus represent overflow of locally synthesized protein (Figure 1). An alternative explanation, however, would be that this phase indicates a two-compartment system governing the release of exogenously derived and sequestrated angiotensinogen according to different kinetics.

To differentiate between these two possibilities, we examined the effects of perfusion with angiotensinogen-rich plasma and treatment with dexamethasone on angiotensinogen release. Although both of these maneuvers raise circulating angiotensinogen levels, only the latter will result in stimulation of local angiotensinogen synthesis. If both early- and late-phase release were simply a function of sequestration and subsequent release of exogenous angiotensinogen, then both experimental conditions should similarly affect the early and late phases of angiotensinogen release. If, however, the rate of angiotensinogen release during the delayed phase depended on local synthesis of angiotensinogen, then no changes would be expected in response to plasma perfusion, whereas dexamethasone exposure should result in sustained increases of angiotensinogen overflow during this phase. Thus, isolated hearts were exposed to a 10-minute perfusion with angiotensinogen-rich plasma prepared from 24-hour nephrectomized rats. In addition, a group of rats was given a 7 mg/kg dose of dexamethasone or an equal volume of saline i.p. 24 hours prior to sacrifice. As expected, both perfusion with angiotensinogen-rich plasma and treatment with dexamethasone resulted in accentuated peak rates of early angiotensinogen release that declined along steeper slopes; this was consistent with the concentration-gradient-driven depletion of a nonreplenished pool, augmented by previous exposure to elevated levels of circulating angiotensinogen. Although plasma perfusion had no effect on delayed phase angiotensinogen release, stimulation of local angiotensinogen synthesis by dexamethasone treatment resulted in a significant and sustained increase of late-phase angiotensinogen release despite the fact that initial rates of release were actually substantially higher after plasma perfusion. These data argue strongly against the notion that late-phase release reflects liberation of previously sequestrated, exogenous angiotensinogen from a second compartment. Instead, they indicate that the source of angiotensinogen released during the delayed phase is local synthesis and that the rate of this release is modulated by regulatory influences affecting the level of local angiotensinogen synthesis.

Intracardiac Activation of Angiotensin Peptides from Cardiac Angiotensinogen

In addition to the demonstration of intracardiac synthesis of angiotensinogen, evidence for the intracardiac expression of the remaining components of the RAS system, that is, renin, the angiotensin-converting enzyme, and the specific angiotensin receptor has meanwhile been presented and is covered later in more detail. Although it is a prerequisite of a biologically active system, a demonstration of the synthesis of elements of the catalytic cascade and precursor molecules does not, in itself, provide direct evidence that these elements interact locally in the expected fashion to produce intracardially-active angiotensin peptides. To test this possibility, we performed a series of functional and kinetic studies.

All the experiments described were again carried out in the isolated, perfused, beating rat heart preparation according to Langendorff. It has not been possible, to date, to measure the unstimulated release of biologically active angiotensin peptides from the perfused rat heart and thus obtain information about whether or not the activity of the cardiac RAS causes peptide spillover into the coronary circulation under baseline conditions. However, we reasoned that stimulation of the catalytic cascade with renin, the component classically viewed as the rate-limiting one, may allow us to at least indirectly assess the capacity of the local system to generate biologically active peptides.

Thus, experiments were conducted in which isolated perfused hearts were exposed to varying concentrations of highly purified hog renin; simultaneously, the coronary sinus effluent was collected in fractions, extracted by c_{18} affinity chromatography, and subsequently assayed by specific radioimmunoassay for A I and A II. The pooled and extracted effluent from a 1-hour perfusion in the absence of renin contained no measurable A I. Similarly, no detectable levels of A I were present in the coronary sinus effluent during the 10-minute collection period preceding the renin-infusion in each experiment. Immediately after the start of the renin infusion, however, A I appeared in the perfusate (Figure 2). Peptide concentrations showed a consistent pattern of a rapid rise, followed by an initially steep and subsequently more gradual decline. Maximum A I release occurred earlier at higher renin concentrations and showed a positive, statistically significant correlation with the concentration of renin infused. Cumulative amounts of released A I were not significantly different at the 3 highest concentrations of infused renin (3.19 $\pm$ 1.21, 4.74 $\pm$ 1.85, and 3.76 $\pm$ 1.14 pmol at renin concentrations of 0.2, 1, and 5 mU/ml) but were lower at renin infusions of 10 and 50 μU/ml(0.11 $\pm$ 0.03 and 0.55 $\pm$ 0.17 pmol/ml).

To test for the specificity of the observed release of A I in response to renin infusions, we simultaneously infused renin at a concentration of 200 μU/ml and the investigational pentapeptide renin-inhibitor, HOE S850057, at a concentration of $5 \cdot 10^{-6}$M (Figure 3). No A I was detectable in the perfusate collected during this first phase of the experiment (Fig. 3). After eight minutes, we stopped the renin-inhibitor but continued the infusion of renin. The fractions of the coronary sinus effluent collected during this second phase of

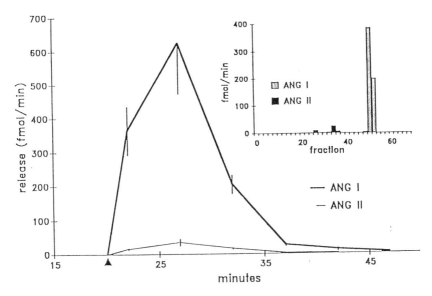

Fig. 2 Representative example of the time course of A I and A II recovery in the coronary sinus effluent of isolated, perfused hearts in response to renin infusion. (Data shown represent infusion of renin at 1 mU/min; arrowhead marks the start of the infusion.) Figure inset shows results of radioimmunoassay for A I and A II performed on HPLC fractions of the coronary sinus effluent sample (from Lindpaintner K, et al.[7]).

the experiment show a steady increase in the amount of released A I, which reached levels not statistically different from those seen with the same dose of renin in the absence of the inhibitor. The slope of the increase in peptide concentration in the perfusate, however, was not as steep as in control experiments without the inhibitor.

Angiotensin II, like A I, was also undetectable in the cardiac perfusate during the 10-minute control period prior to exposure to renin. Similarly, A II promptly appeared in the coronary sinus effluent after the renin infusion was started (Fig. 2). Using simultaneous determinations of A I and A II in the perfusate, we calculated the mean fractional conversion rate of A I to A II as 7.18% ± 1.09%.

To test if the formation of A II was dependent on the classical pathway involving the converting enzyme, we simultaneously infused renin at a concentration of 200 μU/ml and the converting-enzyme inhibitor, captopril, at a concentration of 10^{-6}M. A I levels measured in the perfusate were similar to those found in previous experiments, whereas generation of A II was almost completely suppressed. A lower concentration of the infused converting-enzyme in-

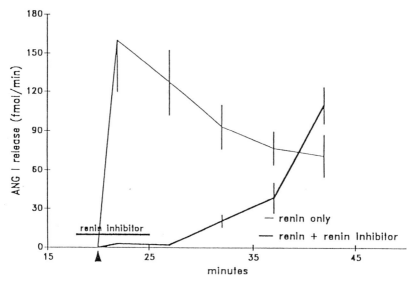

Fig. 3. Angiotensin I formation and release during renin infusion (200 μU/ ml) in the absence and presence of a renin inhibitor, HOE S850057. HOE S850057 infusion was begun 3 minutes prior to starting the renin infusion (indicated by arrowhead) and discontinued 5 minutes thereafter, while the infusion of renin was continued (from Lindpaintner K, et al. [7]).

hibitor resulted in a dose-dependent, progressively less-pronounced attenuation of A II production.

These results demonstrated clearly that the cardiac RAS has the capability to locally activate intracardiac angiotensinogen to the biologically active angiotensin peptides. Undetectable levels of A I in the perfusate before exposure to renin as well as suppression of A I release in the presence of a renin inhibitor strongly argue that the observed effects are mediated specifically by renin. In all experiments in which renin was infused, A I formation peaked early on and decreased steeply thereafter, suggesting the one-time processing of a nonreplenished pool of renin substrate. When renin infusions were maintained for longer time periods, however, an asymptotic plateau of angiotensin release at low rates became evident (because of the limited availability of the purified renin such prolonged infusions were only performed at low concentrations). These findings are in excellent agreement with the previously documented characteristic biphasic kinetics of angiotensinogen release.

Peak A I concentrations measured when renin was infused in physiological concentrations (10 and 50 μU/ml), 0.52 pm and 4.25 pm, respectively, were about one order of magnitude lower than normal plasma levels. This lower level may reflect the limited amount of angiotensinogen available for conversion but may also be due, in part, to the use of a heterologous enzyme rather than a species-specific one. Also, by collecting 10-minute fractions of the coronary sinus effluent, we obtained average values that may not represent true peaks. By measuring only the amount of peptide present in the coronary sinus effluent, we may have further underestimated the amount generated within the heart. Angiotensin I may be processed to A II intracellularly,[14] which limits the amount that reaches the coronary sinus. In addition, A I secreted into the coronary circulation may be subject to reuptake into smooth muscle cells or cardiac myocytes, as suggested by Khairallah et al.[15] Thus, local concentrations at the angiotensin receptor site might be considerably higher than apparent from our measurements and, thus, potentially physiologically significant. In addition to the effects of circulating renin examined in this investigation, local cardiac tissue renin may act on angiotensinogen taken up from the circulating pool or intrinsically produced within the heart.

The observed ratio between A I and A II closely matches previous results obtained in a different system where A I itself was infused.[1] Inhibition of the conversion of A I to A II in the presence of a specific converting-enzyme inhibitor indicates that the reaction was catalyzed by the converting enzyme, perhaps most likely at the luminal surface of the coronary endothelium.[16] However, both vascular smooth muscle cells and cardiac myocytes have been shown to contain the enzyme[14] and must therefore also be considered potential sites of action. As discussed with respect to A I, total amounts of A II may have been underestimated since we did not test for possible further enzymatic degradation of the peptide.

Regulation of Cardiac Angiotensinogen Expression

One of the tenets for the existence of a physiologically relevant cardiac RAS is that it be capable of responding to regulatory signals by modulation of its expression or activity. This can be classically evaluated by either exposing the system to pharmacological manipulation that is known to affect gene expression or by physiological perturbations known to stimulate or inhibit the system.

Using the same protocol as described above, we administered dexamethasone subcutaneously to rats 24 hours prior to sacrifice,

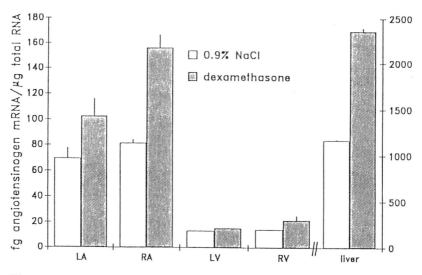

Fig. 4. Effect of dexamethasone treatment (7mg/kg i.p.) on angiotensinogen mRNA concentrations in cardiac and hepatic tissue. In all tissues, there is a statistically significant difference between concentrations between baseline (NaCl sham treatment) and dexamethasone treatment ($p<0.05$) (from Lindpaintner K, et al.[7]).

then excised the hearts, separated the right and left ventricles and atria, homogenized these tissues and extracted RNA. Angiotensinogen mRNA concentrations in the cardiac chambers and liver, as determined by solution-hybridization assay, were comparable to previously measured values.[5] Specificity of the solution-hybridization assay was confirmed by RNAse protection assay. After dexamethasone treatment, angiotensinogen mRNA concentrations were significantly increased ($p>0.05$) in all four cardiac chambers, along with increased hepatic angiotensinogen mRNA concentrations. (Figure 4). The increase was most pronounced in the right and left atrium, followed by the right and left ventricle. This finding is commensurate with the presence of several domains closely related to the putative glucocorticoid and estrogen hormone-responsive elements in the 5'-flanking region of the angiotensinogen gene.[17] Converting-enzyme inhibitor treatment was found to suppress angiotensinogen gene expression in the left ventricle,[12] whereas dietary sodium restriction has been reported to raise cardiac angiotensinogen mRNA levels.[18] The finding that nephrectomy, while inducing increased expression in the liver and suppression in the aorta, adrenal, and lung, did not influence levels of cardiac angiotensinogen mRNA provides further evidence for independent and tissue-specific regulation of cardiac angiotensinogen gene expression.[9]

The recognition that angiotensin does not only have vasoactive properties but may also exert growth-promoting effects[20–23] raised interest in modulation of the activity of the cardiac RAS during pathophysiological states accompanied by increases in cardiac mass. The finding that converting-enzyme inhibition at very low doses, which do not affect systemic hemodynamics, results in prevention or regression of cardiac hypertrophy emphasizes the potential trophic effects of the cardiac RAS;[24] in addition, onset and progression of cardiac hypertrophy have been shown to be associated with enhanced activity of the cardiac RAS.[19,25,26] Baker et al.[19]confirmed upregulation of cardiac angiotensinogen expression in all regions of the heart following the imposition of increased afterload by abdominal aortic constriction in rats, which accompanied development of myocardial hypertrophy. We obtained similar results when investigating the fate of angiotensinogen gene expression in a model of left-ventricular remodeling in the aftermath of an experimentally induced myocardial infraction. The remodeling process, which may be seen as a rapidly occurring hypertrophic adaptation of the noninfarcted left ventricle to compensate for the loss of contractile muscle, had previously been shown to be particularly sensitive to treatment with converting-enzyme inhibitors.[27,28] Experiments were performed in rats 5 days and 25 days after ligation of the left coronary artery or sham operation. Coronary artery ligation resulted in relative infarct sizes averaging 29% and 36% of total left-ventricular mass at 5 days and 25 days and in marked elevations of left-ventricular end-diastolic pressure (LVEDP). Angiotensinogen mRNA levels, measured by solution hybridization assay and confirmed in a second, independent experimental group by RNAse protection assay, were significantly elevated in the noninfarcted portion of the left ventricle at 5 days after infarction when compared to the sham group (22.1 + 3.3 vs. 13.4 ± 2.0 fg/μg total RNA; ratio of densitometric absorbance for angiotensinogen/β-actin: 0.356 ± 0.041 vs. 0.156 ± 0.02) and showed a significant correlation with infarct size (r = 0.93).[6] At 25 days, angiotensinogen gene expression had returned to control values (Figure 5). Similarly, no significant differences in angiotensinogen mRNA levels between animals with and without infarction were found in other cardiac tissues (atria, right ventricle). Plasma renin activity was significantly increased over the baseline in the infarct group at 5, but not at 25, days. The data obtained in the two

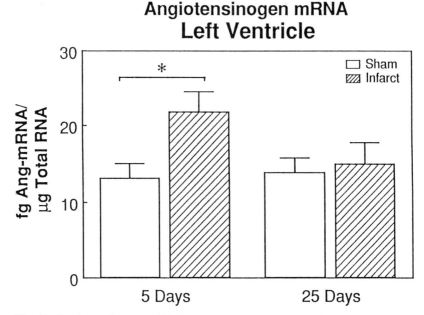

Fig. 5. Angiotensinogen mRNA concentrations (fg/µg total RNA) as determined by solution hybridization assay in the noninfarcted portion of the left ventricle. N = 7 for sham-operated animals at both time points, and n = 8 for animals with infarction at both time points (from Lindpaintner K, et al.[7]).

experimental systems described are consistent with the triggering of enhanced angiotensinogen expression by increases in hemodynamic load by direct (stretch) or indirect (neurohumoral milieu) mechanisms. On the basis of the observed regression or prevention of increases in cardiac mass associated with converting-enzyme inhibition, it is tempting to speculate about an active, growth-promoting role of this upregulation of angiotensinogen. Recent reports implying an untoward influence of angiotensin in ischemic myocardial dysfunction[29] and demonstrating the beneficial effects of converting-enzyme inhibition but the detrimental effects of angiotensin on diastolic function in pressure-overload hypertrophy[25,30] further emphasize the potentially important role that the cardiac RAS may play, particularly where cardiac function is already compromised. It is important to recognize, though, that so far we lack any direct evidence for such a role, and observed changes in the regulation and activity of the cardiac RAS may simply be of secondary nature, representing a biological response to increases in myocardial mass induced by other mechanisms.

Conclusion

The work discussed above provides sound evidence, on the level of molecular-biological as well as protein-biochemical investigations, for the presence of intracardiac angiotensinogen, its conversion within the heart to biologically active peptides, and its differential regulatory response to physiological and pharmacological perturbations. Less is known about the precise cellular localization of cardiac angiotensinogen synthesis and metabolism and about its role in normal and diseased states. Preliminary observations indicate that the range of physiological actions of the RAS is wider than originally perceived, encompassing not only modulation of cardiac and coronary vascular function but also structural and metabolic influences. The need for further investigation and delineation of this system is emphasized by the many parallels that exist between the results obtained in experimental animals and observations made in humans and by the ready availability of a range of potent pharmacological agents through which the system may be modified. Thus, continued efforts toward better characterization of this system stand a high chance not only of providing important new insights into basic physiological and pathological mechanisms but also of having potentially a very direct impact on the clinical practice of cardiovascular medicine.

Summary

The presence of intracardiac synthesis was first postulated on the basis of the finding of significant amounts of angiotensin peptides in the atria and ventricles. More definitive proof for local expression of the protein came forth with the demonstration of specific angiotensinogen mRNA in the heart; in keeping with data on angiotensin peptides, levels were markedly higher in the atria than in the ventricles and tended to be higher on the right side of the heart compared to the left side. The issue of the physiological relevance of the protein was addressed in experiments using isolated hearts that were perfused with renin. Measurements of angiotensin peptides in the collected coronary sinus effluent demonstrated the absence of angiotensin peptides at the outset and rapid appearance of both A I and A II after the start of the renin infusion. This effect was specific: Appearance of both peptides was reversibly inhibited by coadministration of a synthetic renin inhibitor, and appearance of A II, but not of A I, was inhibited in the presence of a converting-enzyme inhibitor. Kinetic studies of angiotensin release revealed a biphasic pattern of angiotensinogen release from the perfused heart, consisting of an initial, brief period during which large, but rapidly declining, amounts of angiotensinogen are released, representing most likely the liberation of protein sequestrated into the myocardium from the circulating pool. This initial period is followed by a delayed, prolonged release of stable, but relatively low, amounts of the protein, representing intracardiac synthesis. Treatment with dexamethasone resulted in significant increases of both angiotensinogen protein and mRNA in all regions of the heart, which indicates the potential for independent modulatory and regulatory potential. Transient, marked increases of angiotensinogen mRNA in the remodeling of the surviving portion of the left ventricle after experimental myocardial infarction point to the potential pathophysiological importance of cardiac angiotensinogen.

References

1. Lindpaintner K, Wilhelm MJ, Jin M, Unger T, Lang RE, Schoelkens BA, et al. Tissue renin-angiotensin systems: focus on the heart. J Hypertens 1987; 5(suppl 2):33–38.
2. Xiang JZ, Schoelkens BA, Ganten D, Unger T. Effects of sympathetic nerve stimulation are attenuated by the converting enzyme inhibitor HOE 498 in isolated rabbit hearts. Clin Exp Hypertens 1984; 6A: 1853–1857.
3. Ohkubo H, Kageyama R, Ujihara M, Hirose T, Inayama S, Nakanishi S. Cloning and sequence analysis of cDNA for rat angiotensinogen. Proc Natl Acad Sci USA 1983; 80:2196–2200.
4. Suzuki F, Lindpaintner K, Keuneke C, Hellman W, Takahashi S, Nakamura Y, et al. Tissue-specific regulation of gene expression for renin and angiotensinogen. Clin Exp Hypertens 1988; A10:1317–1319.
5. Hellmann W, Suzuki F, Ohkubo H, Nakanishi S, Ludwig G, Ganten D. Angiotensinogen gene expression in extrahepatic rat tissues: application of a solution hybridization assay. Naunyn Schmiedeberg's Arch Pharmacol 1988; 338:327–331.
6. Lindpaintner K, Lu W, Niedermaier N, Schieffer B, Just H, Ganten D, et al. Selective activation of cardiac angiotensinogen gene expression in post-infarction ventricular remodeling in the rat. J Mol Cell Cardiol 1993; 25:133–143.
7. Lindpaintner K, Jin M, Niedermeyer N, Wilhelm MJ, Ganten D. Cardiac angiotensinogen and its local activation in the isolated perfused beating heart. Circ Res 1990; 67:564–573.
8. Lindpaintner K, Jin M, Wilhelm MJ, Suzuki F, Linz W, Schoelkens

BA, et al. Intracardiac generation of angiotensin and its physiological role. Circulation 1988; 77(suppl I):I-18–I-23.

9. Campbell DJ, Habener JF. The angiotensinogen gene is expressed and differentially regulated in multiple tissues of the rat. J Clin Invest 1986; 78:31–39.

10. Dzau VJ, Ellison KE, Brody T, Ingelfinger J, Pratt R. A comparative study of the distribution of renin and angiotensinogen messenger ribonucleic acids in rat and mouse tissues. Endocrinology 1987; 120: 2334–2338.

11. Kunapuli SP, Kumar A. Molecular cloning of human angiotensinogen cDNA and evidence for the presence of its mRNA in the rat heart. Circ Res 1987; 60:786–790.

12. Li C, Prakash O, Re RN. Altered regulation of angiotensin gene expression in the left ventricle of the hypertensive rats. Circulation 1989; 80: II-450 (abstract).

13. Drexler H, Lindpaintner K, Lu W, Schieffer B, Ganten D. Transient increase in the expression of cardiac angiotensinogen in a rat model of myocardial infarction and failure. Circulation 1989; 1980:Il-459 (abstract).

14. Hial V, Gimbrone MA, Peyton MP, Wilcox CM, Pisano JJ. Angiotensin metabolism by cultured human vascular endothelial and smooth muscle cells. Microvasc Res 1979; 17:314–329.

15. Khairallah PA, Robertson AL, Davila D. Effect of angiotensin II on DNA, RNA, and protein synthesis. In: Genest J, Koiw E, eds. Hypertension '72. New York: Springer Verlag, 1972, 212–220.

16. Caldwell PRB, Seegal BC, Hsu KC, Das M, Soffer RL. Angiotensin-converting enzyme: vascular endothelial localization. Science 1976; 191: 1050–1051.

17. Ohkubo H, Nakayama K, Tanaka K, Nakanishi S. Tissue distribution of rat angiotensinogen mRNA and structural analysis of its heterogeneity. J Biol Chem 1986; 261:319–323.

18. Dzau VJ. Cardiac renin-angiotensin system: molecular and functional aspects. Am J Med 1988; 84:22–27.

19. Baker KM, Chernin MI, Wixson SK, Aceto JF. Renin-angiotensin system involvement in pressure-overload cardiac hypertrophy in rats. Am J Physiol 1990; 2593:H324–H332.

20. Schelling P, Ganten D, Speck G, Fischer H. Effects of angiotensin II and angiotensin II antagonist saralasin on cell growth and renin in 3T3 and SV3T3 cells. J Cell Physiol 1979; 98:503–513.

21. Taubman MB, Berk BC, Izumo S, Tsuda T, Alexander RW, Nadal-Ginard B. Angiotensin induces c-fos mRNA in aortic smooth muscle: role of Ca2 + mobilization and protein kinase C activation. J Biol Chem 1989; 264:526–530.

22. Naftilan AJ, Pratt RE, Eldrigde CS, Lin HL, Dzau VJ. Angiotensin II induces c-fos expression in smooth muscle via transcriptional control. Hypertension 1989; 13:706–711.

23. Hoh E, Komuro I, Kurabayashi M, Katoh Y, Shibazaki Y, Yazaki Y. The molecular mechanism of angiotensin II-induced c-fos gene expression on rat cardiomyocytes. Circulation 1990; 82:III-351 (abstract).

24. Linz W, Schoelkens BA, Ganten D. Converting enzyme inhibition specifically prevents the development and induces the regression of cardiac hypertrophy in rats. Clin Exp Hypertens 1989; 11:1325–1350.

25. Schunkert H, Dzau VJ, Tang SS, Hirsch AT, Apstein CA, Lorell BH. Increased rat cardiac angiotensin converting enzyme activity and mRNA expression in pressure overload left ventricular hypertrophy: effects on coronary resistance, contractility, and relaxation. J Clin Invest 1990; 86:1913–1920.
26. Fabris B, Jackson B, Kohzuki M, Perich R, Johnston CI. Increased cardiac angiotensin-converting enzyme in rats with chronic heart failure. Clin Exp Pharmacol Physiol 1990; 17:309–314.
27. Pfeffer MA, Pfeffer JM, Steinburg C, Finn P. Survival after an experimental myocardiai infarction: beneficial effects of long-term therapy with captopril. Circulation 1985; 72:406–412.
28. Pfeffer JM, Pfeffer MA, Braunwald E. Influence of chronic captopril therapy on the infarcted left ventricle of the cat. Circ Res 1985; 57: 84–95.
29. Mochizuki T, Eberli FR, Apstein CS, Lorell BH. Exacerbation of ischemic dysfunction by angiotensin II in red cell-perfused rabbit hearts: effects on coronary flow, contractility, and high-energy phosphate metabolism. J Clin Invest 1992; 89:490–498.
30. Eberli FR, Apstein CS, Ngoy S, Lorell BH. Exacerbation of left ventricular ischemic diastolic dysfunction by pressure-overload hypertrophy: modification by specific inhibition of cardiac angiotensin converting enzyme. Circ Res 1992; 70:931–943.

4

Localization and Properties of the Angiotensin-Converting Enzyme and Angiotensin Receptors in the Heart

Jialong Zhuo, Andrew M. Allen,
Hiroshi Yamada, Yao Sun, and
Frederick A.O. Mendelsohn

The renin-angiotensin system (RAS) plays an important role in cardiovascular homeostasis during physiological and pathological states. Apart from its well-described influences on extracellular electrolyte and fluid balance and on peripheral vascular resistance, the active molecule, A II, exerts diverse actions on the heart, including direct, positive inotropic[1–5] and chronotropic effects,[4,5] stimulation of myocyte growth,[6–8] and modulation of myocardial metabolism.[9–11] Although these cardiac actions of A II may directly or indirectly contribute to the regulation of cardiac output in physiological events, under pathophysiological circumstances, however, A II may cause intense coronary vasoconstriction, thus adversely affecting myocardial metabolism and provoking ventricular arrhythmias during ischemic and reperfusion-induced myocardial damage.[9,10] Furthermore, A II stimulated myocyte growth has been implicated in the development of cardiac hypertrophy in hypertension.[6,12–14] Experimental and clinical applications of the angiotensin-converting

Lindpaintner K and Ganten D (editors): *The Cardiac-Renin Angiotensin System,* © Futura Publishing Co., Inc., Armonk, NY, 1994.

enzyme (ACE) inhibitors to block the conversion of inactive A I to the effector A II have been successful in reducing reperfusion arrhythmias,[15-17] increasing coronary blood flow,[10,18,19] improving myocardial metabolism,[10,18] and reducing myocardial hypertrophy.[13,14,20] These observations confirm an important role of the RAS in cardiovascular homeostasis.

Recent evidence suggests the existence of an intrinsic functional tissue RAS in mammalian hearts. All components of the RAS have been localized in the cardiac tissue.[10,21-23] For instance, renin enzymatic activity has been detected in the heart,[24] coexpression of renin and angiotensinogen mRNAs has been demonstrated,[10,25] and intracardiac conversion of A I to A II has been confirmed in the isolated, perfused working heart.[11,26] Also, the ACE[27-29] and A II receptors[30-34] have been identified in cardiac tissue. These studies provide evidence that A II can be generated in the heart and that intracardially formed A II could thereby modulate cardiac function. In view of the increasing interest in local tissue RAS in the heart, we review our recent work and that of others on localization of ACE and A II receptors in rat and human hearts by in vitro autoradiography, and we briefly discuss the regulation of cardiac ACE and A II receptors and their functional significance in cardiac homeostasis during physiological and pathophysiological states.

Distribution of Renin and Its Substrate, Angiotensinogen, in the Heart

Local production of A II in the heart requires the precursor angiotensinogen, the enzyme renin, and the A-I converting enzyme (ACE). Although these components could be delivered to the heart by the circulating plasma, evidence from molecular biological studies indicates that the heart can synthesize the renin substrate, angiotensinogen,[35] and renin.[24] Angiotensinogen- and renin-gene expressions have been demonstrated in the heart, and their distributions are heterogeneous. For example, expression of the angiotensinogen gene occurs predominantly in the atria,[35] and expression of the renin gene appears to be higher in the ventricles.[36] Lindpaintner et al.[26] have recently investigated the source of angiotensinogen released from the isolated, perfused heart, and they found a bimodal pattern of angiotensinogen release from the coronary sinus effluent, with an initial peak followed by a low and stable plateau. These observations suggested that the initial phase of release was due to the washout of circulating angiotensinogen sequestered in the heart, whereas the second low and stable release came from intracardiac synthesis.[26] Nevertheless, the cell types that synthesize cardiac angiotensinogen have not been determined. This is in contrast to cardiac renin since renin has been detected in isolated cardiomyocytes by a specific anti-body, as has renin messenger RNA.[24,37] These observations provide strong evidence for the intracardiac synthesis of renin and angiotensinogen. However, since cardiac angiotensinogen mRNA occurs at only 0.5% of the levels in the liver,[35] and cardiac-renin enzymatic activity was found to be only 0.4% of that demonstrated in the kidney,[38] it is not clear whether locally synthesized angiotensinogen and renin contribute significantly to the intracardiac production of A II and to the physiological control of cardiac function.

Localization of ACE and Angiotensin II Receptors in the Heart by In Vitro Autoradiography

Tissue Preparation

Male Sprague-Dawley rats were killed by decapitation, and the hearts were quickly removed, rinsed in cold saline, and dissected into the atria and ventricles at just below the atrioventricular junction. The chambers were filled with tissue Tek and all parts snap frozen in isopentane dry ice, then stored at $-80°C$. Sections of 10 to 20 μM were cut on cryostat at $-17°C$, thaw-mounted onto gelatin-coated slides, dehydrated for 12 hours under reduced pressure at 4°C, and then stored at $-80°C$ in sealed containers with silica gel until incubation. A human heart was obtained 8 hours postmortem from a patient who died from noncardiac diseases, and frozen sections were cut and processed as described above.

Mapping the Cardiac Angiotensin-Converting Enzyme

Radioligand Preparation

To localize ACE in tissues, we use a specific, tight-binding inhibitor of the enzyme. The inhibitor was radiolabeled to high-specific activity with ^{125}I and permitted precise and sensitive localization of ACE in tissue sections. 351A is a tyrosyl derivative of lisinopril, a potent, specific inhibitor of ACE; 351A was iodinated by the chloramine T method and separated from free ^{125}I by SP Sephadex C25

(Pharmacia LKB, Uppsala, Sweden) column chromatography to yield a product of high specific activity ($>$1,600 μCi/μg).[29] The binding properties of this radioligand have been described previously,[39] and the purity of the radioligand was verified by high-performance liquid chromatography (HPLC).

Binding of [125]I-351A to the Angiotensin-Converting Enzyme in Cryostat Sections of the Heart

The sections of the rat and human hearts were preincubated in 10 mmol sodium phosphate buffer containing 150 mmol NaCl and 0.2% bovine serum albumin (BSA), pH 7.4, for 15 minutes at 20°C and then incubated in the same buffer containing approximately 0.3 μCi/ml of [125]I-351A for 1 hour at 20°C. Nonspecific binding was determined in parallel incubations in the presence of 1 mmol EDTA, which abolishes ACE activity and radioligand binding to ACE.[39] The sections were then processed as described previously.[29]

Mapping Cardiac Angiotensin II Receptors with [125]I-[Sar[1],Ile[8]] A II

Radioligand Preparation

The radioligand we have employed to localize A II receptors in the heart is the antagonist analogue, [125]I-[Sar[1],Ile[8]] A II, which was radioiodinated using the lactoperoxidase-glucose oxidase method and then purified by high-pressure liquid chromatography (HPLC).[40] The binding properties and specific activity have been described previously.[41]

Binding of [125]I-[Sar[1],Ile[8]] A II to Cardiac Angiotensin II Receptors

For localization of A II receptors in the heart, sections were preincubated in a 10 mmol sodium phosphate buffer containing 150 mmol NaCl, 5 mmol Na$_2$EDTA, 0.2 mmol bacitracin, and 0.2% of BSA for 15 minutes to remove endogenous angiotensin and then incubated in fresh buffer containing 0.2 μCi/ml of [125]I-[Sar[1],Ile[8]] A II for 1 hour at room temperature. Nonspecific binding was determined in parallel incubations in the presence of 1 μM of unlabeled A II.[40,41]

Mapping Cardiac Angiotensin II-Receptor Subtypes

Subtypes of A II receptors in the rat heart were mapped by using unlabeled nonpeptide A II receptor antagonists, Losartan and PD 123177, which are specific for AT_1 and AT_2 subtypes, respectively.[42,43] Tissue sections were incubated in the presence of either Losartan (10 µM) or PD 123177 (10 µM) in order to differentiate A II receptor subtypes in the heart. In this regard, AT_1 binding was determined as that displaced by an excess of the AT_1 antagonist, Losartan (10 µM), and AT_2 binding as that displaced by an excess of the AT_2 antagonist, PD 123177 (10 µM). The reducing agent, dithiothreitol (DTT), which has been known to inhibit the AT_1 binding and to enhance the AT_2 binding in various tissues,[44,45] was also used to confirm A II receptor subtypes in the rat heart.

Autoradiography and Quantification of Radioligand Binding

After incubation, the slides were washed four times for 1 minute each in cold buffer without BSA to remove unbound radioligand, dried, and exposed to Agfa Scopix CR3B X-ray film for 2 days for ACE and 3 to 5 weeks for A II receptors. In each cassette, a set of standards, prepared by applying known amounts of ^{125}I-radioactivity to 20 µM sections of rat-brain tissue mounted on gelatin-coated slides 5 mm in diameter, were enclosed. The densities of cardiac ACE and A II receptors were quantified by using a microcomputer imaging device system (Imaging Research Inc., Ontario, Canada) operated by an IBM AT computer with a high-resolution CCD camera.

Distribution of the Angiotensin-Converting Enzyme in Cardiac Tissue

In Vitro Autoradiography

Cardiac Vessels

As shown in Figure 1, panels A to D, (see color plate, p. A3) all of the great vessels arising from the rat heart showed a similar, high density of ACE. These vessels include the ascending (AAO) and descending aorta (DAO), the pulmonary arteries (PA) and veins (PV), inferior vena cava (IVC), and superior vena cava (SVC). These vessels bore ACE in both their adventitial and endothelial layers (Fig. 1). However, the adventitia appeared to have slightly higher ACE densities than the endothelium. The major coronary arteries also had a high density of ACE (Fig. 1).

Cardiac Valves

The highest density of ACE in the rat heart was seen in all heart valves, including the aortic (AV), pulmonary (PV), and mitral and tricuspid valves (V); (Fig. 1, panels E and H). In these valves, ACE was distributed homogeneously through the whole thickness of the leaflets (Fig. 1).

Cardiac Chambers

The distribution of ACE in different cardiac chambers was heterogeneous. ACE density in the right atrium (RA), (Fig. 1, panels D to F) and right atrial appendage (RAP), (Fig. 1, panels B and C) was twice as great as that in the left counterparts (LA), (Fig. 1, panels E to G). However, both the left ventricle (LV) (Fig. 1, panel H) and the right ventricle (RV) (Fig. 1, panels B and D) displayed a similar lower density of ACE.

The densities of ACE in different structures of the rat heart are detailed in Figure 2.

The Cardiac Conduction System

In contrast to A II receptors (discussed later), the cardiac conduction system was devoid of detectable ACE labeling (Figure 3). Direct comparison of autoradiographs (Fig. 3, panels A and B) with photomicrographs obtained from consecutive sections stained for acetylcholinesterase (Fig. 3, panels C and D) or hematoxylin-eosin (Fig. 3, panels E and F) shows that no ACE binding was detected either in the sinoatrial node (Fig. 3, panel A) or in the atrioventricular node (Fig. 3, panel B).[29]

Human Cardiac Tissue

In the human heart, the patterns of ACE distribution differed markedly from those in the rat heart (Fig. 1). In the human, ACE was localized in a similar high density in the left cardiac chambers

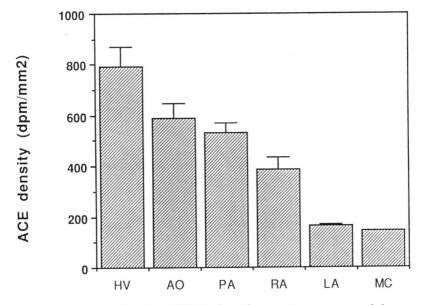

Fig. 2. Bar graphs showing ACE binding density in structures of the rat heart. Abbreviations shown are HV, heart valves; AO, aorta; PA, pulmonary artery; RA, right atrium; LA, left atrium; MC, myocardium.

(Figure 4, panels A and B; see color plate, p. A4) and the right cardiac chambers (panels C and D). Unlike the rat, only a low concentration of ACE was seen in the great vessels including the pulmonary arteries and aorta, and ACE appeared to be localized predominantly to the endothelium (data not shown). Likewise, in the human heart, ACE was present only at low density in the cardiac valves (data not shown).

Characterization of the Cardiac Angiotensin-Converting Enzyme

The properties of cardiac ACE were evaluated in membrane-rich fractions of the atrium, ventricles, and lung by a radioinhibitor-binding assay.[29] Cardiac tissue ACE exhibited a single class of high-affinity binding sites for ^{125}I-351A, but the binding-association constants (K_A) of the radioligand were significantly different in various parts of the rat heart. The atria had higher K_A values and binding-site density for 351A than the ventricles had. Also, binding-site concentrations were higher in the right-sided chambers. The binding

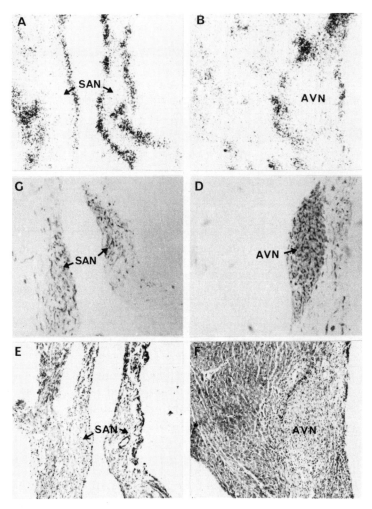

Fig. 3. Bright field of photomicrographs of the sinoatrial node (SAN) and atrioventricular node (AVN) of the rat heart showing that the conduction system is devoid of ACE binding. The left panels show the SAN, and the right panels, the AVN. Panels A and B show autoradiographs of [125]I-351A binding, where silver grains appear as dark regions against a white background; panels C and D show acetylcholinesterase-stained sections, which highlight the SAN and AVN; and panels E and F are adjacent sections stained with hematoxylin-eosin. Magnification: X 50. (from Yamada H, et al.[29]).

of ^{125}I-351A to the right atrium was completely displaced by a series of ACE inhibitors. Identical rank orders of potency were observed in each of the cardiac chambers.[29]

Physiological Role of the Cardiac Angiotensin–Converting Enzyme

The primary function of angiotensin-converting enzyme in the heart is the conversion of biologically inactive A I to the effector molecule, A II. Cardiac ACE activity has been consistently demonstrated in various parts of mammalian hearts, including the atria, ventricles, and coronary artery.[27,46-48] Indirect evidence for intracardiac conversion of A I to A II came from studies using ACE inhibitors in isolated guinea pig atria.[5,49] In the isolated, perfused, beating heart, the intracardiac conversion rate of A I to A II is around 7.2%.[26,50] The production of A II was effectively blocked by the presence of a combination of renin and ACE inhibitors in the perfusate[26] and was significantly enhanced in hypertrophied hearts.[50] Although these studies could be understood as an indication of intracardiac generation of A II, it remains unclear whether A II is formed in the heart mainly by locally synthesized ACE or by blood-delivered ACE. Recently, the messenger RNA for cardiac ACE has been demonstrated in rat hearts with pressure overload-induced left-ventricular hypertrophy and the age-matched controls.[50] The size of cardiac mRNA was found to be identical to that of rat lung mRNA. Increased expression of cardiac mRNA in hypertrophied left ventricles supports involvement of an enhanced cardiac RAS in developing cardiac hypertrophy.[50] Overall, these observations confirm that intracardiac conversion of A I to A II does occur in the heart.

Although mRNAs for angiotensinogen, renin, and ACE and ACE activity in the heart have been demonstrated, specific and anatomical distribution of ACE in the heart has not been previously elucidated. We systematically mapped ACE in the rat heart using in vitro autoradiography.[29] Our results indicate heterogeneous patterns of cardiac ACE distribution with higher densities of ACE in the atria compared with the ventricles and higher levels of binding in the right atrium compared with the left (Fig. 1). Similarly, the characterization of ACE binding in the presence of various ACE inhibitors shows a higher K_A in the atria than in the ventricles (Fig. 4). A further striking finding in our study is that a very dense ACE binding was localized in all valves of the rat heart, followed by the coronary vessels, aorta, and pulmonary arteries (Fig. 1). By contrast, human heart valves contain very low concentrations of ACE. Although the physiological significance of these patterns of cardiac ACE distribution is currently not clear, many sites of ACE localization correlate well with putative sites of A II receptors and intracardiac actions of A II, as revealed by in vitro autoradiography.[29,30] ACE may therefore play an important role in intracardiac formation of A II in these structures.[26,50] However, conversion of A I to A II is not the only role of ACE in modulating cardiovascular function. ACE is known to metabolize many polypeptides such as bradykinin, substance P, neurotensin, and enkephalin by cleaving carboxyl-terminal dipeptides or tripeptides, which all occur in cardiac tissue and have cardiovascular actions.[51-53] It is likely that the physiological and pathophysiological effects of cardiac ACE may at least, in part, be mediated by these polypeptides and/or their metabolites.

In addition, recent evidence indicates that cardiac ACE may not be the only enzyme that is responsible for intracardiac conversion of A I to A II. In mammalian hearts, ACE inhibitors only marginally block the positive inotropic effect of A I on the rat heart.[54] In chronic studies, ACE inhibitors effectively inhibit systemic ACE activity, but plasma A II concentrations usually return shortly to pretreated levels.[55,56] The incomplete inhibition of cardiac and systemic ACEs suggests the existence of other A II-forming enzymes.[57,58] In the human heart, a highly specific chymase has recently been identified as one of the major A II-forming enzymes in cardiac tissue.[54] Although this cardiac chymase shows a high-substrate specificity for conversion of A I to A II, it does not degrade A II, bradykinin, and the vasoactive intestine peptide, thus distinguishing it from cardiac ACE.[54] Therefore, at least two pathways of intracardiac generation of endogenous A II exist in the human heart.

Regulation of the Cardiac Angiotensin–Converting Enzyme in Pathological States

Although physiological modulation of cardiac ACE is not established, the activity of cardiac ACE is markedly altered by angiotensin-converting enzyme inhibition and by cardiovascular disease. We have recently observed that cardiac ACE was largely inhibited after oral administration of ACE inhibitors, zofenopril, captopril, and lisinopril, in all regions of the rat heart.[59] In acute myocardial infarction, produced in rats by ligation of the left coronary artery, ACE concentration in the heart increases rapidly. The rise in cardiac ACE density is particularly marked in the peri-infarct area and in regions adjacent to pericardial inflammation.[60] ACE density remains elevated in myocardial scars for weeks to months following acute myocardial infarction in rats.[61] Although the role of cardiac ACE in the repair process of the infarcted myocardium is not clear, the cardiac RAS and/or bradykinin systems may be involved in this response since ACE is responsible for the formation of A II as well as the breakdown of bradykinin.

Cardiac ACE appears to increase in rat hearts with left-ventricular hypertrophy induced by chronic experimental aortic stenosis. Under this pathological state, a significant increase in the expression of mRNA for ACE has been reported in the hypertrophied left ventricle but not in the nonhypertrophied right ventricle.[50] Cardiac ACE activity increases in parallel with mRNA of cardiac ACE as demonstrated by increased local formation of A II in isolated hearts perfused with A I.[50] ACE density is twofold higher in the myocardium of rats with pressure-overload left-heart hypertrophy, implying an activated cardiac RAS in this tissue.[62] However, a recent report shows that cardiac ACE content is not elevated in the renin-dependent two-kidney, one-clip hypertensive rats and in the low-renin model of DOCA-salt hypertensive rats, although both of these two models of experimental hypertension are accompanied by left-ventricular hypertrophy.[63] The reasons underlying these conflicting findings are not known at present. Nevertheless, the trophic effects of A II on various tissues, including fibroblasts, adrenal cells, vascular smooth muscle, and myocytes, support a role for the peptide in the development of cardiac hypertrophy.[6]

Distribution of Angiotensin II Receptors in Cardiac Tissue

In Vitro Autoradiography

Cardiac Vessels and Valves

The distribution of A II receptors in these structures differed markedly from that of ACE described above. All of the cardiac vessels, including both the aorta and the pulmonary arteries, contained a low to moderate density of binding that was uniform throughout the media and also occurred in some parts of the adventitia (Figure 5; see color plate, p. A5). Curiously, the remnant of arterial duct showed a very high density of A II receptor binding (Fig. 5, panel B).

Atrium and Ventricles

In the rat myocardium, low levels of A II receptors occurred over cardiac muscle throughout both the atrium and the ventricles, but dense punctate binding was seen over the epicardium of the atrium (Fig. 5).

Autonomic Nervous System and Conduction System

In contrast to ACE distribution in the rat heart, the cardiac autonomic nervous system and conduction system displayed regional densities of A II receptor binding (Figure 6; see color plate, p. A6). Dense streaks of A II binding were seen in the vagus and recurrent laryngeal nerves and in the vagal branches to the rat heart. Light binding also occurred in some cholinesterase-negative nerves, and moderate binding was associated with intracardiac ganglion cells situated around the aorta, superior vena cava, and the interatrial septum (Fig. 6, panels D and F). The cardiac conduction system, including the sinus node, the atrioventricular node (panel B), the atrioventricular bundle (Fig. 5, panel A), and left and right bundle branches, showed a moderate density of A II receptors.

The distribution of A II receptor binding in different structures of the rat heart is detailed in Figure 7.

Angiotensin II Receptor Subtypes in the Rat Heart

In our study, the majority of cardiac A II receptors are of the AT_1 subtype (Figure 8; see color plate, p. A7), which are sensitive to the antagonist, Losartan. The addition of an excess of Losartan (10 μM) largely displaced binding of ^{125}I-[Sar^1,Ile^8] A II to the myocardium (80%) and the great vessels (65%), but light binding persisted in the media of the great vessels (Fig. 8, panels E and F). As shown in panels G and H, the AT_2 antagonist, PD 123177 (10 μM), inhibited some of the A II receptor binding, particularly in the walls of the aorta and pulmonary artery, indicating a population of the AT_2 subtype in these structures (35%). Our results contrast with

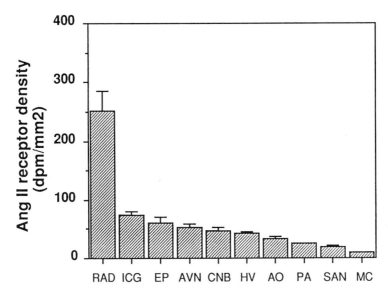

Fig. 7. Bar graph showing the distribution of A II receptor binding in structures of the rat heart. Abbreviations shown in order are RAD, remnant of arterial duct; ICG, intracardiac ganglia; EP, epicardial puncta; AVN, atrioventricular node; CNB, cholinergic nerve bundles; HV, heart valves; AO, aorta; PA, pulmonary arteries; SAN, sinus node; MC, myocardium (from Allen AM, et al.[30]).

those in rabbit ventricular myocardial membranes[64] and in the rat heart,[65] where AT_1 and AT_2 subtypes were reported to represent 50% of total myocardial A II receptors and were distributed throughout the atria and ventricles.

Characteristics of Cardiac Angiotensin II Receptors

Angiotensin II receptors have been identified in the cardiac tissue of many mammalian species, including rats,[28,30,31,66] rabbits,[33,34,67] bovines[68,69] guinea pigs,[70] and humans.[32] Most of these studies have been conducted in either cardiac sarcolemmal membrane fractions[66,68,69] or in cultured cardiomyocytes.[31,33,34] Characterization of A II receptors in these preparations reveals high- and low-affinity binding sites with different binding capacities.[33,69,70] However, the binding dissociation constants (K_d) for these two classes of binding sites are species specific. In rabbit left-ventricular myocardial membranes, a K_d of 4.5 nM and a binding capacity of

53.5 fmol/mg of protein were described for the high-affinity binding sites.[34] In cultured neonatal rat myocytes, the high-affinity sites display a lower K_d (0.65 nM) and a higher B_{max} (245 fmol/mg of protein).[31] By contrast, K_d for the low-affinity binding sites are 5.6 nm with a B_{max} of 720 fmol/mg of protein in cultured neonatal rat myocytes[31] and 433 nm with a B_{max} of 821 fmol/mg of protein in ventricular myocardial membranes of the guinea pig,[70] respectively.

As is the case for A II receptors in the kidney,[40,71] adrenal cortex,[72] and vascular smooth muscle,[73,74] cardiac A II receptors may couple to at least two transduction systems: adenylate cyclase that produces cyclic adenosine monophosphate(cAMP), and phosphatidylinositol 4,5-bisphosphate (PIP_2). Phosphodiesterase (phospholipase C) hydrolyzes PIP_2 to form inositol trisphosphate (IP_3) and diacylglycerol (DAG). In the rat and rabbit myocardial sarcolemma, A II inhibits adenylate cyclase activity in a concentration-dependent manner with K_i ranging from 3 to 6 nM. This inhibitory effect occurs in the presence of guanine nucleotides and can be blocked by the A II antagonist, saralasin, suggesting an A II receptor-mediated response.[66] The fall in cAMP induced by A II in the myocardium may in part mediate intracellular calcium movements, which then exert the cardiac effects of A II.[66,75] However, recent evidence has indicated that the A II-stimulated production of IP_3 is a major second-messenger pathway that initiates the biological actions of A II in cardiac tissue.[70,76–78] Stimulation of phosphatidylinositol turnover by A II has been reported in atrial and ventricular myocytes.[70,77] In cultured neonatal rat heart myocytes and chick myocytes, an A II-induced increase in cytosolic free calcium is accompanied by a parallel rise in inositol phosphate[78] and by an increase in spontaneous contractile frequency of cardiomyocytes.[76] Therefore, there exists a close correlation between A II-stimulated phosphoinositol metabolism, cytosolic calcium activity, and the biological actions of A II in the heart.

The properties of AT_1 and AT_2 A II subtypes in cardiac tissue have not been described. Preliminary observation suggests that AT_1 receptors may mediate A II-induced left-ventricular hypertrophy in rats because Losartan inhibits this trophic cardiac effect of A II both in vivo and in vitro.[23] Whether or not the inotrophic and chronotrophic effects of A II on the heart are also mediated by AT_1 sites is not known. However, on the basis of the findings that physiological actions of A II on the brain, vascular smooth muscle, adrenal, and kidney are all coupled to the AT_1 sites,[79] it is likely that the AT_1 receptor is the functional subtype in cardiac tissue. No physiological effect associated with AT_2 receptors has so far been demonstrated in the heart as well as in other tissues.

Regulation of Cardiac Angiotensin II Receptors

In a manner similar to A II receptors in other tissues, cardiac A II receptors are modulated by ions, guanine nucleotides, and angiotensin itself.[71,40] Monovalent cations (e.g., Na^+, K^+, Li^+) decrease,[33,69] while divalent cations (e.g., Mg^2, Ca^2 Mn^{2+}) increase A II binding to rat and rabbit cardiomyocytes.[31,33,34] The effect of guanine nucleotides on myocardial A II binding has been investigated. In general, guanine nucleotides, including guanine triphosphate and its nonhydrolyzable analogues, reduce agonist binding to A II receptors by increasing the dissociation rate of the bound radioligand and by shifting the receptors from a high-affinity to a low-affinity state.[31,33,34] This effect appears to be dependent upon the presence of divalent cations.[33,34] These observations suggest that divalent cations are important factors for the interactions between A II and its receptors and for cardiovascular responses to A II.

Changes in cardiac A II receptor-binding affinity and receptor number during development have been reported in several mammals.[31,32,72] In the chicken heart, the low-affinity receptor sites shift progressively to the high-affinity sites during ontogeny.[72] Cardiac ventricular A II receptor density is twofold higher in one-day-old rats compared with that in ten-day-old rats and then remains relatively steady thereafter.[32] This developmental influence on cardiac A II receptors occurs throughout most structures of neonatal human hearts, including the atria, ventricles, intraventricular septum, and valves. However, there is no difference in A II receptor density observed in normal and diseased human hearts.[32] The mechanisms underlying the postneonatal developmental changes in cardiac A II receptors is not known. However, recent studies employing nonpeptide A II receptor antagonists, Losartan and PD 123177, to characterize A II receptor subtypes in prenatal and neonatal rat brains and kidneys (Zhuo and Mendelsohn, unpublished observations) reveal that the majority of A II receptors are of the AT_2 subtype before birth, but the receptor density of the AT_2 subtype declines rapidly after birth, and then AT_1 receptors become predominant in some of the specific brain nuclei[41] and in the kidneys of adult rats.[37] Similar shifts of AT_2 to AT_1 subtypes may occur in cardiac tissue during postneonatal development although this issue remains to be confirmed.

Physiological and Pathological Significance of the Cardiac Renin-Angiotensin System

Physiology of the Cardiac Renin-Angiotensin System

Angiotensin II exerts physiological effects on cardiovascular function directly and indirectly. In intact animals, systemic administration of A II is associated with a decrease in cardiac output, an increase in diastolic volume and pressure (particularly in the left ventricle), alterations of heart rate, and a rise in central venous pressure. Since A II facilitates norepinephrine release from sympathetic nerve endings[80-83] and interacts with central nervous and humoral systems affecting cardiovascular homeostasis, changes in cardiac function following systemic administration of A II are believed to be partially mediated by neural and adrenergic transmitters.[72,84] Similarly, the actions of A II on peripheral vascular resistance, aldosterone excretion, renal sodium excretion, and drinking behavior, all of which alter arterial blood pressure and influence body fluid and electrolyte balance, may also modulate cardiac performance.

Localization of A II receptors by us[30] and others[32,33,69,70] has provided an anatomical basis for the direct actions of A II on the heart. In in vitro preparations, such as the isolated perfused heart, atria, papillary muscle strips, or cultured cardiomyocytes, which exclude the possibility of influences from hormonal and autonomic nervous systems, A II exerts direct, positive actions on the myocardial contractility and heart rate in rats,[76,85] dogs,[4] rabbits,[3] cats,[1,86] chickens,[3] and humans.[87] These inotropic and chronotropic effects of A II on the heart in isolated preparations are not affected by a beta-adrenoceptor blockade with propranolol,[4,5] by reserpine pretreatment,[5,88] or by atropine, phentolamine, or indomethacin,[86] but are suppressed by the A II receptor antagonist, saralasin, indicating direct myocardial actions of A II.[3,4,69]

However, there is evidence from morphological and physiological studies that the important actions of A II on cardiac sympathetic and vagus nervous systems contribute to its inotropic and chronotropic effects. Angiotensin II receptors have been localized to human cardiac adrenergic nerves[32] and the conduction system of the rat heart.[28] Our study shows A II receptors in the cardiac autonomic nervous system and the conduction system of the rat.[30] Although neuronal binding of A II is associated with sympathetic, but not parasympathetic, nerve bundles in the human heart, in our study, dense punctate binding is found over parasympathetic nerve bundles and over some cells in intracardiac ganglia that stain for acetylcholinesterase.[30] The rat conduction system, including the sinus node, the atrioventricular node, and the atrioventricular bundles also contains a moderate to high density of A II receptors. The association of A II receptors in cardiac sympathetic nervous structures supports the demonstration that A II potentiates sympathetic nervous activity in the heart by a presynaptic mechanism,[32,49] whereas ACE inhibitors attenuate norepinephrine overflow from isolated, perfused hearts.[89] The demonstration in our study of a high density of A II receptors in cardiac terminals of vagal nerves, intracardiac parasympathetic ganglion cells, and the conduction system[30] is also consistent with previous observations that A II inhibits cardiac vagal efferent activity both centrally and prejunctionally[90–92] and has direct actions on cardiac Purkinje fibers.[93] Therefore, A II can act directly on its receptors located on cardiomyocytes and on cardiac sympathetic and parasympathetic nervous systems to influence cardiac contractility and the heart rate independent of its systemic effects.

The functional significance of an intrinsic RAS in the heart during physiological states remains an important issue to be explored. Although it is clear that the heart can synthesize all components of the system, no unequivocal evidence for direct physiological actions of intracardially formed A II on cardiac function in vivo has been provided. However, indirect evidence from studies using ACE inhibitors and A II antagonists suggests that local A II may have similar actions on the contractility of cardiomyocytes and the heart rate, which have been demonstrated in in vitro preparations.

Pathophysiology of the Cardiac Renin-Angiotensin System

Circulating and cardiac RASs play an important role in the pathophysiology of several cardiovascular diseases, including acute myocardial ischemia, acute and chronic myocardial infarction, chronic congestive heart failure (CHF), and cardiac hypertrophy. During myocardial ischemia, A II may cause intense coronary vasoconstriction and affect myocardial metabolism and electrical properties of the conduction system and cardiomyocytes, thus exerting a deleterious effect on the ischemic heart.[10,18,22,23] The blockade of systemic and intracardiac A II formation with a series of ACE inhibitors reverses these deleterious effects of A II both experimentally and clinically. For instance, in the ischemic, isolated, perfused rat heart, ACE inhibitors have been shown to increase coronary blood flow, improve myocardial metabolism and hemodynamics, and reduce reperfusion arrhythmias.[15,18,94] Additional cardioprotective effects of ACE inhibitors include significant reduction of myocardial infarction size in dogs[95] and prevention or attenuation of left-ventricular remodeling in rats with chronic myocardial infarction.[96-98] These beneficial effects of ACE inhibition on ischemic heart diseases are mainly due to the blockade by ACE inhibitors of direct myocardial and sympathetic facilitatory actions of A II generated intracardially.[22,23] However, there is evidence that bradykinin accumulation within the heart following application of ACE inhibitors may also contribute to the cardioprotective effects of ACE inhibition. In the ischemic, isolated, perfused rat heart, bradykinin is as effective as ACE inhibitors in improving cardiac metabolism and hemodynamic performance, whereas a specific bradykinin antagonist blocks these cardiac responses to ACE inhibition.[99]

The RAS may be activated in patients with severe chronic CHF. In addition to its direct myocardial effects, A II causes extensive peripheral vasoconstriction, thus resulting in increases in systemic vascular resistance (afterload) and decreases in venous capacitance (increases in preload). Angiotensin II also induces sodium and fluid retention in chronic CHF. These adverse effects of A II lead to increases in working load and myocardial oxygen consumption to the failing heart. Therefore, suppression of the RAS may prove to be a therapeutic preference for chronic CHF. Indeed, experimental and clinical observations made during the last decade have shown that ACE inhibition can improve symptoms and signs of chronic CHF, reduce the frequency of ventricular ectopic rhythms,[16] and decrease the mortality rates.[100,101] Thus, ACE inhibitors are more effective than any other vasodilators in treating chronic CHF by reducing both preload and afterload and by blocking the direct myocardial actions of circulating and intracardiac A II.

Recent evidence has suggested that the circulating and cardiac RASs have important influences on the development of cardiac hypertrophy independent of their systemic hemodynamic effects. In addition to its systemic actions and pressor property, A II directly stimulates protein synthesis and cell growth in vascular smooth muscle[6] and in chick heart cells,[7,8] induces oncogene expression, and causes hypertrophy in cultured rat heart myocytes.[102,103] In addition, enhanced expression of proto-oncogenes, including *c-fos, c-myc,* and *c-jun,* by A II has been demonstrated in hypertrophied rat hearts,[104] pointing to a direct trophic action on cardiomyocytes. These actions of A II on cardiac cell growth are further supported by the observation that myocardial hypertrophy in spontaneously hypertensive rats can be prevented or reversed by chronic ACE inhibition.[13,14,20,105] Likewise, increased gene expression of other components of the cardiac RAS, renin and angiotensinogen, together with enhanced cardiac ACE activity in the hypertrophic left ventricle of the rat heart, have also been reported and suggest a potential role for cardiac RAS in the development of cardiac hypertrophy.[50,62]

Conclusion

Components of the RAS have been localized in the mammalian hearts. Direct evidence that shows gene expressions for renin, angiotensinogen, and the angiotensin-converting enzyme in cardiac tissue supports the concept that the heart has the capacity to synthesize the effector, A II. Although the direct physiological role of the cardiac RAS remains to be elucidated, experimental and clinical studies demonstrate (1) the intracardiac formation of A II and localization of its putative receptor sites in the heart; (2) the physiological influences of A II on myocardial contractility and sympathetic nerve activity; and (3) the cardioprotective effects of converting-enzyme inhibitors on several cardiovascular diseases. These studies have established a functional importance of the cardiac RAS in the physiological regulation of cardiovascular homeostasis, as well as in the pathogenesis of ischemic heart diseases, congestive heart failure, and left-ventricular hypertrophy.

Acknowledgements

This work is supported by grants from the National Health and Medical Research Council and the National Heart Foundation of Australia.

Summary

The angiotensin-converting enzyme (ACE) and angiotensin II (A II) receptors in rat and human hearts were localized by quantitative in vitro autoradiography using two potent inhibitors: ^{125}I-351A as the ligand for ACE and ^{125}I-[Sar^1,Ile^8] A II to localize A II receptors. The highest density of ACE in the rat heart occurs on cardiac valve leaflets and the great cardiac vessels. Densities of ACE are high *in both the endothelial and adventitial layers but very low in the media. The coronary arteries also display dense ACE labeling. By contrast, the atrial and ventricular myocardium contain only moderate to low levels of ACE, with relatively higher ACE binding seen in the right-hand-side chambers than in the left-hand-side chambers. The cardiac conduction system, including the SA and the AV nodes, appears to be devoid of ACE binding. In the atrium and ventricle, a single class of high-affinity binding sites is found, with higher binding-association constants (K_A) in the atria than in the ventricles. The distribution of ACE in the human heart differs from that in the rat heart. Human atrial and ventricular myocardium show moderately high densities of ACE labeling, whereas only low concentrations of ACE occur in the great vessels and valves.*

The anatomical distribution of A II receptor binding in the rat heart differs from that of ACE. Angiotensin II receptor-binding sites are sparse in the cardiac valves and the atrial and ventricular myocardium and are closely associated with the media of the great vessels. Most significantly, and in contrast to ACE, A II dense receptor binding is found in parasympathetic nerve bundles and intracardiac ganglia, and moderately dense binding is seen throughout the conduction system of the rat heart. Angiotensin II receptor binding in the myocardium and great vessels is largely displaced by the AT_1 antagonist, Losartan, and is less sensitive to the AT_2 antagonist, PD 123177, indicating a predominant distribution of the AT_1 subtype of A II receptors in these cardiac structures.

Our studies provide anatomical evidence for the localization of ACE and A II receptors in the rat heart. The presence of high densities of ACE in the cardiac valves, great vessels, and the right atrium suggests that these structures are potential sites for intracardiac A II generation and/or metabolism of bradykinin and other vasoactive polypeptides. The distribution of A II receptors reveals sites at which A II could exert its direct inotropic, chronotropic, and trophic effects on cardiac myocytes, as well as on the parasympathetic innervation and conduction system of the heart.

References

1. Koch-Weser J. Myocardial actions of angiotensin. Cir Res 1964; 14: 337--344.
2. Ahmed SS, Levinson GE, Weisse AB, Regan TJ. The effect of angiotensin on myocardial contractility. J Clin Pharmacol 1975; 15: 276–285.
3. Freer RJ, Pappano AJ, Peach MJ, et al. Mechanism for the positive inotropic effect of angiotensin II on isolated cardiac muscle. Cir Res 1976; 39:178–183.

4. Kobayashi M, Furukawa Y, Chiba S. Positive chronotropic and inotropic effects of angiotensin II in the dog heart. Eur J Pharmacol 1978; 50:17–25.
5. Nakashima A, Angus JA, Johnson CI. Chronotropic effects of angiotensin I, angiotensin II, bradykinin, and norepinephrine in guinea pig atria. Eur J Pharmacol 1982; 81:479–485.
6. Schelling P, Fischer H, Ganten D. Angiotensin and cell growth: a link to cardiovascular hypertrophy? J Hypertens 1991; 9:3–15.
7. Baker KM, Aceto JF. Angiotensin II stimulation of protein synthesis and cell growth in chick heart cells. Am J Physiol 1990; 259: H610–H618.
8. Aceto JF, Baker KM. [Sar1]Angiotensin II receptor-mediated stimulation of protein synthesis in chick heart cells. Am J Physiol 1990; 258: H806–H813.
9. Dzau VJ. Implications of local angiotensin production in cardiovascular physiology and pharmacology. Am J Cardiol 1987; 59 :59A–65A.
10. Dzau VJ. Cardiac renin-angiotensin system: molecular and functional aspects. Am J Med 1988; 84:22–27.
11. Lindpaintner K, Wilhelm MJ, Jin M, et al. Tissue renin-angiotensin systems: focus on the heart. J Hypertens 1987; 5(suppl 2):33–38.
12. Robertson AL, Khairallah PA. Angiotensin II: rapid localization in nuclei of smooth and cardiac muscle. Science 1971; 172:1138–1139.
13. Sen S, Tarazi RC, Bumpus FM. Effect of converting enzyme inhibitor (SQ 14225) on myocardial hypertrophy in spontaneous hypertensive rats. Hypertension 1980; 2:169–176.
14. Linz W, Schoelkens BA, Ganten D. Converting enzyme inhibition specifically prevents the development and induces the regression of cardiac hypertrophy in rats. Clin Exp Hypertens 1989; 11:1325–1350.
15. Van Gilst WH, De Graeff PA, Wesseling H, de Langen CDJ.Reduction of reperfusion arrhythmias in the ischemic isolated heart by angiotensin converting enzyme inhibitors: a comparison of captopril, enalapril, and H0E498. J Cardiovasc Pharmacol 1986; 8:722–728.
16. Webster WM, Fitzpatrick MA, Nicholls MG, Ikram H, Wells JE. Effect of enalapril on ventricular arrhythmias in congestive heart failure. Am J Cardiol 1985; 56:566–569.
17. Wesseling H, De Graeff PA, Van Gilst WH, Bel KJ, Kingma JH, de Langen CDJ. Cardiac arrhythmias: a new indication for angiotensin converting enzyme inhibitors. J Human Hypertens 1989; 3:89–95.
18. Linz W, Schoelkens BA, Han Y-F. Beneficial effects of the converting enzyme inhibitor ramipril in ischemic hearts. J Hypertens 1986; 8(suppl 10):S91–S99.
19. Magrini F, Reggiani P, Roberts N, Meazza R, Ciulla M, Zanchetti A. Effect of angiotensin and angiotensin blockade on coronary circulation and coronary reserve. Am J Med 1988; 84:55–60.
20. Nakashima Y, Fouad FM, Tarazi RC. Regression of left ventricular hypertrophy from systemic hypertension by enalapril. Am J Cardiol 1984; 53:1044–1049.
21. Jin M, Wilhelm MJ, Lang RE, Unger T, Lindpaintner K, Ganten D. The endogenous tissue renin-angiotensin systems: from molecular biology to therapy. Am J Med 1987; 84(suppl 3A):28–36.
22. Lindpaintner K, Ganten D. The cardiac renin-angiotensin system. Cir Res 1991; 68:905–921.

23. Baker KM, Booz GW, Dostal DE. Cardiac actions of angiotensin II: role of an intracardiac renin-angiotensin system. Annu Rev Physiol 1992; 54:227–241.
24. Dzau VJ, Re RN. Evidence for the existence of renin in the heart. Circulation 1987; 75(suppl I):I-134–I-136.
25. Kunapuli SP, Kumar A. Molecular cloning of human angiotensinogen cDNA and evidence for the presence of its mRNA in the rat heart. Cir Res 1987; 60:786–790.
26. Lindpaintner K, Jin M, Niedermeyer N, Wilhelm MJ, Ganten D. Cardiac angiotensinogen and its local activation in the isolated perfused beating heart. Cir Res 1990; 67:564–573.
27. Fabris B, Jackson B, Cubela R, Mendelsohn FAO, Johnson CJ. Angiotensin converting enzyme in the rat heart: studies of its inhibition in vitro and ex vivo. Clin Exp Physiol Pharmacol 1989; 16:309–313.
28. Saito K, Gutkind JS, Saavedra JM. Angiotensin II binding sites in the conduction system of rat hearts. Am J Physiol 1987; 253: H1618–H1622.
29. Yamada H, Fabris B, Allen AM, Jackson B, Johnson CI, Mendelsohn FAO. Localization of angiotensin converting enzyme in rat heart. Cir Res 1991; 68:141–149.
30. Allen AM, Yamada H, Mendelsohn FAO. In vitro autoradiographic localization of binding to angiotensin receptors in the rat heart. Int J Cardiol 1990; 28:25–33.
31. Rogers TB, Gaa ST, Allen IS. Identification and characterization of functional angiotensin II receptors on cultured heart myocytes. J Pharmacol Exp Ther 1986; 236:438–444.
32. Urata H, Healy B, Stewart RW, Bumpus FM, Husain A. Angiotensin II receptors in normal and failing human hearts. J Clin Endocrinol Metab 1989; 69:54–66.
33. Wright GB, Alexander RW, Ekstein LS, Gimbrone MA. Characterization of the rabbit ventricular myocardial receptors for angiotensin II: evidence for two sites of different affinities and specificities. Mol Pharmacol 1983; 24:213–221.
34. Baker KM, Campanile CP, Trachte GJ, Peach MJ. Identification and characterization of the rabbit angiotensin II myocardial receptors. Cir Res 1984; 54:286–293.
35. Campbell DJ, Habener JF. The angiotensinogen gene is expressed and differentially regulated in multiple tissues of the rat. J Clin Invest 1986; 78:31–39.
36. Suzuki F, Hellmann W, Paul M, Ludwig G, Lindpaintner K, Ganten D. Renin gene expression in rat tissues: a new quantitative assay method for rat renin mRNA using synthetic cRNA. Clin Exp Hypertens 1988; A10:345–359.
37. Re R. The myocardial intracellular renin-angiotensin system. Am J Cardiol 1987; 59:56A–58A.
38. Wood JM, Baum HP, Carleton J, Dzau VJ. Inhibition of renin-like activity in marmoset tissues by the renin inhibitor CGP 29278. J Hypertens 1987; 5:S67–S69.
39. Mendelsohn FAO. Localization of angiotensin converting enzyme in rat forebrain and other tissues by in vitro autoradiography using 125I-labelled 351A. Clin Exp Physiol Pharmacol 1984; 11:431–436.

40. Zhuo J, Mendelsohn FAO. Intrarenal angiotensin II receptors. In: Nichollas MG, Robertson NR, eds. The Renin-Angiotensin System: Biochemistry, Physiology, Pathophysiology, and Therapeutics. London and New York: Gower Medical Publishing, 1993:25.1–25.14.

41. Zhuo J, Song K, Harris PJ, Mendelsohn FAO. In vitro autoradiography reveals predominantly AT_1 angiotensin II receptors in the rat kidney. Renal Physiol Biochem 1992; 15:231–239.

42. Wong PC, Hart SD, Zaspel A, Chiu AT, Smith RD, Timmermans, PBMWM. Functional studies of nonpeptide angiotensin II receptor subtype-specific ligands: DuP 753 (AII-1) and PD 123177 (AII-2). J Pharmacol Exp Ther 1990; 255:584–592.

43. Bumpus FM, Catt KJ, Chiu AT, et al. Nomenclature for angiotensin receptors. Hypertension 1991; 17:720–721.

44. Chiu AT, McCall DE, Nguyen TT, et al. Discrimination of angiotensin II receptor subtypes of dithiothreitol. Eur J Pharmacol 1989; 170: 117–118.

45. Song K, Zhuo J, Allen AM, Paxinos G, Mendelsohn FAO. Angiotensin II receptor subtypes in rat brain and peripheral tissues. Cardiology 1991; 79(suppl 1):45–54.

46. Cushman DW, Cheung HS. Concentrations of angiotensin-converting enzyme in tissues of the rat. Biochim Biophys Acta 1971; 250:261–265.

47. Sakharov IY, Danilov SM, Dukhanina EA. Affinity chromatography and some properties of the angiotensin-converting enzyme from human heart. Biochim Biophys Acta 1987; 923:143–149.

48. Rosenthal J, von Lutterotti N, Thurnreiter M. Suppression of renin-angiotensin system in the heart of spontaneously hypertensive rats. J Hypertens 1987; 5:S23–S31.

49. Ziogas J, Story DF, Rand MJ. Effects of locally generated A II on noradrenergic transmission in guinea pig isolated atria. Eur J Pharmacol 1985; 106:11–18.

50. Schunkert H, Dzau VJ, Tang SS, Hirsch AT, Apstein C, Lorell B. Increased rat cardiac angiotensin-converting enzyme activity and mRNA levels in pressure overload left ventricular hypertrophy: effects on coronary resistance, contractility and relaxation. J Clin Invest 1990; 86:1913–1920.

51. Erdos EG, Skidgel RA. The unusual substrate and the distribution of human angiotensin I converting enzyme. Hypertension 1986; 8(suppl I):I-34–I-37.

52. Reinecke M, Weihe E, Carraway RE, Leeman SE, Forssmann WG. Localization of neurotensin immunoreactive nerve fibres in the guinea-pig heart: evidence derived by immunohistochemistry, radioimmunoassay, and chromatography. Neuroscience 1982; 7:1785–1795.

53. Wharton J, Polak JM, McGregor GP, Bishop AE, Bloom SR. Localization of substance P-like immunoreactive nerve fibres in the guinea-pig heart. Neuroscience 1981; 6:2193–2204.

54. Urata H, Kinoshita A, Misono KS, Bumpus FM, Husain A. Identification of a highly specific chymase as the major angiotensin Il-forming enzyme in the human heart. J Biol Chem 1990; 265:22348–22357.

55. Nussberger J, Brunner DB, Warber B, Brunner HR. Specific measurement of angiotensin metabolites and in vitro generated angiotensin II in plasma. Hypertension 1986; 8:476–482.

56. Mento PF, Wilkes BM. Plasma angiotensins and blood pressure during

converting enzyme inhibition. Hypertension 1987; 9(supp. III):III-42–III-48.

57. Urata H, Healy B, Stewart RW, Bumpus FM, Husain A. Angiotensin Il-forming pathways in normal and failing human hearts. Cir Res 1990; 66:883–890.

58. Gondo M, Maruta H, Arakawa K. Direct formation of angiotensln II without renin or converting enzyme in the ischemic dog heart. Jpn Heart J 1989; 30:219–229.

59. Sun Y, Mendelsohn FAO. Angiotensin converting enzyme inhibition in heart, kidney, and serum studied ex vivo after administration of zofenopril, captopril, and lisinopril. J Cardiovasc Pharmacol 1991; 18: 478–486.

60. Fabris B, Jackson B, Kohzuki M, Perich R, Johnson CI. Increased cardiac angiotensin-converting enzyme in rats with chronic heart failure. Clin Exp Physiol Pharmacol 1990; 17:309–314.

61. Jackson B, Mendelsohn FAO, Johnson CI.Angiotensin-converting enzyme inhibition: prospects for the future. J. Cardiovasc Pharmacol 1991; 18(suppl 7):S4–S8.

62. Schunkert H, Jackson B, Tang SS, Apstein CS, Lorell BH. Distribution and functional significance of cardiac angiotensin converting enzyme in hypertrophied rat hearts. Circulation 1993; 87:1328–1339.

63. Mooser V, Katopothis A, Casley D, Johnson CI. Cardiac and renal hypertrophy is independent of tissue angiotensin converting enzyme and circulating angiotensin II in hypertensive rats. J Hypertens 1991; 9(suppl 6):S114–S115.

64. Rogg H, Schmid A, de Gasparo M. Identification and characterization of angiotensin II receptor subtypes in rabbit ventricular myocardium. Biochem Biophys Res Commun 1990; 173:416–422.

65. Sechi LA, Grady EF, Griffin CA, Kalinyak JE, Schambelan M. Characterization of angiotensin II receptor subtypes in the rat kidney and heart using the non-peptide antagonists DuP 753 and PD 123177. J Hypertens 1991; 9(supp 6)S224–S225.

66. Anand-Srivastava MB. Angiotensin II receptors negatively coupled to adenylate cyclase in rat myocardial sarcolemma: involvement of inhibitory guanine nucleotide regulatory protein. Biochem Pharmacol 1989; 38:489–496.

67. Rioux F, Park WF, Regoli D. Characterization of angiotensin receptors in rabbit isolated atria. Can J Physiol Pharmacol 1975; 54:229–237.

68. Mukherjee A, Kulkarni PV, Haghani Z, Sutko JL. Identification and characterization of angiotensin II receptors in cardiac sarcolemma. Biochem Biophys Res Commun 1982; 105:575–581.

69. Rogers TB. High affinity angiotensin II receptors in myocardial sarcolemmal membranes. J Biol Chem 1984; 259:8106–8114.

70. Baker KM, Singer HA. Identification and characterization of guinea pig angiotensin II ventricular and atrial receptors: coupling to inositol phosphate production. Cir Res 1988; 62:896–904.

71. Douglas JG. Angiotensin receptor subtypes of the kidney cortex. Am J Physiol 1987; 253:F1–F7.

72. Peach MJ. Molecular actions of angiotensin. Biochem Pharmacol 1981; 30:2745–2751.

73. Alexander RW, Brock TA, Gimbrone MA Jr, Rittenhouse SE. Angio-

tensin increases inositol trisphosphate and calcium invascular smooth muscle. Hypertension 1985; 7:447–451.

74. Anand-Srivastava MB. Angiotensin II receptors negatively coupled to adenylate cyclase in rat aorta. Biochem Biophys Res Commun 1983; 117:420–428.

75. Dosemeci A, Dhallan RS, Cohen NM, Lederer WJ, Rogers TB. Phorbol ester increases calcium current and stimulates the effects of angiotensin II on cultured neonatal rat heart myocytes. Cir Res 1988; 62: 347–357.

76. Allen IS, Cohen NM, Dhallan RS, Gaa ST, Lederer WJ, Rogers TB. Angiotensin II increases spontaneous contractile frequency and stimulates calcium current in cultured neonatal rat heart myocytes: insight into the underlying biochemical mechanisms. Cir Res 1988; 62: 524–534.

77. Leung E, Johnson CI, Woodcock EA. Stimulation of phosphatidylinositol metabolism in atrial and ventricular myocytes. Life Sci 1986; 39: 2215–2220.

78. Baker KM, Singer HA, Aceto JF. Angiotensin II receptor-mediated stimulation of cytosolic free calcium and inositol phosphates in chick myocytes. J Pharmacol Exp Ther 1989; 251:578–585.

79. Smith RD, Chiu AT, Wong PC, Herblin WF, Timmermans PBMWM. Pharmacology of nonpeptide angiotensin II receptor antagonists. Annu Rev Pharmacol Toxicol 1992; 32:135–165.

80. Malik KU, Nasjiletti A. Facilitation of adrenergic transmitter by locally generated A II in rat mesenteric arteries. Cir Res 1975; 38:26–30.

81. Schuermann HJ, Starke K, Werner U. Interaction of inhibitors of noradrenaline uptake and angiotensin on the sympathetic nerves of the isolated rabbit heart. Br J Pharmacol 1970; 39:390–397.

82. Musgrave IF, Majewski H. Effect of phorbol ester and pertussis toxin on the enhancement of noradrenaline release by angiotensin II in mouse atria. Br J Pharmacol 1989; 96:609–616.

83. Boadle MC, Hughes J, Roth RH. Angiotensin accelerates catecholamine biosynthesis in sympathetically innervated tissues. Nature 1969; 222:987–988.

84. Peach MJ. Renin-angiotensin system: biochemistry and mechanism of action. Physiol Rev 1977; 57:313–370.

85. Neyses L, Vetter H. Action of atrial natriuretic peptide and angiotensin II on the myocardium: studies in isolated rat ventricular cardiomyocytes. Biochem Biophys Res Commun 1989; 163:1435–1443.

86. Dempsey PJ, McCallum ZT, Kent KM, Cooper T. Direct myocardial effects of angiotensin II. Am J Physiol 1971; 220:477–481.

87. Moravec CS, Schluchter MD, Paranandi L, Czerska B, Stewart R, et al. Inotropic effects of angiotensin II on human cardiac muscle in vitro. Circulation 1990; 82:1973–1984.

88. Koch-Weser J. Nature of the inotropic action of angiotensin II on ventricular myocardium. Cir Res 1965; 16:230–237.

89. Xiang JZ, Linz W, Becker H, et al. Effects of converting enzyme inhibitors: ramipril and enalapril on peptide action and sympathetic neurotransmission in the isolated heart. Eur J Pharmacol 1984; 113: 215–223.

90. Lumbers ER, McClosky DI, Potter EK. Inhibition by angiotensin II of

baroreceptor-evoked activity in cardiac vagal efferent nerves in the dog. J Physiol 1979; 294:69–80.

91. Potter EK, Reid IA. Intravertebral angiotensin II inhibits cardiac vagal activity in dogs. Neuroendocrinology 1985; 40:493–496.

92. Potter EK. Angiotensin inhibits action of vagus nerve at the heart. Br J Pharmacol 1982; 75:9–11.

93. Kass RS, Blair ML. Effects of angiotensin II on membrane current in cardiac Purkinje fibers. J Mol Cell Cardiol 1981 13:797–809.

94. Michel JB, Lattion A, Salzmann J, et al. Hormonal and cardiac effects of converting enzyme inhibition in rat myocardial infarction. Cir Res 1988; 62:641–650.

95. Ertl G, Kloner RA, Alexander RW, Braunwald E. Limitation of experimental infarct size by an angiotensin converting enzyme inhibitor. Circulation 1982; 65:40–48.

96. Weber KT, Janicki JS. Angiotensin and the remodelling of myocardium. Br J Clin Pharmacol 1989; 28:141S–150S.

97. Pfeffer JM, Lamas GA, Vaughan DE, Parisi AF, Braunwald E. Effect of captopril on progressive ventricular dilatation after anterior myocardial infarction. N Engl J Med 1988; 319:80–86.

98. Pfeffer MA, Braunwald E. Ventricular remodelling after myocardial infarction. Circulation 1990; 81:1161–1172.

99. Schoelkens BA, Linz W, Koenig W. Effects of the angiotensin converting enzyme inhibitor, ramipril, in isolated ischemic rat heart are abolished by a bradykinin antagonist. J Hypertens 1988; 6:S25–S28.

100. Consensus Trial Study Group. Effects of enalapril on mortality in severe congestive heart failure; results of the Cooperative North Scandinavian Enalapril Survival Study. N Engl J Med 1987; 316:1429–1435.

101. Pfeffer MA, Pfeffer JM, Steinburg C, Finn P. Survival after an experimental myocardial infarction: beneficial effects of long-term therapy with captopril. Circulation 1985; 72:406–412.

102. Hori M, Iwai K, Iwakura K, Sato H, Kitabatake A. Angiotensin II stimulates protein synthesis in neonatal rat cardiomyocytes through enhanced Na^+/K^+ exchange. Circulation 1989; 80(suppl II):II-450.

103. Katoh Y, Komuro I, Shibasaki Y, Yanaguchi H, Yazaki Y. Angiotensin II induces hypertrophy and oncogene expression in cultured rat heart myocytes. Circulation 1989; 80(suppl II):II-450.

104. Dzau VJ, Pratt R, Gibbons G, Schunkert H, Lorell B, Ingelfinger J. Molecular mechanism of angiotensin in the regulation of vascular and cardiac growth. J Mol Cell Cardiol 1989; 21(suppl Ill):S7.

105. Linz W, Henning R, Scholkens BA. Role of angiotensin II receptor antagonism and converting enzyme inhibition in the progression and regression of cardiac hypertrophy in rats. J Hypertens 1991; 9(suppl 6):S400–S401.

5

Cloning of the Angiotensin AT$_1$ Receptor and Its Expression in Cardiac Tissue

Kathy K. Griendling and
R. Wayne Alexander

Angiotensin II has direct and indirect actions on the myocardium. It induces a direct, receptor-mediated positive inotropic response in most species, possibly through augmentation of an inward Ca^{2+} current through L-type channels.[1] Angiotensin II may also exert a direct chronotropic effect on cardiomyocytes,[2,3] although its indirect effects on heart rate due to its ability to increase vascular resistance and its influence on sympathetic and parasympathetic tone may be of greater importance. Finally, A II is likely to be involved in the cardiac hypertrophy that is associated with hypertension.[4] This latter action is probably due to a combination of a direct hypertrophic effect on cardiac myocytes as well as a propensity to increase interstitial tissue mass.[5,6] All of these effects are mediated by the A II receptor, the molecule that binds A II at the plasma membrane and initiates second-messenger generation in the interior of the cell.

Angiotensin Receptor Subtypes

In the heart and many other tissues, pharmacological and physiological evidence indicates heterogeneity in the A II receptor popula-

Lindpaintner K and Ganten D (editors): *The Cardiac-Renin Angiotensin System,* © Futura Publishing Co., Inc., Armonk, NY, 1994.

tion. On the basis of differential binding studies, two classes of cardiac A II binding sites have been observed in the myocardium.[7] More recently, the availability of new pharmacological tools, particularly the nonpeptidic A II antagonists, has provided definitive evidence for the heterogeneity of A II receptors. There are two major subtypes of angiotensin receptors, AT_1 and AT_2. New molecular biological evidence has shown that AT_1 receptors can be further subdivided into two subtypes, AT_{1A} and AT_{1B}.[8]

The classification criteria for AT_1 and AT_2 receptors are summarized below. AT_1 receptors are selectively blocked by biphenylimidazoles such as Losartan, whereas AT_2 binding sites are blocked by tetrahydroimidazopyridines typified by PD123177.[9] AT_1 receptors (previously called A II-1, A II-B, and A II$_\alpha$) are more responsive to A II than to A III, are positively coupled to phospholipase C, and may be negatively coupled to adenylate cyclase.[9] AT_2 binding sites (previously called A II-2, A II-A, and A II$_\beta$) bind A II and A III equally well, but the effector to which they are coupled remains elusive. Some evidence suggests that AT_2 binding sites in neuronal cultures may be involved in the modulation of the intracellular content of cyclic guanosine monophosphate (cGMP).[10] In the heart, AT_1 receptors have been shown to mediate inotropic responses [11] and left ventricular cardiac hypertrophy,[12] although the physiological effects of AT_2 receptor activation remain unknown. However, the abundance of AT_2 binding sites in fetal and neonatal rat tissues raises the possibility that they may have a role in development.[13]

Angiotensin II Binding in the Heart

As noted above, early studies of A II binding to the heart indicated that there are at least two binding sites: one high affinity and low capacity, and the other, low affinity and high capacity.[7] Monovalent cations decrease the expression of the high-affinity site and have no effect on the low-affinity site. Divalent cations (Mg^{2+}, Ca^{2+}, Mn^{2+}) and guanine nucleotides also differentially affect the high-affinity sites: Mg^{2+}, by increasing the receptor number, and guanine nucleotides, by reducing the affinity for A II.[7] More recently, binding studies using the AT_1-specific inhibitor Losartan and the AT_2-specific antagonist PD123177 have demonstrated that both AT_1 and AT_2 receptors are widely distributed throughout the heart.[14] Only the AT_1 binding site is sensitive to GTPγS, suggesting that the high-affinity sites described in earlier studies correspond to this receptor.

Cloning of the Angiotensin AT₁ Receptor

Although both AT₁ and AT₂ receptors exist in the heart, only AT₁ receptors have been shown to be functionally important. The recent cloning of the vascular AT₁ receptor has led to a tremendous increase in our understanding of its structure and function. The AT₁ receptor belongs to the superfamily of G-protein-coupled receptors that have seven transmembrane-spanning domains.[15,16] The receptor is a 359 amino acid protein with an M_r of 41 kd,[15,16] but estimates of the molecular weight of the functional receptor range as high as 79 kd.[17] This apparent discrepancy may be due to the fact that the protein is probably glycosylated. There are three potential consensus sites for *N*-glycosylation on the putative extracellular domains (Figure 1).[16] Each of the four extracellular regions also contains a cys-

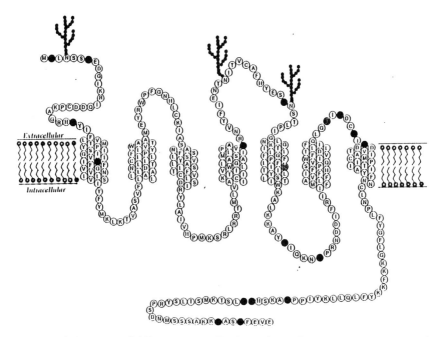

Fig. 1 Schematic of AT₁ receptors. Each circle in the putative structure of the seven-transmembrane-domain AT₁ₐ receptor represents a single amino acid, indicated by the standard one-letter code. Divergence between the AT₁ₐ and the AT₁ʙ receptor is indicated by black (nonconservative changes) and gray (conservative changes) circles. Potential glycosylation sites are depicted by the presence of branched structures representing sugar molecules (from Griendling KK, et al.).[47]

teine residue,[15,16] which may be responsible for the sensitivity of A II binding to sulfhydryl reagents.[18]

Definite subtypes of the AT_1 receptor have been found in the rat and mouse (Fig. 1). Currently, the vascular receptor is classified as AT_{1A}, and the adrenal receptor is denoted as AT_{1B} in the rat. The sequence of the AT_{1B} receptor is 94% identical to that of the AT_{1A} receptor protein in both species. The AT_{1B} receptor mRNA also encodes a protein of 359 amino acids with a M_r of 41 kd. The amino acid differences between the two subtypes are primarily concentrated in the carboxyl terminus of the molecule.[19]

The *mas* oncogene has also been reported to encode an angiotensin binding site,[20] although it shares only a 9% sequence identity with the vascular AT_1 receptor. It is, however, unclear at the present time whether this protein is a unique AT receptor since the pharmacological potency series and antagonist binding are uncharacteristic of AT receptors.

Genomic Analysis of the AT_1 Receptor

Analysis of the AT_1 receptor gene is an area of intense current investigation. Preliminary information indicates that the rat gene contains at least three exons and two introns that collectively span over 80 kb.[21] The entire coding region, a short segment of the 5′ untranslated region and a major portion of the 3′ untranslated region, is contained within the third exon.[21,22] The observation that there are no introns within the receptor protein coding region also holds true for the mouse and human AT_1 receptor genes.[19,23] The gene for the human AT_{1A} receptor encodes a 359 amino acid protein that is 95% identical to the rat and bovine sequences.[23] In this gene, there is an intron/exon junction upstream of the translation initiation codon.[23] Analysis of the 5′ flanking region of the rat gene shows that several potential promoter and regulatory elements are contained in this sequence, including a TATA box, a cap site coding for binding of the small ribosomal subunit to the mRNA, and an SP-1 binding site.[21] There is also some evidence for alternative splicing of this gene since the first report of the cloning of the AT_{1A} receptor showed that the cDNA for the AT_1 receptor hybridized with two sizes of mRNA: 2.3 kb and 3.5 kb.[15]

The first studies of the human genome suggest that only one AT_1 receptor gene may exist in man,[23] but Southern blot analysis of the rat and mouse genome suggests the presence of at least two genes for AT_1 receptors.[19,22] Restriction mapping, differential hybridization, PCR amplification, and sequence analysis of the rat genome indicate that the AT_{1A} and AT_{1B} receptors are encoded by two separate genes, which share a 94% amino-acid sequence identity in the open reading frame but only a 35% identity in the 3' and 5' flanking regions.[22]

Regulation of AT_1 Expression

As with other G-protein coupled receptors, AT_1 receptor expression is controlled both acutely and chronically. When a cell is exposed to A II, the ligand-receptor complex becomes sequestered in the plasma membrane and subsequently internalized.[24–26] The net result is a decrease in the availability of surface receptors. Chronically, the expression of cell surface receptors is influenced by alterations in mRNA levels. Angiotensin II induces homologous downregulation of AT_1 receptors by both inducing internalization[24] and reducing mRNA levels.[27] A 4- to 6-hour treatment with A II reduces AT_{1A} receptor mRNA expression by 50% in both cultured vascular smooth muscle cells and mesangial cells. Elevation of intracellular cyclic AMP, by forskolin or cholera toxin, also causes receptor downregulation at the mRNA level.[27] Dietary depletion of Na^+ increases expression of AT receptors in zona glomerulosa cells[28] but decreases expression in vascular smooth muscle cells by an unclear mechanism. Similarly, dietary K^+ depletion decreases surface vascular AT-receptor expression by altering the rate of recycling of the receptor.[29] The effect that these various phenomena have on receptor expression in cardiac tissue is unknown.

Analysis of the amino acid sequence of the AT_1 receptor suggests other potential, but as yet unproven, regulatory pathways. The presence of three potential sites for protein kinase C phosphorylation in the C terminus of the receptor suggests that phosphorylation by this enzyme may be involved in receptor regulation.[30] Additionally, the tyrosine residues in the cytoplasmic tail of the receptor (Fig. 1) represent potential phosphorylation sites that may be involved in receptor internalization. Posttranscriptional modification is thus likely to be a major contributor to receptor expression.

Regulation of AT_2 binding-site expression is even less well understood. It is clear, however, that expression of this subtype is linked to development. Pharmacologically, AT_2 binding sites are more abundant in embryonic and neonatal tissue than in adult tissue.[13,31–34] In the rat heart, AT_1 and AT_2 receptor expression are both developmentally regulated, peaking 2 days after birth.[14] More detailed studies of AT_2 binding-site expression await identification of its structure.

AT Receptor Subtype Distribution in the Heart

Pharmacological studies of subtype distribution indicate that both AT_1 and AT_2 receptors are widely and evenly distributed throughout the rat atria and ventricles.[14] Both subtypes are found in the septal wall, in the sinoatrial node, and at a very high density in the atrioventricular node.[14] AT_1 receptors have also been identified in the papillary muscle of the rabbit heart.[11] Finally, one study, using a nonsubtype-selective radioligand, found a dense distribution of AT receptors over the parasympathetic nerve bundles and the intracardiac ganglia.[35] Interestingly, the highest density of receptors in this preparation occurred over the remnant of the arterial duct.[35] Undoubtedly, these observations will be extended using molecular biological techniques. The only molecular data available at the present time indicate that the cardiac AT_1 receptor is subtype AT_{1A}, whereas the AT_{1B} subtype is absent from the heart.[8]

Signal Transduction by AT Receptors

The signal transduction pathways utilized by AT_1 receptors have been elucidated in many tissues and in cells transfected with the AT_1 receptor (Figure 2).[15,36] In virtually all systems studied, AT_1 receptors activate phosphoinositide-specific phospholipase C via a guanine nucleotide regulatory protein. Many isozymes of phospholipase C have been identified; however, the subtype activated by calcium mobilizing hormones remains unknown. Phospholipase C cleaves phosphatidylinositol 4,5-bisphosphate (PIP_2) to yield inositol trisphosphate (IP_3) and diacylglycerol. IP_3 mobilizes Ca^{2+} from intracellular stores, and diacylglycerol activates the Ca^{2+}- and phospholipid-dependent enzyme protein kinase C. In many tissues, including the heart, AT_1 receptors are also negatively coupled to adenylate cyclase by G_i, an inhibitory guanine nucleotide regulatory protein.[37] Finally, AT_1 receptors activate phospholipases D[38] and A_2,[39] although whether this coupling occurs in the heart is unknown. Phospholipase D cleaves phosphatidylcholine to generate phosphatidic acid and choline, and phospholipase A_2 action on phosphatidyl-

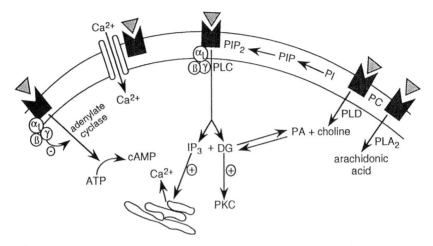

Fig. 2 A II signaling in cardiomyocytes. AT$_1$ receptors have been shown to be positively coupled to phospholipase C, phospholipase D, and phospholipase A$_2$ and negatively coupled to adenylate cyclase. Angiotensin II also stimulates an increase in current through L-type Ca^{2+} channels, an effect that appears to be independent of phospholipase C activation. Abbreviations shown are DG, diacylglycerol; IP$_3$, inositol trisphosphate; $\alpha_i\beta\gamma$, inhibitory guanine nucleotide regulatory protein; PA, phosphatidic acid; PC, phosphatidylcholine; PI, phosphatidylinositol; PIP, phosphatidylinositol 4-phosphate; PIP$_2$, phosphatidylinositol 4,5-bisphosphate; PLA$_2$, phospholipase A$_2$; PLC, phospholipase C; PLD, phospholipase D; PKC, protein kinase C.

choline results in the formation of lysophosphatidylcholine and the release of a free fatty acid, usually arachidonic acid. The role of these latter second messengers in the response of the myocardium to A II is unknown.

The most well studied effect of A II on intracellular signaling in the myocardium is an acute increase in mean diastolic intracellular Ca^{2+} concentration.[40] This is accompanied by an increase in the frequency of Ca^{2+} transients, followed by a significant decrease in their amplitude.[40] Unlike most other tissues in which the increase in intracellular Ca^{2+} in response to A II is a direct consequence of IP$_3$ release, the rise in mean diastolic Ca^{2+} concentration in myocardial tissue appears to parallel, rather than result from, activation of phospholipase C.[41] This is presumably a reflection of the fact that in the heart one of the major actions of A II is to increase current through L-type calcium channels.[1] The subsequent decrease in the amplitude of Ca^{2+} transients following administration of A II can most likely be attributed to a negative feedback mechanism, possibly involving protein kinase C.

The other product of the phosphoinositide signaling pathway, diacylglycerol, has not been investigated extensively in the heart. Stimulation of cardiac myocytes by 12-O-tetradecanoylphorbol-13-acetate (TPA), a phorbol ester that exogenously activates protein kinase C, results in a positive chronotropic effect that is accompanied by increases in L-type Ca^{2+} channel activity and phosphorylation of a discrete set of proteins ranging in weight from 32 to 83 kd.[42] Angiotensin II stimulates phosphorylation of this same set of proteins.[1] The largest, an 83 kd acidic protein, appears to be a specific substrate for protein kinase C. Although the function of these proteins is unknown, the similarity in mechanical and electrical responses of the myocardium to A II and phorbol esters supports the concept that protein kinase C activation may mediate some of the effects of A II.

One of the major unanswered questions concerning the AT_2 binding site is the identification of the signal transduction pathway to which it is coupled. In neuronal cells, AT_2 binding sites are negatively coupled to guanylate cyclase,[10] although this may not be true in all cell systems expressing this protein. It has also been suggested that the coupling of AT_2 binding sites to the particulate guanylate cyclase is mediated by a phosphotyrosine phosphatase.[43] In addition, there appears to be a subpopulation of these binding sites that is sensitive to GTPγS, recently designated AT_{2A} by Tsutsumi and Saavedra.[44] The signaling mechanisms activated by these binding sites remain to be determined conclusively.

Pathophysiology

There has been much recent interest in the therapeutic potential of the specific AT_1 receptor antagonist Losartan for the treatment of cardiac disease. In addition, Losartan has been used to help elucidate which effects of ACE inhibition are due to the reduction of A II generation as compared with the possible effects of increasing bradykinin. Comparison of the effectiveness of ACE inhibitors with Losartan administration in an ovine model of heart failure induced by rapid ventricular pacing indicates that the two agents have similar effects on circulatory hemodynamics.[45] Similar results were obtained in an aortocaval shunt model of high-output heart failure in the rat.[46] Such studies indicate that the efficacy of ACE inhibitors is likely to be related to a diminution of A II formation, rather than to a reduction in the metabolism of bradykinin. These early studies suggest that Losartan has no therapeutic advantage over captopril or enalapril for the treatment of heart failure; however, investigations into this area are just beginning, and a final answer must await further experimental and ultimately clinical verification.

Conclusions and Future Directions

The development of new pharmacological tools and the recent cloning of the AT_1 receptor has opened a new era of investigation into the function and structure of angiotensin receptors. This information will be useful in determining the mechanisms by which AT_1 receptors couple to signaling enzymes. Additionally, the availability of mRNA probes and antibodies will permit studies of the regulation and tissue distribution of these receptors. Cloning, purification, and identification of the signaling pathways to which the AT_2 binding site couples will provide a much-needed impetus for understanding the function of these molecules. Ultimately, such studies could provide the basis for the development of therapeutic molecules that can be specifically targeted to cardiac disease.

Summary

The actions of angiotensin II on the heart are ultimately mediated by the A II receptor. The recent development of subtype-specific pharmacological agents and the cloning of the AT_1 receptor has permitted the direct demonstration of heterogeneity in the angiotensin receptor population in the myocardium. Thus, both AT_1 receptors and AT_2 binding sites have been found in the heart, although only AT_1 receptors have been shown to be functionally coupled to inotropic responses and cardiac hypertrophy.

AT_1 receptors belong to the seven transmembrane-spanning domain family of G-protein coupled receptors. They consist of 359 amino acids with an apparent M_r of 41 kd. Subtypes of AT_1 receptors have now been identified and have been denoted AT_{1A} and AT_{1B}. These subtypes have a 94% sequence identity with each other at the amino acid level. Although there appears to be only one AT_1 receptor gene in humans, there are two genes in the rat and mouse. Expression of AT_1 receptors is controlled acutely by sequestration/internalization of the ligand-receptor complex and chronically by modulation of mRNA levels. Angiotensin II itself, along with agents that increase cyclic AMP concentration, have been shown to alter AT_1 mRNA levels.

Signaling pathways activated by AT_1 receptors in the heart are similar to those in other tissues, with AT_1 receptors positively coup-

ling to phospholipase C and negatively coupling to adenylate cyclase. Although these receptors mediate changes in intracellular Ca^{2+} concentration and flux through Ca^{2+} channels, the mechanisms responsible for these changes remain unclear.

Finally, Losartan, an AT_1-selective antagonist, has recently been investigated for its therapeutic potential in treating heart failure. Its effect is nearly indistinguishable from that of ACE inhibitors; nonetheless, its full therapeutic potential remains to be evaluated.

References

1. Baker KM, Booz GW, Dostal DE. Cardiac actions of angiotensin II: role of an intracardiac renin-angiotensin system. Ann Rev Physiol 1992; 54: 227–241.
2. Kobayashi M, Furukawa Y, Chiba S. Positive chronotropic and inotropic effects of angiotensin II in the dog heart. Eur J Pharm 1978; 50: 17–25.
3. Rogers TB, Gaa ST, Allen IS. Identification and characterization of functional angiotensin II receptors on cultured heart myocytes. J Pharmacol Exp Ther 1986; 236:438–444.
4. Linz W, Schoelkens BA, Ganten D. Converting enzyme inhibition specifically prevents the development and induces the regression of cardiac hypertrophy in rats. Clin Exp Hypertens 1989; 11:1325–1350.
5. Baker KM, Aceto JF. Angiotensin II stimulation of protein synthesis and cell growth in chick heart cells. Am J Physiol 1990; 259: H610–H618.
6. Tan LB, Brilla C, Weber KT. Prevention of structural changes in the heart in hypertension by ACE inhibition. J Hypertens Suppl 1992; 10: S31–S34.
7. Wright GB, Alexander RW, Ekstein LS, Gimbrone MA. Characterization of the rabbit ventricular myocardial receptor for angiotensin II: evidence for two sites of different affinities and specificities. Mol Pharmacol 1983; 24:213–221.
8. Iwai N, Inagami T. Identification of two subtypes in the rat type I angiotensin II receptor. FEBS Lett 1992; 298:257–260.
9. Bumpus FM, Catt KJ, Shiu AT, et al. Nomenclature for angiotensin II receptors: a report of the nomenclature committee of the council for high blood pressure research. Hypertension 1991; 17:720–721.
10. Sumners C, Tang W, Zelezna B, Raizada MK. Angiotensin II receptor subtypes are coupled with distinct signal-transduction mechanisms in neurons and astrocytes from the rat brain. Proc Nat Acad Sci USA 1991; 88:7567–7571.
11. Scott AL, Chang RS, Lotti VJ, Siegl PK. Cardiac angiotensin receptors: effects of selective angiotensin II receptor antagonists, DUP 753 and PD 121981, in rabbit heart. J Pharm Exp Ther 1992; 261:931–935.
12. Dostal DE, Baker KM. Angiotensin II stimulation of left ventricular hypertrophy in adult rat heart: mediation by the AT_1 receptor. Am J Hypertens 1992; 5:276–280.

13. Milan MA, Carvallo P, Izumi S-I, et al. Novel sites of expression of functional angiotensin II receptors in the late gestation fetus. Science 1989; 244:1340–1342.
14. Sechi LA, Griffin CA, Grady EF, Kalinyak JE, Schambelan M. Characterization of angiotensin II receptor subtypes in rat heart. Circ Res 1992; 71:1482–1489.
15. Murphy TJ, Alexander RW, Griendling KK, Runge MS, Bernstein KE. Isolation of a cDNA encoding the vascular type-I angiotensin II receptor. Nature 1991; 351:233–236.
16. Sasaki K, Yamano Y, Bardhan S, et al. Cloning and expression of a complementary DNA encoding a bovine adrenal angiotensin II type-1 receptor. Nature 1991; 351:230–232.
17. Catt KJ, Carson MC, Hausdorff WP, et al. Angiotensin II receptors and mechanisms of action in adrenal glomerulosa cells. J Steroid Biochem 1987; 27:915–927.
18. Gunther S. Characterization of angiotensin II receptor subtypes in rat liver. J Biol Chem 1984; 259:7622–7629.
19. Sasamura H, Hein L, Krieger JE, et al. Cloning, characterization, and expression of two angiotensin receptor (AT-1) isoforms from the mouse genome. Biochem Biophys Res Commun 1992; 185:253–259.
20. Jackson TR, Blair LAC, Marshall J, Goedert M, Hanley MR. The *mas* oncogene encodes an angiotensin II receptor. Nature 1988; 335:437–440.
21. Langford K, Frenzel K, Martin BM, Bernstein KE. The genomic organization of the rat AT_1 angiotensin receptor. Biochem Biophys Res Commun 1992; 183:1025–1032.
22. Elton TS, Stephan CC, Taylor GR, et al. Isolation of two distinct type I angiotensin II receptor genes. Biochem Biophys Res Commun 1992; 184:1067–1073.
23. Furata H, Guo D-F, Inagami T. Molecular cloning and sequencing of the gene encoding human type-1 angiotensin II receptor. Biochem Biophys Res Commun 1992; 183:8–13.
24. Griendling KK, Delafontaine P, Rittenhouse SE, Gimbrone MA Jr, Alexander RW. Correlation of receptor sequestration with sustained diacylglycerol accumulation in angiotensin II-stimulated cultured vascular smooth muscle cells. J Biol Chem 1987; 262:14555–14562.
25. Ullian ME, Linas SL. Role of receptor cycling in the regulation of angiotensin II surface receptor number and angiotensin II uptake in rat vascular smooth muscle cells. J Clin Invest 1989; 84:840–846.
26. Anderson KM, Murahashi T, Dostal DE, Peach MJ. Morphological and biochemical analysis of angiotensin II internalization in cultured rat aorta smooth muscle cells. Am J Physiol 1993; 264:C179–C188.
27. Iwai N, Inagami T. Regulation of the expression of the rat angiotensin II receptor mRNA. Biochem Biophys Res Commun 1992; 182:1094–1099.
28. Aguilera G, Schirar A, Baukal A, Catt KJ. Angiotensin II receptors: properties and regulation in adrenal glomerulosa cells. Circ Res 1980; 46(suppl I):118–127.
29. Linas SL, Marzec-Calvert R, Ullian ME. K^+ depletion alters angiotensin II receptor expression in vascular smooth muscle cells. Am J Physiol 1990; 258:C849–C854.
30. Bernstein KE, Alexander RW. Counterpoint: molecular analysis of the angiotensin II receptor. Endocr Rev 1992; 13:381–386.

31. Grady EF, Sechi LA, Griffin CA, Schambelan M, Kalinyak JE. Expression of AT_2 receptors in the developing rat fetus. J Clin Invest 1991; 88:921–933.
32. Millan MA, Jacobowitz DM, Aguilera G, Catt KJ. Differential distribution of AT_1 and AT_2 angiotensin II receptor subtypes in the rat brain during development. Proc Nat Acad Sci USA 1991; 88:11440–11444.
33. Viswanathan M, Tsutsumi K, Correa FM, Saavedra JM. Changes in expression of angiotensin receptor subtypes in the rat aorta during development. Biochem Biophys Res Commun 1991; 179:1361–1367.
34. Tsutsumi K, Saavedra JM. Characterization and development of angiotensin II receptor subtypes (AT_1 and AT_2) in rat brain. Am J Physiol 1991; 26:R209–R216.
35. Allen AM, Yamada H, Mendelsohn FA. In vitro autoradiographic localization of binding to angiotensin receptors in the rat heart. Int J Cardiol 1990; 28:25–33.
36. Griendling KK, Tsuda T, Berk BC, Alexander RW. Angiotensin II stimulation of vascular smooth muscle. J Cardiovas Pharm 1989; 14(suppl. 6):S27–S33.
37. Anand-Srivastava MB. Angiotensin II receptors negatively coupled to adenylate cyclase in rat myocardial sarcolemma: involvement of inhibitory guanine nucleotide regulatory protein. Biochem Pharm 1989; 38: 489–496.
38. Lassègue B, Griendling KK, Murphy TJ, Alexander RW. Regulation of angiotensin II receptor expression in vascular smooth muscle cells. FASEB J 1992; 6:A1859.
39. Schlondorff D, DeCandido S, Satriano JA. Angiotensin II stimulates phospholipases C and A_2 in cultured rat mesangial cells. Am J Physiol 1987; 253:C113–C120.
40. Kem DC, Johnson EI, Capponi AM, et al. Effect of angiotensin II on cytosolic free calcium in neonatal rat cardiomyocytes. Am J Physiol 1991; 261:C77–C85.
41. Baker KM, Singer HA, Aceto JF. Angiotensin receptor-mediated stimulation of cytosolic-free calcium and inositol phosphates in chick myocytes. J Pharm Exp Ther 1989; 251:578–585.
42. Dosemeci A, Dhallan RS, Cohen NM, Lederer WJ, Rogers TB. Phorbol ester increases calcium current and simulates the effects of angiotensin II on cultured neonatal rat heart myocytes. Circ Res 1988; 62:347–357.
43. Bottari SP, King IN, Reichlin S, et al. The angiotensin AT_2 receptor stimulates protein tyrosine phosphatase activity and mediates inhibition of particulate guanylate cyclase. Biochem Biophys Res Commun 1992; 183:206–211.
44. Tsutsumi K, Saavedra JM. Heterogeneity of angiotensin II AT_2 receptors in the rat brain. Mol Pharmacol 1992; 41:290–297.
45. Fitzpatrick MA, Rademaker MT, Charles CJ, et al. Angiotensin II receptor antagonism in ovine heart failure: acute hemodynamic, hormonal and renal effects. Am J Physiol 1992; 263:H250–H256.
46. Qing G, Garcia R. Chronic captopril and Losartan (Dup 753) administration in rats with high-output heart failure. Am J Physiol 1992; 263: H833–H840.
47. Griendling KK, Murphy TJ, Alexander RW. Molecular biology of the renin-angiotensin system. Circulation, 1993; 87: 1816–1828.

6

Regulation of Cardiac Second Messengers by Angiotensins

George W. Booz, David E. Dostal, and Kenneth M. Baker

Introduction

Angiotensin II has multiple direct and indirect actions on the heart, which affect heart rate, contractility, cell growth, and extracellular matrix remodeling.[1–5] The direct cardiac actions of A II are mediated by specific cell surface receptors that have been identified on all major cell types of the heart and are linked by guanine nucleotide binding proteins (G-proteins) to second-messenger generation. Studies characterizing the A II receptor are described elsewhere.[1,6,7] The purpose of this review is to provide an overview of studies that have examined second-messenger generation in cardiac cells in response to A II. The first part of the review deals with individual cell types in the heart and describes various responses attributable to A II that are of physiological and pathophysiological importance in cardiac function. Where established, the involvement of a particular second messenger in a cellular response is discussed. Effects of A II on aortic vascular smooth muscle cells (VSMC) are included since no comparable studies have been performed on VSMC of coronary arteries. Studies do indicate, however, that small resistance vessels are a target for the physiological and pathophysiological actions of A II.[4,8–10] Moreover, numerous studies have demonstrated that all of the known in vivo biological responses to A II result from the generation of a defined group of second messengers,[1,6,11,12] suggest-

Lindpaintner K and Ganten D (editors): *The Cardiac-Renin Angiotensin System,* © Futura Publishing Co., Inc., Armonk, NY, 1994.

ing that any differences between VSMC of large conduction vessels and resistance vessels in this regard are likely to be quantitative. The second part of this review focuses on individual second messengers and provides evidence for their generation by A II. The way in which a second messenger may affect a particular cellular response is discussed. In some cases, the putative involvement of a second messenger in other cellular responses is mentioned. Admittedly, much of this section is speculative, reflecting in part the descriptive nature that has characterized most of the studies to date on second-messenger generation by A II. Only now with recent advances in molecular biology can we hope to gain some insight into the exact processes by which A II affects second-messenger generation and how different signaling pathways are integrated to produce a final cellular response.

Physiological and Pathophysiological Actions of Angiotensin

Angiotensin II has a wide variety of direct and indirect actions on the cardiovascular system.[1-3] Multiple indirect actions are mediated in part through its influence on various cardiovascular regulatory sites in the brain, modulation of the activity of sympathetic neurons, and stimulation of aldosterone synthesis and release. Direct cardiovascular actions of A II include chronotropic and inotropic effects on the myocardium, effects on cardiac metabolism and growth, and vasoconstriction of blood vessels. Autoradiographic studies have shown that receptors for A II are widely distributed in the human heart, being present in the myocardium, as well as on coronary vessels and sympathetic nerves.[13] Studies on cultured cells and isolated membrane preparations have established that cardiomyocytes, VSMC, cardiac fibroblasts, and endothelial cells all possess G-protein-coupled A II receptors that are linked to a particular biological response by second-messenger generation.[6,11,14-18] Angiotensin II receptors can be classified into two groups[1,11] on the basis of data obtained using nonpeptide receptor antagonists and on the basis of their differential sensitivity to dithiothreitol and whether or not they couple to G-proteins. The AT_1 class of receptors mediate all known biological actions of A II and bind the nonpeptide receptor antagonist Losartan. Cardiomyocytes possess two types of AT_1 receptors, which differ in affinity for A II and may represent subtypes that couple to different second-messenger pathways.[1] The AT_2 class of receptors, present as well on cardiomyocytes, VSMC, and cardiac fibroblasts have no known biological function in these cell types but may play some role in fetal development.[11] For rat neonatal cardiac fibroblasts, the number of AT_2 binding sites decreases with passage (K. Baker, unpublished observation).

Studies on cultured cardiomyocytes, cardiac fibroblasts, and VSMC have shown that A II is a trophic agent as well, enhancing gene expression and inducing hypertrophic and/or proliferative cell growth([8–10,15,19–22]; K. Baker, unpublished data). This observation, together with recent evidence showing that the myocardium[23–25] and vasculature[10] both possess a local RAS, lends support to the notion that circulating or locally generated A II may contribute to the ventricular remodeling and compensatory hypertrophy seen after myocardial infarction and in some forms of hypertension. Such a possibility was originally suggested by clinical studies demonstrating the efficacy of ACE inhibitors in the treatment of heart failure, myocardial ischemia, and hypertension.[1]

Cardiomyocytes

Inotropic and Chronotropic Effects

Angiotensin II has direct and indirect positive inotropic effects on cardiac muscle. Indirect inotropic and chronotropic effects of A II result, in part, from its modulatory actions on neurotransmitter release and reuptake at sympathetic nerve terminals by means of prejunctional A II receptors.[26,27] Prolongation of the action potential and increased Ca^{2+} influx may explain the augmentation of sympathetic transmitter release by A II, although the second-messenger system that is activated by these receptors is not yet established. Evidence against the involvement of either adenosine $3',5'$-cyclic monophosphate (cyclic AMP)[28] or protein kinase C (PKC) has been reported.[29] The direct positive inotropic effect of A II that is observed on the cardiac muscle of most species, including humans, is due to activation of voltage-sensitive, L-type (slow) Ca^{2+} channels.[1] The direct inotropic action of A II is dose dependent and is blocked or attenuated by A II receptor antagonists, demonstrating that it is a receptor-mediated response. With the possible exception of the hamster heart,[30] the half-maximal contractile response occurs at concentrations of A II close to the K_d for the high-affinity A II binding site.[1] A positive inotropic effect has also been reported for A III,[31] while a direct inotropic effect of A I is less certain.[1] Studies showing that A I is inotropic may, in part, reflect its conversion to A II by ACE or heart chymase.[30,32-34]

Two species that show no inotropic response to A II are the guinea pig[35,36] and adult rat.[37] Guinea pig atrial and ventricular cardiomyocytes were shown to have Losartan-sensitive A II receptors that couple to phospholipid hydrolysis[35] (K. Baker, unpublished observation), suggesting that there is a subtype of the AT_1 receptor, not expressed by cardiomyocytes of this species, that couples to activation of L-type Ca^{2+} channels but not to phospholipase C (PLC) activation. A low number of A II receptors may, in part, explain the lack of a positive inotropic response in the adult rat heart,[38] although a positive inotropic response to A II was reported for cultured adult rat ventricular myocytes.[39,40] Angiotensin II was shown not to have a positive inotropic effect on cultured neonatal rat cardiomyocytes, although it did augment Ca^{2+} current in voltage-clamped cells.[41] In this preparation, A II exerted a delayed negative inotropic effect, which was attributed to A II receptor-mediated activation of PKC.[41,42] This observation raises the possibility that other intracellular events triggered by A II in cardiac cells of this species, such as a PKC-mediated reduction in the amplitude of the intracellular Ca^{2+} transient,[43] may serve to counteract an initial increase in Ca^{2+} entry brought about by its activation of Ca^{2+} channels.

Angiotensin II may exert opposing effects on heart rate: a reflex slowing of the heart, resulting from its hypertensive action and baroreceptor stimulation, and an increase in heart rate by various sympathoadrenal mechanisms and centrally mediated reduction in vagal tone.[1,3] In addition, there is evidence that A II may exert a direct chronotropic effect on cardiomyocytes, which could conceivably contribute to the high incidence of ventricular arrhythmias in chronic congestive heart failure syndromes in which there are often elevated circulating levels of A II. Studies suggesting that A II does have a direct, albeit small, positive chronotropic action were reported for both dog and rat hearts.[44,45] Recently, A II was shown to stimulate the spontaneous beating rate of cultured neonatal rat cardiomyocytes with an ED_{50} that was similar to the K_d for the high-affinity binding site.[14,41,42] Both binding and chronotropic actions of A II were inhibited by receptor antagonists. The chronotropic action of A II likely resulted from an enhancement of Ca^{2+} and Na^+ channel activity in the sarcolemma. In addition to augmenting Ca^{2+} current, A II was shown to increase the frequency of opening, and the rates of activation and inactivation, of voltage-dependent Na^+ channels in patch-clamped neonatal rat ventricular myocytes when applied outside the patch.[46] Preliminary evidence indicated that the A II effect on Na^+ channels was mediated by PKC.[46]

Growth Effects

A number of recent in vivo studies have implicated A II in the etiology of cardiac hypertrophy assocated with hypertension, by both afterload-dependent and -independent mechanisms,[1,2,47–50] and in addition, in the rapid perinatal growth of the left ventricle in the neonatal pig.[51,52] The notion that A II is a direct stimulus for hypertrophic growth of cardiomyocytes was substantiated by in vitro studies showing that A II can stimulate protein synthesis and induce cellular hypertrophy of cultured chick myocytes.[15,19] The hypertrophic action of A II, which was blocked by a specific A II receptor antagonist, was not secondary to A II-stimulated increases in contractile activity since it was observed in depolarized, nonbeating cells as well.[19] Total RNA levels in myocytes were increased at 12 hours following exposure to A II,[19] with increases at 3 hours in mRNA levels of the proto-oncogene *c-fos* (K. Baker, unpublished data). Increased *c-fos* expression has been observed in cultured neonatal rat cardiomyocytes in response to other agents that induce hypertrophy,[53] and is an early event in the hypertrophic response of cardiac myocytes to pressure overload in vivo.[54] Although the role of *c-fos* is not fully understood, the induction of *c-fos* seems to be important in the transition from quiescence into the cell cycle and is common to both hypertrophic and proliferative responses. Circumstantial evidence supports the idea that the activation of PKC by A II is responsible for enhanced *c-fos* expression.[53] Although it has been suggested that increases in intracellular Ca^{2+} may play a separate, or synergistic, role in cardiac hypertrophy or *c-fos* expression,[4,8,53] both A II and [Sar^1,Ile^8]A II were shown to stimulate increases in cytosolic free Ca^{2+} in cultured embryonic chick myocytes, yet [Sar^1,Ile^8]A II blocked the growth effects of A II.[19] The *c-fos* protein and the protein product of another proto-oncogene, *c-jun*, form a heterodimeric complex (AP-1) that binds to a specific DNA consensus sequence (AP-1 binding site or 12-O-tetradecanoylphorbol 13-acetate (TPA) responsive element, TRE) of target genes to stimulate their transcription. Angiotensin II may enhance gene transcription as well by PKC-mediated posttranslational modification of pre-existing AP-1, as suggested by studies on VSMC.[55]

Vascular Smooth Muscle

Vasoconstriction

The intravenous administration of A II causes an immediate, dose-dependent rise in blood pressure because of increased systemic resistance. This vasopressor action of A II, which has been well studied using vascular strips and perfused arteries, results from both a direct effect of A II on VSMC, as well as from various indirect effects mediated through the sympathetic nervous system.[7] Studies on cultured VSMC have shown that A II induces a rapid, transient increase in intracellular free Ca^{2+}, resulting for the most part from inositol 1,4,5-triphosphate (IP_3)-induced release of Ca^{2+} from the sarcoplasmic reticulum.[17,56,57] The transient rise in intracellular Ca^{2+} correlates temporally with initiation of contraction in vascular strips exposed to A II and is likely responsible for the initiation of contraction through Ca^{2+}/calmodulin-dependent phosphorylation of the myosin light chain.[12,17] Activation of PKC by the diacylglycerol (DG) branch of the PLC-initiated cascade of intracellular signals may then feed back to inhibit further IP_3 formation.[17,56,57] In rat VSMC, A II induces a biphasic increase in DG: an initial, transient rise in DG, likely produced during IP_3 formation, followed by a sustained increase.[57,58] It has been proposed that the sustained formation of DG, and the resultant activation of PKC, may be responsible for the prolonged contraction of VSMC that is induced by some vasopressor agents.[57,59] The two phases of A II-induced DG formation appear to be differentially regulated. Although the initial rise in DG, like IP_3 formation, is attenuated by activators of PKC, the second, sustained phase is not.[57,58] The basis for this differential regulation is not known, although receptor internalization appears to be involved, in as much as it is necessary for the sustained phase of DG formation.[58] A recent study on mesangial cells indicated that PKC-α is selectively involved in inhibiting A II-induced IP_3 formation in those cells;[60] whether a specific PKC isoform plays a similar role in VSMC has not been reported.

Growth Effects

Numerous in vivo studies have implicated A II in the adaptive changes that occur in the vasculature during chronic hypertension, suggesting that A II is a trophic agent for VSMC.[4,8] Studies examining the growth effects of A II on cultured rat aortic VSMC have shown that A II exerts a hypertrophic effect with some induction of polyploidy, reflecting the situation in chronic hypertension.[20,22] In aortic VSMC from the spontaneously hypertensive rat (SHR), A II exerts a small proliferative as well as hypertrophic effect.[61,62] A proliferative effect of A II was also reported for VSMC of human aorta[63] and rat mesenteric resistance arteries.[9,64] The ED_{50} for the trophic effects of A II on VSMC was reported to be near the K_d of the AT_1 receptor, which may represent a high concentration for circulating A II. The existence of a local RAS in the vasculature, however, would make the question of what is a physiological concentration of A II irrelevant.[10] In addition to stimulating VSMC hypertrophy or proliferation, A II has been shown to stimulate collagen[65] and glycoconjugate[62] synthesis by VSMC, which may contribute to extracellular matrix remodeling associated with certain types of hypertension.

The trophic effects of A II on VSMC may be mediated through an induction of autocrine growth factors.[10,21,66] In cultured rat aortic VSMC, A II has been shown to cause a delayed increase in the mRNA and medium concentrations of the platelet-derived growth factor (PDGF),[66,67] transforming growth factor-β (TGF-β),[21,66,68] and endothelin.[69] Antisense oligonucleotides to PDGF mRNA were found to attenuate A II-induced hypertrophy of rat aortic VSMC.[70] It has been suggested that A II may activate an antiproliferative pathway in this preparation, mediated by PKC-dependent TGF-β production.[10] Coincubation of these cells with anti-TGF antibody markedly enhanced A II-stimulated DNA synthesis and cell number. Different findings, however, were recently reported for cultured aortic SHR-derived VSMC perhaps because of strain differences or "phenotypic modulation."[21] In this preparation, the A II-induced increases in DNA synthesis, which were associated with a nondetectable increase in cell number, were inhibited by treatment with an anti-TGF-β antibody. More important, however, A II was found to increase the mitogenic response of SHR-derived VSMC to epidermal growth factor (EGF) and PDGF, an effect that was partially mediated by autocrine secretion of TGF-β. This finding may, in part, explain the excessive VSMC mitogenesis that occurs after vascular injury associated with angioplasty.

In rat aortic VSMC, A II activates protein synthesis in a Ca^{2+}-dependent manner.[20] Protein synthesis did not require activation of PKC or Na^+/H^+ exchange,[20] although A II was reported to enhance ribosomal S6 kinase by an amiloride-sensitive pathway.[71] The mechanism by which increased intracellular Ca^{2+} triggers protein synthesis and cellular hypertrophy has not been defined but may involve the activation of Ca^{2+}/calmodulin-dependent kinases with perhaps an indirect activation of tyrosine kinases. Angiotensin II has also been shown to increase levels of mRNA for the proto-oncogene *c-fos* in rat aortic VSMC in a concentration-dependent manner, with maximum levels of *c-fos* mRNA observed at approximately 100 nm A II.[72,73] Induction of *c-fos*, which could be blocked by a competitive inhibitor of the A II receptor, was rapid, with maximum levels at approximately 30 minutes.[72,73] By using the nuclear runoff transcription assay, it was demonstrated that A II stimulated the transcription rate of the *c-fos* gene.[73] Angiotensin II-induction of *c-fos* mRNA was shown to occur by both Ca^{2+}- and PKC-dependent pathways, with maximum induction requiring both.[72] Antisense oligonucleotides to *c-fos* were found to block A II-induced stimulation of protein synthesis in VSMC.[74]

Angiotensin II has been shown to stimulate the expression of other proto-oncogenes in VSMC as well, including *c-jun* and *c-myc*.[10,61,67] Transfection of VSMC with an expression vector containing a triple tandem repeat of SV40-TRE linked to a reporter gene demonstrated that A II is capable of enhancing the expression of genes that contain an AP-1 binding sequence via a PKC-dependent pathway.[55] Angiotensin II can also stimulate transcription of genes that do not contain an AP-1 binding site, such as the gene for PDGF-A chain.

Endothelial Cells

Recent studies have shown that endothelial cells possess all of the components of a local RAS and thus may be an important source of A II as a paracrine growth factor for VSMC, fibroblasts, or cardiomyocytes.[75] In addition, A II has been shown to induce the synthesis and release of endothelin from cultured bovine endothelial cells.[18] Endothelin itself is a potent growth factor and thus may serve to amplify the trophic effects of A II on vessels and the myocardium. Elevated circulating levels of A II have also been linked to structural abnormalities of coronary endothelial cells, leading to alterations in vascular permeability.[76]

Cardiac Fibroblasts

Contrary to an earlier report that neonatal rat cardiac fibroblasts do not possess receptors for A II,[14] we have found that these cells do, in fact, have a G-protein-linked AT_1 receptor that couples to growth. A 48 hour exposure to a protease-resistant analog of A II, [Sar^1]A II (1 μM) resulted in an increase in cardiac fibroblast protein of 29.4 ± 1.9%, total DNA of 13.7 ± 5.4%, and protein/DNA ratio of 12.5 ± 4.5% (SEM; N = 3). Cell number was increased by 32.1 ± 9.0% (N = 3). The AT_1 receptor antagonist Losartan (10 μM) inhibited the A II-stimulated increases in protein and DNA by 26% and 25%, respectively, whereas the PKC inhibitor, staurosporine (0.1 nM), and downregulation of PKC activity completely blocked the responses. Radioligand competition binding studies showed that cardiac fibroblasts have a single class of high-affinity (IC_{50} = 1.14 ± 0.2 nM) binding sites (B_{max} 784 ± 133 fmol/mg protein) that are 92% Losartan sensitive. Dissociation of the labeled agonist was increased by nonhydrolyzable analogs of GTP, indicating that the receptors couple to a G-protein. The receptors also couple to increases in intracellular Ca^{2+}, the inhibition of which prevented the growth effects of A II. These results suggest that the growth effects of A II on cardiac fibroblasts may be linked to PKC activation and Ca^{2+} mobilization and, in part, were mediated through a non-AT_1 receptor. Others have subsequently reported studies on cardiac fibroblasts, which in general support these findings.[77] Such in vitro studies showing that A II has a direct growth effect on cardiac fibroblasts are significant in light of a recent in vivo study demonstrating that A II, as well as aldosterone, may play a more important role than hemodynamic changes in the remodeling of the right and left ventricles in some forms of hypertension.[78] Moreover, we have recently reported that both cultured rat cardiac fibroblasts and myocytes possess all the components of a local RAS and show high intracellular levels of A II, supporting the concept that the intracardiac generation of A II may have paracrine or autocrine growth effects on these cells.[23,24] Given the existence of a nuclear A II receptor or a direct effect of A II on gene transcription,[79] A II may have intracrine effects on growth as well.

Transmembrane Signaling by Angiotensins

All of the known physiological actions of A II are mediated through the AT_1 class of A II receptors, which are reported to be linked via G-proteins to PLC, L-type Ca^{2+} channels, or adenylyl cyclase (Figure 1; see color plate, p. A8). Circumstantial evidence suggests that the AT_1 class of receptors represents a heterogenous group that couple to different signal transduction pathways. Coupling to Ca^{2+} channels is thought to be responsible for the chronotropic and inotropic actions of A II on cardiomyocytes. Activation of PLC, with hydrolysis of inositol phospholipids and the generation of IP_3 and DG, is important for the vasopressor actions of A II on VSMC and for A II-induced growth and gene expression. Through AT_1 receptors, A II may also indirectly activate other signaling transduction pathways, such as tyrosine kinases and prostaglandins.[11,12,80,81]

Inositol Phosphates

Angiotensin II has been shown to stimulate PLC activity in neonatal rat and chick cardiomyocytes, resulting in the hydrolysis of phosphatidylinositol 4,5-bisphosphate and a sustained increase in levels of inositol 4 (or 1)-monophosphate and inositol 1,4-bisphosphate.[16,41,82,83] In neonatal rat cardiomyocytes, phosphoinositide hydrolysis was not an indirect consequence of A II-induced increases in inward Ca^{2+} current, I_{Ca}, since increased inositol phosphate production occurred in the presence of a Ca^{2+} channel blocker.[41] At present, the physiological role that such water soluble inositol phosphates play in cardiac function is unknown, although conceivably they may function as second messengers.[84-86] The A II stimulation of PLC also resulted in a transient increase in IP_3,[16,82] which in skinned or permeabilized cardiac cells, was shown to release Ca^{2+} from the sarcoplasmic reticulum.[87,88] Angiotensin II was reported to induce a short-lived increase in the intracellular Ca^{2+} of neonatal rat cardiomyocytes, principally by releasing Ca^{2+} from the sarcoplasmic reticulum by an extracellular Ca^{2+}-independent mechanism (ostensibly via IP_3 formation).[43] It is unlikely, however, that IP_3-induced Ca^{2+} release makes any significant contribution to the positive inotropic actions of A II based on the following observations: (1) in chick cardiomyocytes, A II-induced increases in cytosolic Ca^{2+} were dependent on external Ca^{2+}, they occurred before the stimulated peak in IP_3, and unlike A II activation of PLC, could not be blocked by pertussis toxin;[16] and, (2) the guinea pig heart contains an A II receptor that couples to inositol phosphate production but not to an inotropic response.[35]

In rat VSMC, internalization of the A II-receptor complex results in a shift, of undefined importance, in the substrate for PLC hydrolysis from phosphatidylinositol 4,5 bisphosphate and phosphatidylinositol 4-phosphate to phosphatidylinositol and, possibly, phosphatidylcholine.[57,58] Protein kinase C activation has been reported to prevent hydrolysis of the former two phosphoinositides, but not phosphatidylinositol.[57,58] As mentioned, A II-induced IP_3 generation in VSMC is responsible for initiating contraction by releasing Ca^{2+} from the sarcoplasmic reticulum.

Protein Kinase C

The activation of PLC by A II would be expected to generate DG, the endogenous activator of PKC, and in fact, a brief exposure to A II was observed to increase the activity of membrane-associated PKC in neonatal rat cardiomyocytes (K. Baker, unpublished data). In addition, others have shown that A II and the PKC activator, TPA, phosphorylate the same set of proteins in these cells.[42] Activation of PKC is likely responsible for the growth effects of A II on cardiomyocytes since phorbol esters that activate PKC have been shown to induce hypertrophy of neonatal rat cardiomyocytes and to increase the nuclear activities of PKC, RNA polymerase I, and the transcriptional rate of ribosomal DNA.[89] Angiotensin II-induced PKC activity might result in enhanced gene expression by several mechanisms, including the following: (1) activation of transcription factors; (2) phosphorylation of nuclear lamins, an event associated with A II activation of PKC in cultured VSMC;[90] and (3) activation of the plasma membrane Na^+/H^+ exchanger.[91] The latter event, resulting in an increase in intracellular pH, was reported to be an early signal regulating the growth of fibroblasts,[92] but was shown not to be important for A II-stimulated protein synthesis[20] or *c-fos* expression[72] in cultured rat aortic VSMC.

Protein kinase C may also be an important inhibitory regulator of A II-induced activation of PLC in VSMC[56] and cardiomyocytes.[82] Short-term treatment of cultured neonatal rat ventricular cardiomyocytes with TPA resulted in a loss of PLC activation by A II and other Ca^{2+} mobilizing agonists, a heterologous pattern of receptor desensitization.[82] Under the same conditions, the AlF_4-stimulated response, acting presumably through G-protein activation, was not affected, suggesting that TPA inhibition occurred upstream from G-proteins or PLC, possibly at the level of the receptor. Several serine and threonine residues that are potential targets for PKC phosphorylation exist in the cytoplasmic domains of the AT_{1A} receptor, recently cloned from rat aortic VSMC.[93] In contrast, homologous desensitization of the A II receptor in this preparation was shown not to involve PKC, although it too appeared to occur at the level of the receptor and did not involve a loss of surface binding sites.[82] In chick cardiomyocytes[15] and rat VSMC,[58] internalization of the A II receptor complex was documented and may explain in part homologous desensitization in these cells.[94] Internalization of the A II-receptor complex was not a consequence of PKC activation in VSMC.[58] In these cells, internalization of the A II-receptor complex was shown to be responsible for the sustained phase of DG accumulation and thus may be important in mediating the long-term effects of A II on growth and gene expression. Although evidence is scant, receptor internalization may be involved in delivering A II to the nucleus or perinuclear region of the cell, where it could activate a nuclear pool of PKC and/or directly activate gene transcription.[79] In support of this idea, radiolabeled A II that was perfused into rat hearts was shown to localize to the perinuclear region of cardiac and vascular myocytes.[95]

Angiotensin II was reported to produce a dose-dependent delay in relaxation in rat ventricular cardiomyocytes[39,40] and human atrial trabeculae.[96] In human and hamster cardiac muscles, a dose-dependent decrease in resting tension accompanied the increase in developed tension in response to A II.[96] These observations remain unexplained but may represent a contribution of the DG/PKC pathway to the inotropic actions of A II. Protein kinase C activation may mediate all of the observed actions of A II on contractility of rat neonatal cardiomyocytes: a chronotropic action through activation of Ca^{2+} and Na^+ channels, followed by a negative inotropic action through putative inactivation of Ca^{2+} channels, reduced Ca^{2+} release from the sarcoplasmic reticulum, or decreased sensitivity of myofilaments toward Ca^{2+}.[41] Endothelin, another vasoactive peptide, was shown to exert a positive inotropic effect in rat ventricular myocytes in part by stimulating sarcolemmal Na^+/H^+ exchange by a PKC-dependent pathway, which resulted in intracellular alkalinization and sensitization of cardiac myofilaments to Ca^{2+}.[97] Angiotensin II has been shown to stimulate Na^+/H^+ exchange in VSMC, raising intracellular pH, by both PKC-dependent and -independent mechanisms.[4,9,17] The effect of A II on the Na^+/H^+ exchange of cardiomyocytes, however, has not been reported.

Tyrosine Kinase

Numerous studies have implicated tyrosine kinase activity in the control of cell proliferation, including the observation that the receptors for several growth factors, e.g., EGF and PDGF, exhibit ligand-activated tyrosine kinase activity.[92,98] Although the AT_1 receptor itself does not have tyrosine kinase activity, a study on WB rat liver epithelial cells showed that the A II-induced mobilization of Ca^{2+} stimulated a rapid and transient increase in the phosphotyrosine content of a subset of EGF-sensitive proteins.[80] In glomerular mesangial cells, A II was also demonstrated to enhance the tyrosine phosphorylation of a subset of EGF-targeted protein but in this case by PKC-dependent and -independent (perhaps involving phospholipase A_2) mechanisms.[81] Whether such A II-induced tyrosine kinase activity plays any role in its mitogenic effect on cardiac fibroblasts or VSMC has not been explored.

Calcium Channels

The positive inotropic action of A II on ventricular and atrial tissue results from an augmentation of I_{Ca} through L-type Ca^{2+} channels.[12,36,99] In rabbit atria that were partially depolarized so as to inactivate voltage-sensitive Na^+ channels, the A II-induced contractile response was preceded by a slow-rising action potential.[36] Both the contractile response and slow action potential were blocked by inhibitors of L-type Ca^{2+} channels but not by a Na^+ channel blocker. Comparable studies have been reported for the rabbit papillary muscle, bovine Purkinje muscle, and chick ventricle.[36,99–101] Although the basis for how A II increases I_{Ca} has not been established, it is likely that A II increases the number of functional Ca^{2+} channels in the sarcolemma and/or the probability of a channel being open, as has been shown for β-adrenergic agonists.[102] The molecular mechanism that couples the A II receptor to the L-type Ca^{2+} channel is also unknown, although two lines of circumstantial evidence suggest that the mechanism is distinct from that for activation of PLC as follows: (1) in chick cardiomyocytes, A II was shown to couple to PLC via a pertussis toxin-inhibitable G-protein, whereas A II-induced increases in cytosolic Ca^{2+}, which were dependent on external Ca^{2+}, did not involve this G-protein;[16] and (2), the high-affinity A II binding site of the guinea pig heart couples to inositol phosphate production but not to an inotropic response.[35] It is also possible that cardiomyocytes possess two (or more) subtypes of the AT_1 receptor, one subtype coupling to inositol phosphate production and another to activation of L-type Ca^{2+} channels. It should be noted that no direct evidence showing that the A II receptor couples to the L-type Ca^{2+} channel via a G-protein has been reported.

Cyclic AMP

In some tissues (liver, kidney, and adrenal), A II receptors that are Losartan sensitive and thus classified as AT_1 inhibit adenylyl cyclase activity.[6,11] Studies on the A II receptor of the liver indicate that there may be subtypes of the AT_1 receptor that either activate PLC or inhibit adenylyl cyclase or that the coupling of a single AT_1 receptor subtype to a signal transduction pathway is determined by the availability of a particular G-protein.[6,103] In rat fetal skin fibroblasts, A II was reported to stimulate cyclic AMP production through an AT_1 receptor.[104] Whether A II has any effect on adenylyl cyclase of cardiac fibroblasts has not been examined. Angiotensin II has no direct effect on adenylyl cyclase of VSMC, although it has been suggested that A II may indirectly activate adenylyl cyclase (and guanylate cyclase) through prostaglandin formation.[6,12] The situation regarding cardiomyocytes is as yet unsettled. The A II enhancement of contractile force by heart muscle is not accompanied by a shortening of time to peak tension, arguing against an A II-induced increase in cyclic AMP.[96,105] Recently, the A II receptors of rat and rabbit sarcolemma were reported to inhibit adenylyl cyclase through the guanine nucleotide binding protein, G_i, suggesting that the inotropic actions of A II may be partly mediated by opposing cyclic AMP-stimulated Ca^{2+} uptake by the sarcoplasmic reticulum.[106] Some form of coupling between the cardiac A II receptor and adenylyl cyclase is supported by the observations that A II inhibited isoprenaline-stimulated cyclic AMP accumulation in nonhypertrophic ventricular myocytes of Dahl S rats and enhanced the effect of isoprenaline on hypertrophic myocytes of Dahl R rats.[107] Other studies, however, have failed to demonstrate any coupling, negative or positive, of the A II receptors of neonatal rat myocytes[41] or rabbit ventricular myocardium[108] to adenylyl cyclase.

Prostaglandins

The vasconstrictor effect of A II on the coronary circulation is much less marked than observed in the peripheral vasculature, possibly because the A II-induced synthesis of vasodilator prostaglandins, most likely by VSMC, counteracts its pressor action[5,96,109] (and references therein). Besides a direct autocrine effect in inducing VSMC relaxation, prostaglandins have inhibitory effects on the sympathetic nervous system as well.[5] Angiotensin II may activate phospholipase A_2, thereby releasing arachidonic acid from membrane phospholipids and producing prostaglandins, either through an elevation in intracellular Ca^{2+} or through activation of PKC.[60,110]

Future Perspectives

Research over the last two decades has established that A II exerts multiple functional and/or trophic effects on every major cell type in the heart and cardiovascular system via the AT_1 class of G-protein linked membrane receptors that are coupled to several second-messenger pathways. Recent advances in recombinant DNA techniques offer the immediate prospects of identifying multiple subtypes of the AT_1 receptor and will help define how these receptors function at the molecular level. This knowledge may lead to the development of more selective and potent receptor antagonists. In the next few years, we should gain a better understanding of what role the AT_2 receptor plays, especially in fetal development, what its intracellular signals are, and how the signaling pathways of the AT_1 and AT_2 receptors may interact. The next few years should also see the cloning and characterization of other angiotensin-related receptors, such as the recently identified receptor for [des-Asp^1-des-Arg^2]A II.[111] From the standpoint of understanding the role of A II in normal and pathological cardiac development, the most difficult, but surely most rewarding, challenge of the immediate future will be defining in detail the intracellular events whereby A II affects gene transcription and cell growth and how these events are functionally integrated with those of other growth factors.

Acknowledgements

The authors appreciate the privilege of discussing various aspects of the manuscript with Drs. H. A. Singer, T. J. Thekkumkara, K. C. Chang, and W. Schorb. The authors thank Dr. Schorb and Ms. K. Conrad for their invaluable assistance in carrying out and interpreting some of the fibroblast studies and M. B. Shoop for producing Figure 1. This research was supported in part by grants from the National Institutes of Health (K.M.B., HL44883, and HL44379), the American Heart Association (K.M.B., 900607), the Pennsylvania Affiliate of the American Heart Association (KMB and DED), the Geisinger Clinic (KMB, DED, GWB) and the Mars Foundation (KMB).

Summary

Angiotensin II has multiple direct and indirect actions on the heart, which affect contractility, metabolism, vasoconstriction of blood *vessels, extracellular matrix remodeling, and cell growth. Angiotensin II has direct inotropic and chronotropic effects on cardiomyocytes, is a potent vasopressor via an action on vascular smooth muscle, and induces synthesis and release of endothelin from endothelial cells and production of vasodilator prostaglandins from smooth muscle. Recent studies have demonstrated that A II is a growth factor for cardiac cells as well. The peptide has been implicated in the left-ventricular hypertrophy associated with hypertension and induces hypertrophy of cultured cardiomyocytes. Angiotensin II also has hypertrophic or proliferative growth effects on vascular smooth muscle, which underlie the adaptive changes in the vasculature produced by hypertension. Recently, A II was shown to have a proliferative effect on cultured cardiac fibroblasts, supporting the hypothesis that these cells participate in the A II-induced remodeling of the cardiac interstitium associated with a variety of physiological and pathophysiological conditions. The direct actions of A II are mediated by specific cell surface receptors that are linked via G-proteins to phospholipase C, L-type Ca^{2+} channels, or adenylyl cyclase. Activation of phospholipase C leads to formation of inositol 1,4,5-triphosphate, which can release Ca^{2+} from intracellular stores, and diacylglycerol, which activates protein kinase C. Angiotensin II may also activate indirectly other signaling transduction pathways, such as tyrosine kinases, which may play a role in the control of cell proliferation, and prostaglandins. Although protein kinase C and/or Ca^{2+} have been implicated in A II-induced gene transcription and cell growth, the exact intracellular pathways involved await future identification.*

References

1. Baker KM, Booz GW, Dostal DE. Cardiac actions of angiotensin II: role of an intracardiac renin-angiotensin system. Annu Rev Physiol 1992; 54:227–241.
2. Morgan HE, Baker KM. Cardiac hypertrophy: mechanical, neural, and endocrine dependence. Circulation 1991; 83:13–25.
3. Baker KM. Cardiac actions of angiotensin. J Vasc Med Biol 1991; 3: 30–37.
4. Schelling P, Fischer H, Ganten D. Angiotensin and cell growth: a link to cardiovascular hypertrophy? J Hypertens 1991; 9:3–15.
5. Lindpainter K, Ganten D. The cardiac renin-angiotensin system: an appraisal of experimental and clinical evidence. Circ Res 1991; 68: 905–921.
6. Peach MJ, Dostal DE. The angiotensin II receptor and the actions of angiotensin II, J Cardiovasc Pharmacol 1990; 16(suppl 4):S25–S30.
7. Wright GB, Alexander RW, Gimbrone MA. Cardiovascular angioten-

sin receptors. In: Haft JI and Karliner JS, eds. *Receptor Science in Cardiology.* Mt. Kisco, New York: Futura Publishing Co., 1984, pp. 163–203.

8. Heagerty AM. Angiotensin II: vasoconstrictor or growth factor? J Cardiovasc Pharmacol 1991; 18(suppl 2):S14–S19.

9. Lyall F, Morton JJ, Lever AF, Cragoe EJ. Angiotensin II activates Na^+-H^+ exchange and stimulates growth in cultured vascular smooth muscle cells. J Hypertens 1988; 6(suppl 4):S438–S441.

10. Pratt RE, Itoh H, Gibbons GH, Dzau VJ. Role of angiotensin in the control of vascular smooth muscle growth. J Vasc Med Biol 1991; 3: 25–29.

11. Smith RD, Chiu AT, Wong PC, Herblin WF, Timmermans PBMWM. Pharmacology of nonpeptide angiotensin II receptor antagonists. Annu Rev Pharmacol Toxicol 1992; 32:135–165.

12. Peach MJ. Molecular actions of angiotensin. Biochem Pharmacol 1981; 30:2745–2751.

13. Urata H, Healy B, Stewart RW, Bumpus FM, Hussain A. Angiotensin II receptors in normal and failing human hearts. J Clin Endocrinol Metab 1989; 69:54–66.

14. Rogers TB, Gaa ST, Allen IS. Identification and characterization of functional angiotensin II receptors on cultured heart myocytes. J Pharmacol Exp Ther 1986; 236:438–444.

15. Aceto JF, Baker KM. [Sar¹]angiotensin II receptor-mediated stimulation of protein synthesis in chick heart cells. Am J Physiol 1990; 258: H806–H813.

16. Baker KM, Singer HA, Aceto JF. Angiotensin II receptor mediated stimulation of cytosolic free calcium and inositol phosphates in chick myocytes. J Pharmacol Exp Ther 1989; 251:578–585.

17. Griendling KK, Tsuda T, Berk BC, Alexander RW. Angiotensin II stimulation of vascular smooth muscle cells: secondary signalling mechanisms. Am J Hypertens 1989; 2:659–665.

18. Emori T, Harita Y, Ohta K, Shichiri M, Marumo F. Secretory mechanism of immunoreactive endothelin in cultured bovine endothelial cells. Biochem Biophys Res Commun 1989; 160:93–100.

19. Baker KM, Aceto JF. Angiotensin II stimulation of protein synthesis and cell growth in chick heart cells. Am J Physiol 1990; 259: H610–H618.

20. Berk BC, Vekshtein V, Gordon HM, Tsuda T. Angiotensin II-stimulated protein synthesis in cultured vascular smooth muscle cells. Hypertension 1989; 13:305–314.

21. Stouffer GA, Owens GK. Angiotensin II-induced mitogenesis of spontaneously hypertensive rat-derived cultured smooth muscle cells is dependent on autocrine production of transforming growth factor-β. Circ Res 1992; 70:820–828.

22. Geisterfer AAT, Peach MJ, Owens GK. Angiotensin II induces hypertrophy, not hyperplasia, of cultured rat aortic smooth muscle cells. Circ Res 1988; 62:749–756.

23. Dostal DE, Rothblum KC, Chernin MI, Cooper GR, Baker KM. Intracardiac detection of angiotensinogen and renin: evidence for a localized renin-angiotensin system in neonatal rat. Am J Physiol 1992; C838–C850.

24. Dostal DE, Rothblum KC, Conrad KM, Cooper GR, Baker KM. Detec-

tion of angiotensin I and II in cultured rat cardiac myocytes and fibro-blasts: evidence for local production. Am J Physiol 1992; C851–C863.

25. Cherin MI, Candia AF, Stark LL, Aceto JF, Baker KM. Fetal expression of renin, angiotensinogen, and atriopeptin genes in chick heart. Clin Exp Hypertens 1990; A12:617–629.

26. Starke K. Regulation of noradrenaline release by presynaptic receptor systems. Rev Physiol Biochem Pharmacol 1977; 77:1–124.

27. Zimmerman BG. Adrenergic facilitation by angiotensin: does it serve a physiological function? Clin Sci 1981; 60:343–348.

28. Costa M, Majewski H. Facilitation of noradrenaline release from sympathetic nerves through activation of ACTH receptors, β-adrenoceptors and angiotensin II receptors. Br J Pharmacol 1988; 95:993–1001.

29. Musgrave IF, Majewski H. Effect of phorbol ester and pertussis toxin on the enhancement of noradrenaline release by angiotensin II in mouse atria. Br J Pharmacol 1989; 96:609–616.

30. Hirakata H, Fouad-Tarazi FM, Bumpus FM, et al. Angiotensins and the failing heart. Enhanced positive inotropic response to angiotensin I in cardiomyopathic hamster heart in the presence of captopril. Circ Res 1990; 66:891–899.

31. Baker KM, Campanile CP, Trachte GJ, Peach MJ. Identification and characterization of the rabbit angiotensin II myocardial receptor. Circ Res 1984; 54:286–293.

32. Baker KM, Khosla MC. Cardiac and vascular actions of decapeptide angiotensin analogs. J Pharmacol Exp Ther 1986; 239:790–796.

33. Meulemans AL, Andries LJ, Brutsaert DL. Does endocardial endothelium mediate positive inotropic response to angiotensin I and angiotensin II? Circ Res 1990; 66:1591–1601.

34. Urata H, Kinoshita A, Misono KS, Bumpus FM, Husain A. Identification of a highly specific chymase as a major angiotensin II-forming enzyme in the failing heart. J Biol Chem 1990; 265:22348–22357.

35. Baker KM, Singer HA. Identification and characterization of guinea pig angiotensin II ventricular and atrial receptors: coupling to inositol phosphate production. Circ Res 1988; 62:896–904.

36. Freer RJ, Pappano AJ, Peach MJ, et al. Mechanism for the positive inotropic effect of angiotensin II on isolated cardiac muscle. Circ Res 1976; 39:178–183.

37. Doggrell SA. The effects of atriopeptin and angiotensin on the rat right ventricle. Gen Pharmacol 1989; 20:253–257.

38. Sen I, Rajasekaran AK. Angiotensin II-binding protein in adult and neonatal rat heart. J Mol Cell Cardiol 1991; 23:563–572.

39. Neyses L, Vetter H. Action of atrial natriuretic peptide and angiotensin II on the myocardium: studies in isolated rat ventricular cardiomyocytes. Biochem Biophys Res Commun 1989; 163:1435–1443.

40. Neyses L, Vetter H. Isolated myocardial cells: a new tool for the investigation of hypertensive heart disease. J Hypertens 1990; 8(suppl 4): S99–S102.

41. Allen IS, Cohen NM, Dhallan RS, Gaa ST, Lederer WJ, Rogers TB. Angiotensin II increases spontaneous contractile frequency and stimulates calcium current in cultured neonatal rat heart myocytes: insights into the underlying biochemical mechanisms. Circ Res 1988; 62: 524–534.

42. Dösemeci A, Dhallan RS, Cohen NM, Lederer WJ, Rogers TB. Phorbol

ester increases calcium current and stimulates the effects of angiotensin II on cultured neonatal rat heart myocytes. Circ Res 1988; 62: 347–357.

43. Kem DC, Johnson EIM, Capponi AM, et al. Effect of angiotensin II on cytosolic free calcium in neonatal rat cardiomyocytes. Am J Physiol 1991; 261:C77–C85.

44. Knape JTA, van Zwieten PA. Positive chronotropic activity of angiotensin II in the pithed normotensive rat is primarily due to activation of cardiac β_1-adrenoreceptors. Naunyn-Schmiedeberg's Arch Pharmacol 1988; 338:185–190.

45. Kobayashi M, Furukawa Y, Chiba S. Positive chronotropic and inotropic effects of angiotensin II in the dog heart. Eur J Pharmacol 1978; 50:17–25.

46. Moorman JR, Kirch GE, Lacerda AE, Brown AM. Angiotensin II modulates cardiac Na^+ channels in neonatal rat. Circ Res 1989; 65: 1804–1809.

47. Dostal DE, Baker KM. Angiotensin II stimulation of left ventricular hypertrophy in adult rat heart: mediation by the AT_1 receptor. Am J Hypertens 1992; 5:276–280.

48. Dostal DE, Baker KM, Peach MJ. Growth promoting effects of angiotensin II in the cardiovascular system. In: Maggi M and Greenen V eds. Horizons in Endocrinology, Vol II, New York: Raven Press, 1991, 265–272.

49. Baker KM, Chernin MI, Wixson SK, Aceto JF. Renin-angiotensin system involvement in pressure-overload cardiac hypertrophy in rats. Am J Physiol 1990; 259:H324–H332.

50. Peeler TC, Baker KM, Esmurdoc CF, Chernin MI. Angiotensin converting enzyme inhibition in Dahl salt-sensitive rats. Cell Mol Biochem 1991; 104:45–50.

51. Beinlich CJ, White GJ, Baker KM, Morgan HE. Angiotensin II and left ventricular growth in newborn pig heart. J Mol Cell Cardiol 1991; 23:1031–1038.

52. Beinlich CJ, Baker KM, White GJ, Morgan HE. Control of growth in the neonatal pig heart. Am J Physiol 1991; 261:3–7.

53. Chein KR, Knowlton KU, Zhu H, Chein S. Regulation of cardiac gene expression during myocardial growth and hypertrophy: molecular studies of an adaptive physiological response. FASEB J 1991; 5: 3037–3046.

54. Izumo S, Nadal-Ginard B, Mahdavi V. Proto-oncogene induction and reprogramming of cardiac gene expression produced by pressure overload. Proc Natl Acad Sci USA 1988; 85:339–343.

55. Takeuchi K, Nakamura N, Cook NS, Pratt RE, Dzau VJ. Angiotensin II can regulate gene expression by the AP-1 binding sequence via a protein kinase C-dependent pathway. Biochem Biophys Res Commun 1990; 15:1189–1194.

56. Brock TA, Rittenhouse SE, Powers CW, Ekstein LS, Gimbrone MA, Alexander RW. Phorbol ester and 1-oleoyl-2-acetylglycerol inhibit angiotensin activation of phospholipase C in cultured vascular smooth muscle cells. J Biol Chem 1985; 260:14158–14162.

57. Griendling KK, Rittenhouse SE, Brock TA, Ekstein LS, Gimbrone MA, Alexander RW. Sustained diacylglycerol formation from inositol phos-

pholipids in angiotensin II-stimulated vascular smooth muscle cells. J Biol Chem 1986; 261:5901–5906.

58. Griendling KK, Delafontaine P, Rittenhouse SE, Gimbrone MA, Alexander RW. Correlation of receptor sequestration with sustained diacylglycerol accumulation in angiotensin II-stimulated cultured vascular smooth muscle cells. J Biol Chem 1987; 262:14555–14562.

59. Rasmussen H, Barrett PQ. Calcium messenger system: an integrated view. Physiol Rev. 1984; 64:938–984.

60. Huwiler A, Fabbro D, Pfeilschifter J. Possible regulatory functions of protein kinase C-α and -ε isoenzymes in rat renal mesangial cells. Stimulation of prostaglandin synthesis and feedback inhibition of angiotensin II-stimulated phosphoinositide hydrolysis. Biochem J 1991; 279:441–445.

61. Paquet J-L, Baudouin-Legros M, Brunelle G, Meyer P. Angiotensin II-induced proliferation of aortic myocytes in spontaneously hypertensive rats. J Hypertens 1990; 8:565–572.

62. Scott-Burden T, Hahn AWA, Resink TJ, Bühler FR. Modulation of extracellular matrix by angiotensin II: stimulated glycoconjugate synthesis and growth in vascular smooth muscle cells. J Cardiovasc Pharmacol 1990; 16(suppl 4):S36–S41.

63. Campbell-Boswell M, Robertson AL. Effects of angiotensin II and vasopressin on human smooth muscle cells in vitro. Exp Mol Pathol 1981; 35:265–276.

64. Owens GK, Schwartz SM, McCanna M. Evaluation of medial hypertrophy in resistance vessels of spontaneously hypertensive rats. Hypertension 1988; 11:198–207.

65. Kato H, Suzuki H, Tajima S, et al. Angiotensin II stimulates collagen synthesis in cultured vascular smooth muscle cells. J Hypertens 199; 9:17–22.

66. Hahn AWA, Resink TJ, Bernhardt J, Ferracin F, Bühler FR. Stimulation of autocrine platelet-derived growth factor AA-homodimer and transforming growth factor β in vascular smooth muscle cells. Biochem Biophys Res Commun 1991; 178:1451–1458.

67. Naftilan AJ, Pratt RE, Dzau VJ. Induction of platelet-derived growth factor A-chain and c-myc gene expressions by angiotensin II in cultured rat vascular smooth muscle cells. J Clin Invest 1989; 83: 1419–1424.

68. Gibbons GH, Pratt RE, Dzau VJ. Transforming growth factor: beta expression modulates the bifunction of growth response of vascular smooth muscle cells to angiotensin II [abstract]. Clin Res 1990; 38: 287a.

69. Hahn AW, Resink TJ, Scott-Burden T, Powell J, Dohi Y, Bühler FR. Stimulation of endothelin mRNA and secretion in rat vascular smooth muscle cells: a novel autocrine function. Cell Regul 1990; 1:649–659.

70. Itoh H, Pratt RE, Dzau VJ. Antisense oligonucleotides complementary to PDGF mRNA attenuate angiotensin II-induced vascular hypertrophy [abstract]. Hypertension 1990; 16:325.

71. Scott-Burden T, Resink TJ, Baur U, Bürgin M, Bühler FR. Amiloride sensitive activation of S_6 kinase by angiotensin II in cultured vascular smooth muscle cells. Biochem Biophys Res Commun 1988; 151: 583–589.

72. Taubman MB, Berk BC, Izumo S, Tsauda T, Alexander RW, Nadal-Ginard B. Angiotensin II induces *c-fos* mRNA in aortic smooth muscle. Role of Ca^{2+} mobilization and protein kinase C activation. J Biol Chem 1989; 264:526–530.

73. Naftilan AJ, Pratt RE, Eldridge CS, Lin HL, Dzau VJ. Angiotensin II induces *c-fos* expression in smooth muscle via transcriptional control. Hypertension 1989; 13:706–711.

74. Rainer RS, Eldridge CS, Gilliland GK, Naftilan AJ. Antisense oligonucleotide to *c-fos* blocks the angiotensin II-induced stimulation of protein synthesis in rat aortic smooth muscle cells [abstract]. Hypertension 1990; 16:326.

75. Tang S-S, Stevenson L, Dzau VJ. Endothelial renin-angiotensin pathway; adrenergic regulation of angiotensin secretion. Circ Res 1990; 66:103–108.

76. Weber KT, Brilla CG. Pathological hypertrophy and cardiac interstitium: fibrosis and renin-angiotensin-aldosterone system. Circulation 1991; 83:1849–1865.

77. Zhou G, Brilla CG, Weber KT. Angiotensin II-mediated stimulation of collagen synthesis in cultured cardiac fibroblasts [abstract]. FASEB J 1992; 6:A1914.

78. Brilla CG, Pick R, Tan LB, Janicki JS, Weber KT. Remodeling of the rat right and left ventricles in experimental hypertension. Circ Res 1990; 67:1355–1364.

79. Booz GW, Conrad KM, Hess AL, Singer HA, Baker KM. Angiotensin II binding sites on hepatocyte nuclei. Endocrinology 1992; 130: 3639–3641.

80. Huckle WR, Prokop CA, Dy RC, Herman B, Earp S. Angiotensin II stimulates protein-tyrosine phosphorylation in a calcium-dependent manner. Mol Cell Biol 1990; 10:6290–6298.

81. Force T, Kyriakis JM, Avruch J, Bonventre JV. Endothelin, vasopressin, and angiotensin II enhance tyrosine phosphorylation by protein kinase C-dependent and -independent pathways in glomerular mesangial cells. J Biol Chem 1991; 266:6650–6656.

82. Abdellatif MM, Neubauer CF, Lederer WJ, Rogers TB. Angiotensin-induced desensitization of the phosphoinositide pathway in cardiac cells occurs at the level of the receptor. Circ Res 1991; 69:800–809.

83. Baker KM, Aceto JF. Characterization of avian angiotensin II cardic receptors: coupling to mechanical activity and phosphoinositide metabolism. J Mol Cell Cardiol 1989; 21:375–382.

84. Sylvia V, Curtin G, Norman J, Stec J, Busbee D. Activation of a low specific activity form of DNA polymerase α by inositol-1,4-bisphosphate. Cell 1988; 54:651–658.

85. Tsai M-H, Yu C-L, Wei F-S, Stacey DW. The effect of GTPase activating protein upon Ras is inhibited by mitogenically responsive lipids. Science 1989; 243:522–526.

86. Tsai M-H, Yu C-L, Stacey DW. A cytoplasmic protein inhibits the GTPase activity of H-Ras in a phospholipid-dependent manner. Science 1990; 250:982–985.

87. Fabioto A. Inositol (1,4,5)-triphosphate-induced release of Ca^{2+} from the sarcoplasmic reticulum of skinned cardiac cells [abstract]. Biophys J 1986; 49:190a.

88. Nosek TM, Williams MF, Aeigler ST, Godt RE. Inositol triphosphate enhances calcium release in skinned cardiac and skeletal muscle. Am J Physiol 1986; 250:C807–C811.

89. Allo SN, McDermott PJ, Carl LL, Morgan HE. Phorbol ester stimulation of protein kinase C activity and ribosomal DNA transcription: role in hypertrophic growth of cultured cardiomyocytes. J Biol Chem 1991; 266:22003–22009.

90. Tsuda T, Alexander RW. Angiotensin II stimulates phosphorylation of nuclear lamins via a protein kinase C-dependent mechanism in cultured vascular smooth muscle cells. J Biol Chem 1990; 265:1165–1170.

91. Moolenaar WH. Effects of growth factors on intracellular pH regulation. Annu Rev Physiol 1986; 48:363–376.

92. Rozengurt E. Early signals in the mitogenic response. Science 1986; 234:161–166.

93. Murphy TJ, Alexander RW, Griendling KK, Runge MS, Bernstein KE. Isolation of a cDNA encoding the vascular type-1 angiotensin II receptor. Nature 1991; 351:233–236.

94. Ullian ME, Linas SL. Angiotensin II surface receptor coupling to inositol triphosphate formation in vascular smooth muscle cells. J Biol Chem 1990; 265:195–200.

95. Robertson AL, Khairallah PA. Angiotensin II: rapid localization in smooth and cardiac muscle. Science 1971; 172:1138–1139.

96. Moravec CS, Schluchter MD, Paranandi L, et al. Inotropic effects of angiotensin II on human cardiac muscle in vitro. Circulation 1990; 82: 1973–1984.

97. Krämer BK, Smith TW, Kelly RA. Endothelin and increased contractility in adult rat ventricular myocytes: role of intracellular alkalosis induced by activation of the protein kinase C-dependent Na^+-H^+ exchanger. Circ Res 1991; 68:269–279.

98. Carpenter G, Cohen S. Epidermal growth factor. J Biol Chem 1990; 265:7709–7712.

99. Kass RS, Blair ML. Effects of angiotensin II on membrane current in cardiac Purkinje fibers. J Mol Cell Cardiol 1981; 13:797–809.

100. Bonnardeaux JL, Regoli D. Action of angiotensin and analogues on the heart. Can J Physiol Pharmacol 1974; 52:50–60.

101. Rioux F, Park WF, Regoli D. Characterization of angiotensin receptors in rabbit isolated atria. Can J Physiol Pharmacol 1975; 54:229–237.

102. Sperelakis N. Regulation of calcium slow channels of cardiac muscle by cyclic nucleotides and phosphorylation. J Mol Cell Cardiol 1988; 20:75–105.

103. Bauer PH, Chiu AT, Garrison JC. DuP 753 can antagonize the effects of angiotensin II in rat liver. Mol Pharmacol 1991; 39:579–585.

104. Johnson C, Aguilera G. Changes in angiotensin II receptor subtypes and coupling to adenylate cyclase in cultured fetal fibroblasts [abstract]. FASEB J 1991; 5:A872.

105. Dempsey PJ, McCallum ZT, Kent KM, Cooper T. Direct myocardial effects of angiotensin II. Am J Physiol 1971; 220:477–481.

106. Anand-Srivastava MB. Angiotensin II receptors negatively coupled to adenylate cyclase in rat myocardial sarcolemma: involvement of inhibitory guanine nucleotide regulatory protein. Biochem Pharmacol 1989; 38:489–496.

107. Sunga PS, Rabkin SW. Reversal of angiotensin II effects on the cyclic adenosine 3,',5' monophosphate response to isoprenaline in cardiac hypertrophy. Cardiovasc Res 1991; 25:965–968.

108. Wright GB, Alexander RW, Ekstein LS, Gimbrone MA Jr. Characterization of the rabbit ventricular myocardial receptor for angiotensin II: evidence for two sites of different affinities and specificities. Mol Pharmacol 1983; 24:213–221.

109. Gunther S, Cannon PJ. Modulation of angiotensin II coronary vasoconstriction by cardiac prostaglandin synthesis. Am J Physiol 1980; 238: H895–H901.

110. Farago A, Nishizuka Y. Protein kinase C in transmembrane signalling. FEBS Lett 1990; 268:350–354.

111. Hanesworth J, Harding J. Investigation of the AIV receptor in rabbit heart membranes [abstract]. FASEB J 1992; 6:A1577.

7

Characterization and Localization of Angiotensin Receptors in Central and Autonomic Nervous Systems Regulating Heart Function

Juan M. Saavedra, Mohan Viswanathan, and Kazuto Shigematsu

The role of A II in cardiovascular control and in the pathogenesis and maintenance of experimental and genetic hypertension is well established.[1] The effects of A II on cardiac function are complex and are probably exerted on different anatomical and physiological levels. For example, A II can influence the heart rate via multiple mechanisms[2] such as the release of catecholamines from the adrenal medulla[3] and cardiac sympathetic nerve terminals,[4,5] the stimulation of peripheral sympathetic ganglia,[6] and a centrally mediated reduction in vagal tone.[7]

We focus here on the localization, characterization, and possible role of A II receptors in cardiac function. Our presentation advances additional evidence for the concept of the presence of local A II systems,[8] which affect tissue function, in addition to the classical or "hormonal" role of circulating A II. We studied A II receptors localized in the heart conduction system, peripheral sympathetic ganglia innervating the heart, and in the nucleus of the solitary tract in the brain, which forms part of the baroreceptor reflex mechanisms. This

Lindpaintner K and Ganten D (editors): *The Cardiac-Renin Angiotensin System*, © Futura Publishing Co., Inc., Armonk, NY, 1994.

approach highlights the concept of A II as a modulator of cardiac function at multiple levels of regulation.

Angiotensin II Receptors in the Heart Conduction System

In the heart, A II exerts positive inotropic and chronotropic actions.[9-12] These effects of A II can be mediated by specific A II receptors located in the cardiomyocytes, which have been well characterized.[11,13-15] More recently, however, we have shown that, at least in the rat, specific A II receptors are selectively concentrated in the heart conduction system.[16] This finding raised the possibility that the chronotropic effects of A II could be mediated by direct actions on the specialized conduction system of the heart. This possibility was supported by Lambert et al.[17] who demonstrated that in the dog, A II has direct, positive chronotropic actions when injected into the sinus node artery.

Recently, A II receptors have been classified into two main subtypes, AT_1 and AT_2.[18-20] AT_1 receptors seem to mediate all main known effects of A II, such as vasoconstriction and elevation of blood pressure,[19] whereas the function of AT_2 receptors is currently unknown.[20] Losartan ((2-n-butyl-4-chloro-5-hydroxymethyl-1- 1-[2'-(1H-tetrazol-5-yl) biphenyl-4-yl)methyl]imidazole) is a selective inhibitor of AT_1 receptors and is currently being tested as an antihypertensive compound in humans.[21] For this reason, it was of interest to elucidate the subtype of A II receptors present in the conduction system of the rat heart.

To study A II receptors in the heart conduction system, we dissected the atrioventricular (AV) and sinoatrial (SA) nodes under a stereomicroscope.[16] The presence of the AV and SA nodes was determined in the tissue sections by staining for acetylcholinesterase activity.[22] After identification of the AV and SA nodes, the total number of A II receptors[16] and the relative concentration of the A II receptor subtypes[23] was analyzed by autoradiography as described earlier.[24] The A II agonist, $[^{125}I][Sar^1]$A II was used as the ligand. Consecutive sections were incubated with 5×10^{-10}M $[^{125}I][Sar^1]$ A II (total binding), 10^{-5}M PD 123177 (1-(4-amino-3-methylphenyl)methyl-5- diphenylacetyl-4, 5, 6, 7 -tetrahydro-1H-imidazo[4,5-c]pyridine-6-carboxylic acid-2HCl), (AT_1 receptors), 10^{-5}M Losartan (AT_2 receptors), or 5×10^{-6}M unlabeled A II (nonspecific binding).[23]

Specific A II binding was highly localized to the AV and SA

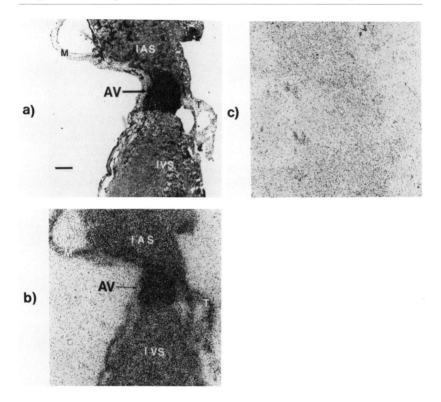

Fig. 1. Autoradiographic localization of angiotensin II (A II) binding in the conduction system of rat hearts. (a): acetylcholinesterase staining. Sections contain the atrioventricular node. (b): total A II binding. Sections adjacent to A were incubated in the presence of 3 nM ^{125}I-Sar^1-A II. (c):nonspecific binding. Sections adjacent to (a) were incubated like those in (b) with the addition of 5 μM unlabeled A II. IAS: interatrial septum; IVS: interventricular septum; M: mitral valve leaflet; T: tricuspid valve leaflet; AV: atrioventricular node (from Saito K, et al.[16]).

nodes (Figure 1). Much lower numbers of A II receptors were localized to the heart muscle and to the cardiac endothelium in both the epicardium and the endocardium (Fig.1). Incubation of consecutive heart sections containing the AV and SA node in the presence of selective displacers of the A II receptor subtypes AT$_1$ and AT$_2$ revealed that binding to all A II receptors was displaced by Losartan but not by PD 123177 (Figure 2) (Table 1).

A number of previous studies have suggested the participation of A II in the in vivo regulation of the heart rate,[2] including the release of catecholamines from the adrenal medulla [3] and cardiac

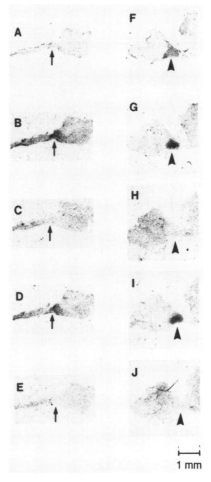

1 mm

Fig. 2. Autoradiographic characterization of A II receptor subtypes in the rat conduction system. A–E: sinoaortic node. F–J: atrioventricular node. A and F: acetylcholinesterase staining. B and G: total A II binding. Sections adjacent to A and E were incubated in the presence of 5×10^{-10}M ^{125}I-Sar^{1}A II. C and H: A II AT$_2$ receptors. Adjacent sections were incubated like those in B and G in the presence of 10^{-5}M Losartan. Note that the AT$_1$ selective antagonist totally displaces A II binding. D and I: A II AT$_1$ receptors. Adjacent sections were incubated like those in B and G in the presence of 10^{-5}M PD 123177. Note the absence of displacement of A II binding by the AT$_2$ selective compound. E and J: nonspecific binding. Adjacent sections were incubated like those in B and G in the presence of 5×10^{-6}M unlabeled A II. Note total displacement of A II binding.

Table 1
Angiotensin II Receptor Subtypes in SA Node and
AV Node of Rats

	Specific Binding	AT_1	AT_2
		fmol/mg protein	
SA node	17.3 ± 1	18.4 ± 2	ND
AV node	15.1 ± 3	15.3 ± 2	ND

Values are mean ± SEM obtained from 7 rats, measured individually. AT_1: specific binding not displaced by 10^{-5}M PD 123177; AT_2: specific binding not displaced by 10^{-5} Losartan. ND: not detectable.

sympathetic nerve terminals,[4,5] stimulation of peripheral sympathetic ganglia,[6] and a centrally mediated reduction in vagal tone.[7] In addition, A II exerts positive chronotropic actions in isolated atrial preparations,[11] and high-affinity A II receptors have been found in spontaneously beating cultured neonatal rat myocytes.[25] Thus, there is the additional possibility of a direct chronotropic effect of A II in the heart. Our results demonstrating the presence of large numbers of A II receptors selectively localized in the heart conduction system supports this hypothesis. In a previous study,[16] we reported that the SA artery irrigating the SA node contains high levels of ACE. Taken together, these data indicate the possibility of a local formation of A II that acts in a paracrine or autocrine manner in the regulation of the heart rate.[16,26]

Our results indicate that all A II receptors in the AV and SA nodes are of the AT_1 subtype. Our data contain the first indication of a possible role for AT_1 receptors, and therefore of their antagonist Losartan, on the regulation of the heart rate. Whether this finding bears clinical importance could only be decided after the current clinical trials of hypertensive patients with Losartan are completed.[21]

Angiotensin II Receptors in Peripheral Sympathetic Ganglia

One of the mechanisms by which A II regulates cardiac function is stimulation of sympathetic activity at the peripheral sympathetic ganglion level, resulting in facilitation of ganglionic transmission,[27-29] probably by direct stimulation of adrenergic ganglion cells.[30] The sympathetic ganglia, including the stellate ganglia, which provide most of the innervation to the rat heart, contain high affinity A II binding sites.[31] In the sympathetic ganglia, A II receptors were associated with the principal ganglion cells.[31] In the superior cervical ganglia, A II stimulates phosphoinositide hydrolysis as a mechanism of signal transduction[32] (Figure 3). Because of the

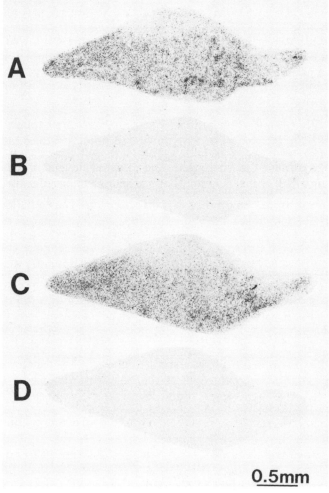

0.5mm

Fig. 3. Autoradiography of A II receptors in rat superior cervical ganglia. Consecutive sections from superior cervical ganglia of 8-week-old rats were incubated in the presence of 5×10^{-10}M ^{125}I-Sar^1-A II. A: total binding; B: incubated as in A in the presence of 10^{-5}M Losartan; C: incubated as in A in the presence of 10^{-5}M PD.123177; D: incubated as in A in the presence of 5×10^{-6}M unlabeled A II (from Strömberg C, et al.[32]).

sensitivity of A II binding to guanine nucleotides, it was concluded that probably the ganglionic AT_1 binding sites were G protein-linked.[32] These observations indicated that the AT_1 binding sites in sympathetic ganglia could be considered physiologically active receptors.[32] It has recently been established that the A II receptors in peripheral sympathetic ganglia belong to the AT_1 subtype [32] (Figure 4). In the spontaneously hypertensive rat (SHR), a model of genetic hypertension, Pinto et al.[33,34] demonstrated the presence of increased numbers of A II receptors. Such an increase in the number of ganglionic A II receptors could represent the enhanced response of neural structures to circulating A II. The actions of A II in sympathetic ganglia are short-lived because of the rapid development of tachyphylaxis.[30] This indicates that A II may only augment efferent sympathetic activity for short periods of time, and that the actions of A II in sympathetic ganglia would be important mainly in acute alterations of sympathetic function. During stress, for example, plasma renin activity is enhanced, indicating that probably A II synthesis is increased and plasma levels of the peptide are high.[35] Increased sympathetic response to circulating A II, mediated through increased A II receptors in the sympathetic ganglia, could be partially responsible for the increased release of peripheral catecholamines observed in stressed SHR.[36] The participation of the neural A II system in the regulatory mechanisms of hypertension is not unlikely since the brain A II system is stimulated in hypertension[37] and the increase in the number of ganglionic A II receptors in SHR is abolished by preganglionic denervation.[34]

Angiotensin II Receptors in Brain Cardioregulatory Areas

In addition to the conduction system of the heart and the peripheral sympathetic ganglia, there is a close association of A II receptors with central structures involved in the control of autonomic function, including the paraventricular nucleus (PVN), the parabrachial nucleus, the nucleus of the solitary tract (NTS) (Figures 5 and 6) rostral and caudal ventrolateral medulla, the intermediate cell column of the spinal cord, the nodose ganglion, and the nerve trunk of the vagus nerve.

Phillips [38] proposed that presynaptic A II receptors mediate the central baroreflex inhibitory action of A II by inhibiting transmitter release at the level of the NTS, the first synapse in the baroreceptor pathway.[39] In the NTS, A II receptors also mediate the peptide stim-

IP₁-accumulation

(% increase over control)

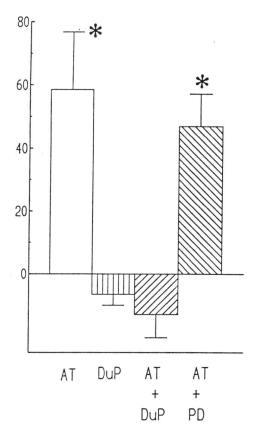

Fig. 4. Stimulation of inositol-1-phosphate accumulation by A II (10^{-6}M) or Losartan (DuP) (10^{-6}M) and the effect of Losartan or PD 123177 (10^{-5}M) on A II-induced stimulation in rat superior cervical ganglia. Each bar represents the mean ± SEM of five ganglia measured individually. * $p < 0.05$ vs control, 6748 ± 985 dpm/ganglion (from Strömberg C, et al.[32]).

ulation of the peripheral sympathetic system. Microinjections of A II in the NTS increase blood pressure, an effect blocked by hexamethonium.[40–42] This increase is probably due to dampening of the relay synapse of the baroreceptor reflex since inhibition of the reflex overcomes the decrease in heart rate that normally occurs when blood pressure is raised and has been interpreted as a tonic effect

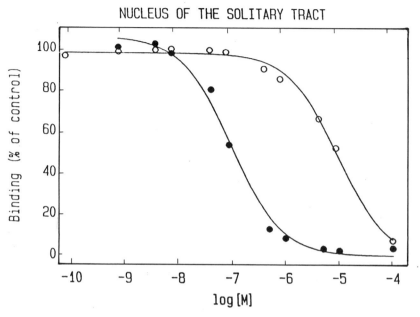

Fig. 5. A II receptor subtypes in the nucleus of the solitary tract. Consecutive sections of the rat brain stem containing the nucleus of the solitary tract were incubated with 5×10^{-10}M ^{125}I-Sar^1-A II with or without selective displacers. Closed circles: consecutive sections incubated with increasing concentrations of Losartan. Open circles: consecutive sections incubated with increasing concentrations of CGP 42112A (CIBA-Geigy, Basel, Switzerland).

of A II.[43] Without the decrease in heart rate, blood pressure rises even further.

Other investigators suggested that A II acts in the resetting of the baroreflex.[44] The source of the partial control of the sympathetic outflow by the NTS may be the PVN.[45] In addition, A II receptors in the NTS are associated with vagal afferent nerve fascicles in the medulla oblongata.[46] The receptors originate in the nodose ganglion overlying cell bodies,[47] and they reach the brain stem by transport through the vagus nerve.[46–51] These findings indicate peripheral actions of A II on visceral sensory function or on peripheral vagal motor action, as has been proposed for the heart. This suggests that A II has actions related to the control of both sympathetic and parasympathetic efferent activity. This hypothesis is supported by the finding of large numbers of A II receptors in the cardiac parasympathetic ganglia.[16]

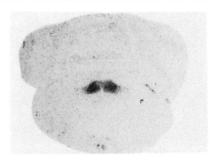

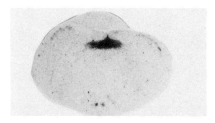

Fig. 6. Autoradiography of A II receptors in the rat brain stem. Figures represent autoradiograms of coronal sections of the rat brain stem incubated with 3×10^{-9}M ^{125}I-Sar^1-A II. Upper figure: coronal section, bregma: -13.3. Lower figure: coronal section, bregma: -13.8 (from Paxinos G and Watson C[61]).

The responses to A II in brain stem sites situated in close proximity are sometimes different. For example, A II produces hypotension when injected into the dorsal nucleus of the vagus nerve,[52] probably by activation of the parasympathetic system, resulting in bradycardia.[53]

The hypothesis that AII plays a role in the control of heart function and hypertension is supported by a large body of experimental data, which indicates that in genetic hypertension, there is a high expression of brain components of the A II system.[26] For example, SHR show higher brain A II receptor numbers in selected brain areas involved in cardiovascular control (Table 2).[54-60] These observations, together with the observation of an increased number of A II receptors in peripheral sympathetic ganglia, indicate that the enhanced A II effects could be exerted at different levels.[33,34] Since all the central structures connected to cardiovascular control express only AT$_1$ receptors,[26] we can conclude at this point that the central

Table 2
Angiotensin II Receptor Concentrations in Brain Stem Nuclei of
4-Week-Old and 14-Week-Old Spontaneously Hypertensive Rats
(SHR) and Wistar-Kyoto (WKY) Rats

	Age in Weeks	Apparent Concentration (fmol/mg protein)
Nucleus of the solitary tract (NTS)		
WKY	4	74 ± 4
SHR	4	111 ± 8*
WKY	14	92 ± 4
SHR	14	126 ± 8*
Area postrema (AP)		
WKY	4	74 ± 9
SHR	4	86 ± 8
WKY	14	105 ± 4
SHR	14	119 ± 8
Inferior olive (IO)		
WKY	4	103 ± 12
SHR	4	100 ± 8
WKY	14	40 ± 5
SHR	14	44 ± 5

All values are presented as mean ± SEM. Brain sections were incubated with 3 nmol/l ^{125}I Sar^{1}A II. Groups consisted of six to eight animals, assayed individually. * Significantly different from age-matched WKY rats (from Gutkind JS and Kurihara M[57]).

and peripheral regulation of cardiac function by A II is predominantly, if not exclusively, a property of AT_1 receptor stimulation.

In conclusion, A II AT_1 receptors are located in all central and peripheral structures that contribute to the regulation of heart function. Angiotensin II effects could be exerted at multiple levels within the central nervous system, at the level of the peripheral sympathetic ganglia, and on the heart conduction system itself. Selective blockade of AT_1 with Losartan will provide a new tool to further analyze the effects of A II in the regulation of heart function.

Summary

Angiotensin II has been accepted as a major contributor to the regulation of blood pressure and cardiac function. Using quantitative *autoradiography, we report the localization and characterization of angiotensin receptors regulating heart function. We found that angiotensin receptors are present in brain areas involved in the control of autonomic function, in peripheral sympathetic ganglia, and in the heart conduction system. In all these areas, angiotensin receptors belong to the AT_1 subtype; that is, binding is selectively displaced by the specific AT_1 receptor antagonist Losartan. There is a higher expression of angiotensin receptors in the nucleus of the solitary tract and in peripheral sympathetic ganglia in genetically (spontaneously) hypertensive rats compared to normotensive rats. Our results indicate that an increased number of angiotensin receptors in cardioregulatory areas may play a role in genetic hypertension. A specific role for AT_1 receptors in the regulation of cardiac rhythmicity directly at the level of the heart conduction system could also be postulated.*

References

1. Page IH. Hypertension Mechanisms. New York: Grune & Stratton Inc., 1987.
2. Nishith SD, Davis LD, Youmans WB. Cardioaccelerator action of angiotensin. Am J Physiol 1962; 202:237–240.
3. Feldberg W, Lewis GP. The action of peptides on the adrenal medulla: release of adrenaline by bradykinin and angiotensin. J Physiol Lond 1964; 171:98–108.
4. Starke K. Action of angiotensin on uptake, release and metabolism of ^{14}C-noradrenaline by isolated rabbit hearts. Eur J Pharmacol 1971; 14:112–123.
5. Lanier SM, Malik KU. Attenuation by prostaglandins of the facilitatory effect of angiotensin II at adrenergic prejunctional sites in the isolated Krebs-perfused rat heart. Circ Res 1982; 51:594–601.
6. Aiken JW, Reit E. Stimulation of the cat stellate ganglion by angiotensin. J Pharmacol Exp Ther 1968; 159:107–114.
7. Lee WB, Ismay MJ, Lumbers ER. Mechanisms by which angiotensin II affects the heart rate of the conscious sheep. Circ Res 1980; 47:286–292.
8. Dzau VJ, Pratt RE. Renin-angiotensin system: biology, physiology, and pharmacology. In: Fozzard HA, Haber E, Jennings RB, Katz AM, Morgen HE, eds. New York: Raven Press, 1986, 1631–1662.
9. Freer RJ, Pappano AJ, Peach MJ, et al. Mechanism for the positive inotropic effect of angiotensin II on isolated cardiac muscle. Circ Res 1976; 39:178–183.
10. Kass P, Blair ML. Effects of angiotensin II on membrane current in cardiac Purkinje fibers. J Mol Cell Cardiol 1981; 13:797–809.
11. Kobayashi M, Furukawa Y, Chiba S. Positive chronotropic and inotropic effects of angiotensin II in the dog heart. Eur J Pharmacol 1978; 50:17–25.
12. Turker RK. Evidence for a prostacyclin-mediated chronotropic effect of angiotensin II in the isolated cat right atria. Eur J Pharmacol 1982; 83:271–275.

13. Baker KM, Campanile CP, Trachte GJ, Peach MJ. Identification and characterization of the rabbit angiotensin II myocardial receptor. Circ Res 1984; 54:286–293.
14. Rogers TB. High affinity angiotensin II receptors in myocardial sarcolemmal membranes. J Biol Chem 1984; 259:8106– 8114.
15. Wright GB, Alexander RW, Ekstein LS, Gimbrone MA. Characterization of the rabbit ventricular myocardial receptor for angiotensin II. Mol Pharmacol 1983; 24:213–221.
16. Saito K, Gutkind JS, Saavedra JM. Angiotensin II binding sites in the conduction system of rat hearts. Am J Physiol 1987; 253:H1618–H1622.
17. Lambert C, Godin D, Fortier P, Nadeau R. Direct effects in vivo of angiotensin I and II on the canine sinus node. Can J Physiol Pharmacol 1991; 69:389–392.
18. Bumpus FM, Catt KJ, Chiu AT, et al. Nomenclature for angiotensin receptors: a report of the Nomenclature Committee of the Council for High Blood Pressure Research. Hypertension 1991; 17:720–721.
19. Chiu AT, Herblin WF, McCall DE, et al. Identification of angiotensin II receptor subtypes. Biochem Biophys Res Commun 1989; 165:196–203.
20. Whitebread S, Mele M, Kamber B, de Gasparo M. Preliminary biochemical characterization of two angiotensin II receptor subtypes. Biochem Biophys Res Commun 1989;163:284–291.
21. Smith RD, Chiu AT, Wong PC, Herblin WF, Timmermans PBMWM. Pharmacology of nonpeptide angiotensin II receptor antagonists. Annu Rev Pharmacol Toxicol 1992; 32:135–165.
22. Karnovsky MJ. The localization of cholinesterase activity in rat cardiac muscle by electron microscopy. J Cell Biol 1964; 23: 217–232.
23. Viswanathan M, Tsutsumi K, Correa FMA, Saavedra JM. Changes in expression of angiotensin receptor subtypes in the rat aorta during development. Biochem Biophys Res Commun 1991; 179: 1361–1367.
24. Nazarali AJ, Gutkind JS, Saavedra JM. Calibration of [^{125}I] brain paste standards for use in quantitative receptor autoradiography. J Neurosci Methods 1989;30:247–253.
25. Rogers TB, Gaa ST, Allen IS. Identification and characterization of functional angiotensin II receptors on cultured heart myocytes. J Pharmacol Exp Ther 1986; 236:438–444.
26. Saavedra JM. Brain and pituitary angiotensin. Endocr Rev 1992; 13: 329–380.
27. Brown DA, Constanti A, Marsh S. Angiontensin mimics the actions of muscarinic agonists on rat sympathetic neurons. Brain Res 1980; 193: 614–619.
28. Dun NJ, Nishi S, Karczmar AG. An analysis of the effect of angiotensin II on mammalian ganglion cells. J Pharmacol Exp Ther 1978; 204: 669–675.
29. Trendelenburg U. Observations on the ganglionic-stimulating action of angiotensin and bradykinin. J Pharmacol Exp Ther 1966; 154:418–425.
30. Reit E. Actions of angiotensin on the adrenal medulla and autonomic ganglia. Fed Proc 1972; 31:1338–1343.
31. Castren E, Kurihara M, Gutkind JS, Saavedra JM. Specific angiotensin II binding sites in the rat stellate and superior cervical ganglia. Brain Res 1987; 422:347–351.
32. Strömberg C, Tsutsumi K, Viswanathan M, Saavedra JM. Angiotensin

II AT$_1$ receptors in rat superior cervical ganglia: characterization and stimulation of phosphoinositide hydrolysis. Eur J Pharmacol Mol Pharmacol 1991; 208:331–336.

33. Pinto JEB, Nazarali AJ, Saavedra JM. Angiotensin II binding sites in the superior cervical ganglia of spontaneously hypertensive and Wistar-Kyoto rats after preganglionic denervation. Brain Res 1988; 475: 146–150.

34. Pinto JEB, Nazarali AJ, Saavedra JM. Angiotensin II binding sites in the superior cervical ganglia of spontaneously hypertensive and Wistar-Kyoto rats after preganglionic denervation. Am J Hypertens 1989; 2: 647–649.

35. Jindra A, Kvetnansky R, Belova TI, Sudakov KV. Effect of acute and repeated immobilization stress on plasma renin activity, catecholamines and corticosteroids in Wistar and August rats. In: Usdin E, Kvetnansky R, Kopin IJ, eds. Catecholamines and Stress: Recent Advances. Amsterdam, Holland: Elsevier, 1980, 249–254.

36. Grobecker H, Saavedra JM, McCarty R, Chiueh CC, Kopin IJ. Dopamine-β-hydroxylase activity and catecholamine concentrations in plasma: experimental and essential hypertension. Postgrad Med J 1977; 53 (suppl. 3):43–48.

37. Ganten D, Hermann K, Bayer C, Unger T, Lang RE. Angiotensin synthesis in the brain and increased turnover in hypertensive rats. Science 1983; 221:869–871.

38. Phillips MI. Functions of angiotensin in the central nervous system. Ann Rev Physiol 1987; 49:413–435.

39. Palkovits M, Zaborszky L. Neuroanatomy of central cardiovascular control. Nucleus tractus solitari: afferent and efferent neuronal connections in relation to the baroreceptor reflex arc. Prog Brain Res 1977; 47:1–34.

40. Casto R, Phillips MI. Cardiovascular actions of microinjections of angiotensin II in the brain stem of rats. Am J Physiol 1984; 246:R811–R816.

41. Casto R, Phillips MI. Mechanism of pressor effects by angiotensin in the nucleus tractus solitarius of rats. Am J Physiol 1984; 247:R575–R581.

42. Casto R, Phillips MI. Neuropeptide action in nucleus tractus solitarius: angiotensin specificity and hypertensive rats. Am J Physiol 1985; 249: R341–R347.

43. Campagnole-Santos MJ, Diz DI, Ferrario CM. Baroreceptor reflex modulation by angiotensin II at the nucleus tractus solitari. Hypertension 1988; 11 (suppl I):I167–I171.

44. Reid IA, Chou L. Analysis of the action of angiotensin II on the baroreflex control of heart rate in conscious rabbits. Endocrinology 1990; 126:2749–2756.

45. Swanson LW, Sawchenko PE. Hypothalamic integration: organization of the paraventricular and supraoptic nuclei. Annu Rev Neurosci 1983; 6:269–324.

46. Diz DI, Barnes KL, Ferrario CM. Contribution of the vagus nerve to angiotensin II binding sites in the canine medulla. Brain Res Bull 1986; 17:497–505.

47. Lewis SJ, Allen AM, Verberne AJM, Figdor R, Jarrott B, Mendelsohn FAO. Angiotensin II receptor binding in the rat nucleus tractus solitarii is reduced after unilateral nodose ganglionectomy or vagotomy. Eur J Pharmacol 1986; 125:305–307.

48. Speth RC, Dinh TT, Ritter S. Nodose ganglionectomy reduces angiotensin II receptor binding in the rat brain stem. Peptides 1987; 8:677–685.
49. Allen AM, Chai SY, Sexton PM, et al. Angiotensin II receptors and angiotensin converting enzyme in the medulla oblongata. Hypertension 1987; 9 (suppl III):III198–III205.
50. Allen AM, Lewis SJ, Verberne AJM, Mendelsohn FAO. Angiotensin receptors and the vagal system. Clin Exp Hypertens 1988; 10:1239(A).
51. Diz DI, Ferrario CM. Bidirectional transport of angiotensin II binding sites in the vagus nerve. Hypertension 1988; 11:I139–I143.
52. Diz DI, Barnes KL, Ferrario CM. Hypotensive actions of microinjections of angiotensin II into the dorsal motor nucleus of the vagus. J Hypertens 1984; 1 (suppl 3):53–56.
53. Rettig R, Healy DP, Printz MP. Cardiovascular effects of microinjections of angiotensin II into the nucleus tractus solitarii. Brain Res 1986; 364:233–240.
54. Saavedra JM, Correa FMA, Plunket LM, Israel A, Kurihara M, Shigematsu K. Binding of angiotensin and atrial natriuretic peptide in brain of hypertensive rats. Nature 1986; 320:758–760.
55. Saavedra JM, Kurihara M, Israel A. Alterations in angiotensin and atrial natriuretic peptide receptors in brain nuclei of spontaneously hypertensive rats. J Hypertens 1986; 4:S395–S397.
56. Saavedra JM, Correa FMA, Kurihara M, Shigematsu K. Increased number of angiotensin II receptors in the subfornical organ of spontaneously hypertensive rats. J Hypertens 1986;4:S27–S30.
57. Gutkind JS, Kurihara M, Castren E, Saavedra JM. Increased concentration of angiotensin II binding sites in selected brain areas of spontaneously hypertensive rats. J Hypertens 1988; 6:79–84.
58. Plunket LM, Saavedra JM. Increased angiotensin II binding affinity in the nucleus tractus solitarius of spontaneously hypertensive rats. Proc Natl Acad Sci USA 1985; 82:7721–7724.
59. Gehlert DR, Speth RC, Wamsley JK. Quantitative autoradiography of angiotensin II receptors in the SHR brain. Peptides 1986; 7:1021–1027.
60. Hwang BH, Harding JW, Liu DK, Hibbard LS, Wieczorek CM, We JY. Quantitative autoradiography of ^{125}I-[Sar^1,Ile^8]-angiotensin II binding in the brain of spontaneously hypertensive rats. Brain Res Bull 1986; 16:75–82.
61. Paxinos G, Watson C. The Rat Brain in Stereotoxic Coordinates. New York: Academic Press, 1986.

8

The Renin-Angiotensin System As a Growth Regulator in Cardiovascular and Non-Cardiovascular Tissues

Richard N. Re

Introduction

The renin-angiotensin system (RAS) is widely appreciated as a major determinant of intravascular volume, vascular tone, and cardiovascular homeostasis.[1] Over the last 20 years, however, abundant evidence has accumulated to indicate that, in addition to a kidney-based renin-angiotensin system, a variety of local renin cascades exist in multiple tissues.[2-17] That is, one or more components of the RAS have been either identified in specific tissues or have been demonstrated to be synthesized in specific nonrenal tissues. In some instances, the generation of the effector protein, A II, by non-renal tissues has been demonstrated. As a general rule, however, the physiological function of these local systems is not clear. In the brain, local generation of A Il likely subserves important effects relating to sympathetic nervous system tone, vasopressin release, and thirst.[18] In the pituitary, adrenal, and ovary, local hormonal regulation and physiological action seem likely.[8,14-17] In the vascular wall, renin taken up from plasma likely generates A I and A II in situ with subsequent delivery to the circulation.[19-21] Thus, in

Lindpaintner K and Ganten D (editors): *The Cardiac-Renin Angiotensin System,* © Futura Publishing Co., Inc., Armonk, NY, 1994.

these examples, putative actions of the local system can be suggested on the basis of known physiological principles. However, in other cases, the function of these systems, if any, is unclear, although in theory one could consider local systems as playing a role in local vasoconstriction, neuroregulation, and, as recent data suggests, cellular growth.

The idea that the RAS is a growth regulatory system is not new. Kharallah and coworkers demonstrated in the 1970s that the infusion of A II into animals is associated with enhanced cardiac synthesis of DNA, RNA, and protein.[22] Gantin demonstrated that A II is mitogenic at high concentrations for cultured 3T3 cells, and Campbell-Boswell demonstrated a mitogenic effect of A II on vascular smooth muscle cells (VSMC) grown in the presence of serum.[23,24] More recently, Owens demonstrated that when arterial smooth muscle cells are cultured in a defined medium, hypertrophy is, in general, produced by the addition of A II rather than hyperplasia.[25] Dzau and coworkers have suggested that specific autocrine loops dictate whether proliferation or hypertrophy will result after exposure of VSMC to A II.[26] These studies and other data suggest that A II is an important growth factor in the cardiovascular system.

The possibility that A II is a growth factor makes the observation that local renin systems exist more relevant. For example, over ten years ago we reported that cultured aortic smooth muscle cells are capable of synthesizing renin in culture.[3] This finding does not bear on the question of the role of this local renin production given the fact that quantitative arguments suggest that most (though not necessarily all) of the renin in the large vessels is taken up from plasma.[21] Our results, however, raise the possibility that under certain circumstances (for example, following vascular injury or in the case of VSMC located in smaller resistance arterioles) VSMC are capable of synthesizing renin and possibly activating the renin-angiotensin cascade in situ. Thus, the local system operative in the resistance vessels, or even in the large vessels, could play a role in vascular remodeling, given the growth regulatory properties of angiotensin. Perhaps even more relevant to physiology is the existence of a renin system in vascular endothelial cells.[27] Similarly, some years ago we reported the presence of renin in cardiac myocytes.[4-6] Although a local RAS could in theory play a role in enhancing cardiac inotropy and in regulating cardiac nerve function, the recent accumulating evidence indicating that A II can induce hypertrophy not only in neonatal but also in adult cardiac myocytes, suggests that this system may play a role in left-ventricular hypertrophy (LVH).[28-31] The known capacity of converting-enzyme inhibitors to regress or prevent hypertension-related LVH is, of course, consistent with this hypothesis.

Thus, considerable evidence indicates that multiple local RASs exist, and it appears that one role of such systems may be the regulation of cellular growth.

Cardiovascular Tissue

As discussed above, we and others have reported the existence of components of the RAS in cardiovascular tissues. Indeed, evidence exists to support the presence of, or the synthesis of, renin, angiotensinogen, converting enzyme, and A II in cardiac tissue. Ogihara and coworkers have found a correlation between tissue A II levels in the hearts of experimental animals and the presence of LVH.[30] In these studies, regression of LVH using converting-enzyme inhibitors was paralleled by a decrease in tissue A II concentrations. The effect did not appear to be related to circulating A II concentrations. Although these results could be interpreted as an epiphenomenon, they are suggestive of a role for the cardiac angiotensin system in LVH. These results are also consistent with prior results indicating that converting-enzyme inhibitors can reduce left-ventricular mass in the absence of blood pressure changes, whereas other drugs, such as direct vasodilators, reduce blood pressure without rapidly changing mass.[31-33] All these results, then, suggest that an effect of A II on LVH exists at least in the experimental animal, and that a local system may well play an important role. In preliminary experiments, we have demonstrated what we believe to be a disregulation of angiotensinogen gene expression in the left ventricles of spontaneously hypertensive rats (SHR) as compared to normal Wistar-Kyoto animals (WKY).[34] When animals were treated with high doses of the converting-enzyme inhibitor to reduce any A II-mediated stimulation of angiotensinogen gene transcription to a minimum, the ventricles of SHR contained a greater abundance of angiotensinogen mRNA than did their WKY controls. This result suggests a primary disregulation of angiotensinogen gene regulation in the left ventricles of these animals and raises the possibility that an inappropriate production of angiotensinogen in SHR leads to inappropriate local levels of A Il and hypertrophy in these animals. The ability of converting-enzyme inhibitors to regress or prevent LVH in SHR is consistent with these findings.

However, it must be noted that recent evidence indicates that in humans the majority of A II generation in the heart is the result of a "convertase" or "chymase" rather than a converting-enzyme activity.[35] Because converting-enzyme inhibitors do not affect convertase, one would expect the effect of these agents on the cardiac production of A II in humans to be smaller than in rats. Nonetheless, clinical evidence indicates that converting-enzyme inhibitors are effective in regressing hypertrophy in humans, and this suggests that the 10% or so of A II generated in the heart by the converting enzyme itself may be functionally significant.

In addition to the evidence indicated above suggesting that A II has a trophic action on VSMC in culture, whole animal experiments utilizing vascular injury followed by converting-enzyme administration, indicate that these pharmacological agents are capable of suppressing postinjury vascular proliferation.[36,37] This effect is seen only at high doses of converting-enzyme inhibitors but is marked. A similar observation has been reported in the Watanabe hypercholesterolemic rabbit.[37] These data then suggest that A II plays an important role in vascular proliferation induced either by injury or hyperlipidemia. Although it is not clear whether these results will be duplicated in humans, it must be recognized that the doses of converting-enzyme inhibitor required are quite large, and it is unlikely that clinically tolerable doses will produce this effect in humans. In any event, however, the observation in animals is intriguing.

Recently, we studied cultured human mesangial cells, or cells that play an important role in the development of chronic renal insufficiency in diabetes and other disorders. Chronic renal insufficiency in diabetes is associated with hypertrophy and proliferation of mesangial cells as well as the elaboration of an enlarged mesangial matrix compartment by these cells. In our studies, we demonstrated that in the presence of insulin, converting-enzyme inhibitors were capable of reducing maximal mesangial cell proliferation. Angiotensin II under these circumstances increased mesangial cell proliferation.[38] These data strongly suggest that A II is a trophic factor for human mesangial cells. We were unable to demonstrate converting-enzyme activity associated with mesangial cells, but utilizing reverse transcription followed by polymerase chain reaction, we were able to detect angiotensinogen mRNA in these cells. Moreover, an antisense oligonucleotide directed against the angiotensinogen mRNA reduced mesangial cell proliferation in the presence of insulin.[39] The coadministration of A II to cells exposed to the antisense oligonucleotide resulted in a restoration of thymidine incorporation into DNA. This result indicates a role for locally produced angiotensinogen in the regulation of mesangial cell proliferation and indicates that the local mesangial cell RAS can act as an autocrine regulator of growth. Thus, A II, in the presence of insulin, augments mesangial cell proliferation. We believe that the angiotensinogen substrate for local angiotensin production could be provided either by the serum or by the mesangial cells themselves. The converting enzyme necessary to convert A I to A II is likely derived from the serum because we are unable to detect any converting-enzyme activity in association with the mesangial cells, although it may be present in small concentrations.

Thus, our findings suggest that a local RAS in the mesangium functions in a paracrine or autocrine fashion to regulate cell proliferation and perhaps other cellular functions such as contraction and protein synthesis. These findings then argue that the RAS could play an important role in diabetes and other forms of chronic renal disease. This suggestion obtains support from evidence that converting-enzyme inhibitors do appear to slow chronic renal failure in several animal models.[40]

In sum then, it appears that the RAS at the systemic level and/or at the local level likely plays a role in the regulation of cardiovascular tissue proliferation and modeling. Additional clinical observations, such as the fact that converting-enzyme inhibitors are capable of preventing postmyocardial infarction ventricular dilatation, are consistent with this view.[41]

Non-Cardiovascular Tissues

In recent years, evidence has accumulated to indirectly suggest novel growth regulatory actions of A II. For example, the peptide has been shown to possess the capacity to induce neovascularization and vessel ingrowth in a rabbit cornea test model, suggesting an important role for A II in neovascularization.[42] This idea derives some indirect support from the finding of immunohistochemically detectable renin in the vessels supplying several forms of human tumors, including lung cancers.[43] Although it is not clear that any or all of the renin found in these tumor vessels is synthesized locally, or that renin acts to produce local A II with subsequent neovascularization of the tumor tissue itself, these observations are nonetheless provocative and raise the possibility that A II functioning as a stimulus for neovascularization can play an important role in some forms of neoplasia.

Of potentially even more interest is the observation that the human *mas* oncogene encodes a protein that confers enhanced growth responsiveness to A II upon cells into which it is transfected.[44] This phenomenon likely explains why cells transformed with *mas* grow more aggressively in vivo (where they are exposed to endogenous A II) than in vitro. Indeed, it appears that *mas* is one member of a family of genes that confers this enhanced growth sensitivity to A II. Because *mas* was derived from human tumor cells, this observation again raises the possibility that A II may play a role in the growth regulation of human cancer.

In the 1970s, Inagami et al. demonstrated the presence of functioning RASs in some murine neuroblastoma cell lines.[13] Because of this demonstration and recent evidence suggesting the potential for A II in the growth of noncardiovascular tissues, we investigated the possibility that the growth of human neuroblastoma cells could be A II sensitive. We cultured human SHSY5Y neuroblastoma cells and demonstrated that the addition of A II at 10^{-8}M and 10^{-6}M resulted in about a 25% increase in thymidine incorporation into DNA.[45-48] Converting-enzyme inhibitors reduced thymidine incorporation to a comparable degree. We could detect the converting enzyme in washed cells and, therefore, it is possible that the observed converting-enzyme inhibitor effect could have resulted from inhibition of low levels of the converting enzyme in the serum of the culture medium or from inhibition of endogenous converting enzyme synthesized by the cells. Of note is that both the peptide A II antagonist, saralasin, and the nonpeptide AT_1 A II antagonist, DuP753, also blunted thymidine incorporation into DNA. Surprisingly, the AT_2 receptor antagonist PD123177 also was effective in reducing proliferation in this system. Thus, inhibition of either the AT_1 or AT_2 receptor subtype appears to be effective. We are uncertain if this inhibition represents crosstalk between the two receptors or the unexpected inhibition of one receptor subtype by concentrations of inhibitor for the other subtype used under the conditions of this experiment.

In additional experiments, we again used antisense oligonucleotides designed to prevent translation of the angiotensinogen message.[39] In these experiments, antisense oligos, but not sense oligos, suppressed neuroblastoma cell thymidine incorporation by more than 25%. The coadministration of 10^{-6} A II to cells exposed to the antisense oligo resulted in a restoration of thymidine incorporation into DNA, strongly suggesting that the effect of the antisense oligo resulted from inhibition of endogenous generation of A II. Of note is that when the basic fibroblast growth factor (bFGF) was administered to these cells, thymidine incorporation increased to an amount comparable to that seen following the administration of A II. In the presence of the antisense oligo, the administration of bFGF had only a minimal effect on thymidine incorporation into DNA. Finally, when control murine L929 cells were exposed to A II, no increase in thymidine incorporation was seen, and no effect of either the sense or antisense oligo was detected. The bFGF produced an increase in thymidine incorporation into DNA by these cells.

These data indicate that the inhibition of the translation of angiotensinogen mRNA results in a decrease of A II production by the neuroblastoma cells with a resultant reduction in cell proliferation. This effect can be offset by the coadministration of exogenous A II, but not by the coadministration of other growth factors. These data strongly argue that not only is A II a growth factor for human neuroblastoma cells but that A II functions in an autocrine manner in regulating the growth of these cells. This observation potentially has important significance for the treatment of neuroblastoma and other human cancers, especially those associated with A II receptors and/or endogenous RASs. It may well be that the converting-enzyme inhibitors and A II antagonists will find a role in the treatment of neoplastic disease. Because these agents are relatively nontoxic and well understood, they may well provide a novel and well-tolerated mode of therapy for diseases as diverse as neuroblastoma and adrenal cell carcinoma.

Intracrine Angiotensin II Action

In the early 1970s, Kharallah and coworkers presented autoradiographic evidence suggesting that A II gains access to cell interiors and localizes in cell nuclei and mitochondria.[22] Over the ensuing years, we have developed evidence to confirm this hypothesis and to extend it. We detected high-affinity specific A II receptors associated with chromatin and further demonstrated that A II binding to chromatin at these locations is associated with conformational changes in chromatin comparable to those seen during gene activation.[49–53] Further, we detected a direct effect of A II on RNA polymerase activity. On the basis of these and other findings in our laboratory, we hypothesized that A II, and perhaps other peptides, could act in what we termed an intracrine fashion,[54] or an intracellular mode of peptide hormone action. We envisioned A II functioning in an intracrine mode after either intracellular synthesis with release to the cytoplasm and nuclear compartment or following binding to external membrane receptors with subsequent internalization and dissociation of peptides or peptide fragments from the receptor. Over recent years, considerable evidence supporting both A II intracrine action and the intracellular actions of other peptides has accumulated.[55-61] Thus, there is evidence to suggest that many peptide hormones operate in the intracellular milieu, and this in turn suggests that intracrine action may be an important arena for therapeutic intervention. One could hypothesize that A II intracrine action is involved in the regulation of the synthesis of the components of the RAS by those cells that contain local renin systems. Moreover, it is possible that A II, operating in an intracrine fashion, helps direct the metabolic and growth-promoting activities of this octapeptide. These possibilities are intriguing in that they offer new targets for therapeutic intervention.

Conclusion

In the century since Tigerstedt and Bergmann isolated renin, and in the 60 years since Goldblatt demonstrated the role of this circulating enzyme in the genesis of renovascular hypertension, the RAS has come to be seen as a cornerstone of cardiovascular homeostasis. Over the last two decades, however, it has become clear that our concept of the RAS must be expanded to include local synthesis of the components of this system and the effects of A II on the growth of cardiovascular, noncardiovascular, and malignant tissues. It now appears that the RAS can function as a circulating hormonal cascade, as well as operate in autocrine, paracrine, and intracrine modes. The RAS potentially plays a role in physiological activities as diverse as embryogenesis, neovascularization, atherosclerosis, renal insufficiency, and neoplasia. As such, the RAS is an exciting target for study and therapeutic intervention.

Summary

In recent years, the components of the renin-angiontensin system (RAS) have been identified in a variety of tissues, and an ability to regulate the growth of some target cells has been ascribed to A II. This finding raises the possibility that locally or systemically produced angiotensin could serve a growth regulatory function in cardiovascular and noncardiovascular tissues.

In the cardiovascular system, components of the RAS, either locally produced or taken up from plasma, have been identified in the vascular endothelium, the vascular wall, the myocardium, and in a variety of locations within the kidney. Direct or indirect evidence links

A II with hypertrophy or hyperplasia in vascular smooth muscle cells, cardiac hypertrophy, and mesangial cell proliferation. Indirect evidence links A II to myocardial hypertrophy in animals and humans, and additional evidence suggests a role for A II in neovascularization. Thus, a case can be made for the argument that A II can serve as a growth regulatory peptide in a variety of tissues.

At the same time, however, it is extremely difficult to determine the precise physiological role of A II in growth regulation or to determine to what extent local, as opposed systemically generated, A II is operative. In order to address this issue, we have undertaken studies utilizing antisense oligonucleotides directed against angiotensinogen mRNA. These oligonucleotides have the capacity to reduce or eliminate A II synthesis in cells to which they are administered. The administration of these oligonucleotides to cultured human mesangial cells or to cultured human neuroblastoma cells results in a significant decrement in cellular proliferation. This result demonstrates that the local RAS regulates growth in these cells. Thus, A II likely functions as an autocrine or paracrine growth-regulatory factor. Finally, our laboratory has developed data that strongly indicate that A II can also operate intracellularly in what we have termed an intracrine fashion.

Taken together, these findings and others make clear that our concept of the RAS must be expanded to include local synthesis of the components of this system and the effects of A II on the growth of cardiovascular, noncardiovascular, and even malignant tissues.

References

1. Re RN. The renin-angiotensin systems. Med Clin North Am 1987; 71: 5.
2. Re RN. The cellular biology of the renin-angiotensin systems. Arch Intern Med 1984; 144:2037–2041.
3. Re RN, Fallon TJ, Dzau VS, Quay S, Haber E. Renin synthesis by cultured arterial smooth muscle cells. Life Sci 1982; 30:99–106.
4. Dzau VJ, Re RN. Evidence for the existence of renin in the heart. Circulation 1987; 75(suppl I):I134–I136.
5. Jin M, Wilhelm MJ, Lang RE, Unger T, Lindpaintner K, Ganten D. Endogenous tissue renin-angiotensin systems from molecular biology to therapy. Am J Med 1988; 84(suppl 3A):28–36.
6. Re RN. The myocardial intracellular renin-angiotensin system. Am J Cardiol 1987; 59:56A–58A.
7. Lynch K, Simnad V, Ben-Ari E, Garrison J. Localization of preangiotensinogen messenger RNA sequences in the rat brain. Hypertension 1986; 8:540–543.
8. Horiba N, Nomura K, Shizume K. Exogenous and locally synthesized

angiotensin II and glomerulosa cell function. Hypertension 1990; 15: 190–197.

9. Ganten D, Schelling P, Vecsei P, et al. Iso-renin of extrarenal origin: the tissue angiotensinase system. Am J Med 1976; 60:760–772.

10. Felix D, Harding JW, Imboden H. The hypothalamic-angiotensin system: location and functional considerations. Clin Exp Hypertens 1988; [A]10 (suppl 1):45–62.

11. Cassis LA, Saye J, Peach MJ. Location and regulation of rat angiotensinogen messenger RNA. Hypertension 1988; 11:591–596.

12. Campbell D, Habener J. Angiotensinogen gene is expressed and differentially regulated in multiple tissues of the rat. J Clin Invest 1986; 78: 31–39.

13. Clemens DL, Clauser E, Celio MR, Inagami T. Generation of angiotensin by cultured neuroblastoma and glioma cells. Brain Res 1986; 364: 205–211.

14. Aguilera EP, Hyde CL, Catt KJ. Angiotensin II receptors and prolactin release in pituitary lactotrophs. Endocrinology 1980; 111:1045–1049.

15. Glorioso N, Atlas SA, Laragh JH, Jewelewicz R, Sealey J. Prorenin in high concentrations in human ovarian follicular fluid. Science 1987; 233:1424–1427.

16. Hseuh Wa. Renin in the female reproductive system. Cardiovasc Drugs Therapeutics 1987; 2:473–477.

17. Horiba N, Nomura K, Shizume K. Exogenous and locally synthesized angiotensin II and glomerulosa cell functions. Hypertension 1990; 15: 190–197.

18. Buckley JP. The central effects of the renin-angiotensin system. Clin Exp Hypertens 1988; [A]10:1–16.

19. Swales JD, Abramovici A, Beck F, Bing RF, Loudon M, Thurston H. Arterial wall renin. J Hypertens 1983; 1(suppl 1):17–22.

20. Admiraal PJJ, Derkx FHM, Danser AHJ, Pieterman H, Schalekamp MADH. Metabolism and production of angiotensin I in different vascular beds in subjects with hypertension. Hypertension 1990; 15:44–55.

21. Swales JD, Abramovici A, Beck F, Bing RF, Loudon M, Thurston H. Arterial wall renin. J Hypertens 1983; 1(suppl 1):17–22.

22. Khairallah PA, Robertson AL, Davila D. Effects of angiotensin II on DNA, RNA and protein synthesis. In: Genest J, Koiw E, eds. Hypertension '72. New York: Springer-Verlag, 1972: 212–220.

23. Ganten D, Schelling P, Flugel RM. Effect of angiotensin and an angiotensin antagonist on isorenin and cell growth in 3T3 mouse cells. Intern Res Commun Med Sci 1975; 3:327–330.

24. Campbell-Boswell M, Robertson A. Effects of angiotensin II and vasopressin on human smooth muscle cells in vitro. Exp Mol Path 1981; 35: 265–276.

25. Geisterfer A, Peach MJ, Owens GK. Angiotensin II induces hypertrophy, not hyperplasia of cultured rat aortic smooth muscle cells. Circ Res 1988; 62:749–756.

26. Naftilin AJ, Hsaio LL, Pratt RE, Dzau VJ. Stimulation of platelet derived growth factor A-chain expression by angiotensin II in cultured smooth muscle cells. Circulation 1988a (suppl II)78:II-4.

27. Dzau VJ. Significance of the vascular renin-angiotensin pathway. Hypertension 1988; 8:553–559.

28. Baker KM, Chernin MI, Wixson SK, Aceto JF. Renin-angiotensin system involvement in pressure-overload cardiac hypertrophy in rats. Am J Physiol 1990; 259:H324–H332.

29. Dostal DE, Baker KM. Angiotensin II stimulation of left ventricular hypertrophy in adult rat heart: mediation by the AT_1 receptor. Am J Hypertens 1992; 5:276–280.

30. Nagano M, Higaki J, Mikami H, Nakamura M, Higashimori K, Katahira K, et al. Converting enzyme inhibitors regressed cardiac hypertrophy and reduced tissue angiotensin II in spontaneously hypertensive rats. J Hypertens 1991; 9:595–599.

31. Linz W, Schölkens BA, Ganten D. Converting enzyme inhibition specifically prevents the development and induces regression of cardiac hypertrophy in rats. Clin Exp Hypertens 1989; 11:1325–1350.

32. Pfeffer JM, Pfeffer MA, Mersky I, Braunwald E. Regression of left ventricular hypertrophy and prevention of left ventricular dysfunction by captopril in the spontaneously hypertensive rat. Proc Natl Acad Sci USA 1982; 79:3310–3314.

33. Schelling P, Fischer H, Ganten D. Angiotensin and cell growth: a link to cardiovascular hypertrophy. J Hypertens 1991; 9:3–15.

34. Re RN, Li C, Prakash O. Role of angiotensin II in cardiovascular growth regulation. J Vasc Med Biol 1991; 3:22–24.

35. Urata H, Kinoshita A, Bumpus FM, Graham RM, Husain A. Tissue specific expression of human heart chymase. Program of the 14th Scientific Meeting of the International Society of Hypertension. Madrid, Spain 1992; S9.

36. Powell JS, Clozel J-P, Muller RKM, et al. Inhibitors of angiotensin-converting enzyme prevent myointimal proliferation after vascular injury. Science 1989; 254:186–188.

37. Chobanian AV, Haudenschild CC, Nickerson C, Drago R. Antiatherogenic effect of captopril in the watanabe heritable hyperlipidemic rabbit. Hypertension 1990; 15:327–331.

38. Bakris GL, Re RN. Endothelin modulates angiotensin II-induced mitogenesis of human mesangial cells. Am J Physiol 264 (Renal Fluid Electrolyte Physiol 33) 1993: F937–F942.

39. Cook JL, Chen L, Bhandaru S, Bakris GL, Re RN. The use of antisense oligonucleotides to establish autocrine angiotensin growth effects in human neuroblastoma and mesengial cells. Antisense Research and Development 1992; 2:199–210.

40. Tolins JP, Shultz P, Raji L. Mechanisms of hypertensive glomerular injury. Am J Cardiol 1988; 62:54G–58G.

41. Pfeffer JM, Pfeffer MA, Fletcher PJ, Braunwald E. Progressive ventricular remodeling in rat with myocardial infarction. Am J Physiol 1991; 260:H1406–H1414.

42. Fernandez LA, Twickler J, Mead A. Neovascularization produced by angiotensin II. J Lab Clin Med 1985; 105:141–145.

43. Taylor GM, Cook HT, Sheffield EA, Hanson C, Peart WS. Renin in blood vessels in human pulmonary tumors: an immunohistochemical and biochemical study. Am J Pathol 1988; 130:543–551.

44. Jackson TR, Blair AC, Marshall J, Goedert M, Hanley MR. The *mas* oncogene encodes an angiotensin receptor. Nature 1988; 335:437–440.

45. Chen L, Re RN, Prakash O, Mondal D. Angiotensin-converting enzyme

inhibition reduces neuroblastoma cell growth rate. Proc Soc Exp Biol Med 1991; 196:280–283.

46. Chen L, Re RN, Prakash O, Mondal D. Converting enzyme inhibition reduces neuroblastoma cell growth rate. Clin Res 1989; 37:940A.

47. Chen L, Re RN. Angiotensin and the regulation of neuroblastoma cell growth. Am J Hypertens 1991; 4:82A.

48. Chen L, Prakash O, Re RN. The interaction of insulin and angiotensin II on the regulation of human neuroblastoma cell growth. Molecular and Chemical Neuropathology 1993; 18:189–196.

49. Re RN, MacPhee AA, Fallon JT. Specific nuclear binding of angiotensin II. Clin Sci 1981; 61:245s–247s.

50. Re RN, LaBiche RA, Bryan SE. Nuclear-hormone mediated changes in chromatin solubility. Biochem Biophys Res Commun 1983; 110:61–68.

51. Re RN. Changes in nuclear initiation sites after the treatment of isolated nuclei with angiotensin II. Clin Sci 1982; 63:191s–193s.

52. Re RN, Vizard DL, Brown T, Bryan B. Angiotensin receptors in chromatin fragments generated by micrococcal nuclease. Biochem Biophys Res Commun 1984; 119:220–227.

53. Re RN, Parab M. Effect of angiotensin II on RNA synthesis by isolated nuclei. Life Sci 1984; 34:647–651.

54. Re RN. The cellular biology of angiotensin: paracrine, autocrine, and intracrine actions in cardiovascular tissues. J Mol Cell Cardiol 1989; 21(suppl 5):63–69.

55. Bouche G, Gus N, Prats H, et al. Basic fibroblast growth factor enters the nucleolus and stimulates the transcription of ribosomal genes in ABAE cells undergoing G_0 G_1 transition. Proc Natl Acad Sci 1987; 84: 6770–6774.

56. Burwen SJ, Jones AL. The association of polypeptide hormones and growth factors with the nuclei of target cells. Trends In Biological Sciences 1987; 12:159–162.

57. Frankel, AD, Pabo CO. Cellular uptake of the *tat* protein from human immunodeficiency virus. Cell 1988; 55:1189–1193.

58. Millan MA, Millan JC. Nuclear localization of radiolabeled A II in isolated rat adrenal glomerulosa cells. Program and Abstracts of the 70th Annual Meeting of the Endocrine Society 1988; p.51.

59. Rakowicz-Szulzynskce E, Rodeck U, Herlyn M, Koproswki H. Chromatin-binding of epidermal growth factor, nerve growth factor and platelet-derived growth factor in cells bearing appropriate surface receptors. Proc Natl Acad Sci, USA 1986; 83:3728–3732.

60. Miller DS. Stimulation of RNA and protein synthesis by intracellular insulin. Science 1988; 240:506–511.

61. Kiron MAR, Soffer RL. Purification and properties of a soluble angiotensin II-binding protein from rabbit liver. J Biol Chem 1989; 264: 4138–4142.

Myocardial Fibrosis: Structural Basis for Pathological Remodeling and the Role of the Renin-Angiotensin-Aldosterone System

Scott E. Campbell, Christian G. Brilla, and
Karl T. Weber

Introduction

Myocardial failure is a worldwide health problem of major and ever-increasing proportions. For patients with advanced symptomatic heart failure, despite optimal use of available palliative medical therapy, survival is significantly impaired. Insights into the pathogenesis and pathophysiology of myocardial failure are needed to reverse these disturbing trends and to establish pharmacological strategies that prevent or perhaps even reverse myocardial failure. Where might the clues needed to unravel this puzzle be found? An examination of associated risk factors proves illuminating in this regard.

Left-ventricular hypertrophy (LVH) and an elevation in plasma hormones of the renin-angiotensin-aldosterone system (RAAS) and the adrenergic nervous system have each been associated with an

Lindpaintner K and Ganten D (editors): *The Cardiac-Renin Angiotensin System,* © Futura Publishing Co., Inc., Armonk, NY, 1994.

increased risk of adverse cardiovascular events. In patients both with and without documented systemic hypertension, for example, LVH is a major risk factor associated with the appearance of symptomatic heart failure and sudden cardiac death.[1–3] This is true for the Framingham cohort, a predominantly white suburban community, as well as for black Americans in urban locations.[4–6] At the same time, and independent of LVH, an elevation in plasma aldosterone or aldosterone secretion relative to dietary sodium and plasma renin activity predisposes hypertensive patients to adverse cardiovascular outcomes, such as myocardial infarction.[7,8] In patients with symptomatic heart failure, increased plasma aldosterone (ALDO) worsens an already poor prognosis.[9] Could it be that these seemingly unrelated observations are, in fact, causally related, and how might this be so?

One explanation that brings these risk factors, LVH and aldosterone, together (see Figure 1) resides in the adverse structural remodeling of the myocardium, coronary, and systemic circulations, which is expressed as an abnormal accumulation of fibrous tissue

RISK FACTORS FOR ADVERSE CARDIOVASCULAR

EVENTS, INCLUDING MORTALITY

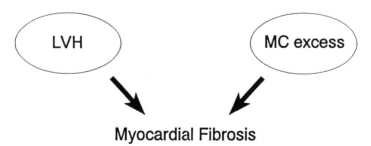

Fig. 1. Left ventricular hypertrophy (LVH) and elevations in the plasma concentration of mineralocorticoid (MC) hormones relative to dietary sodium intake, representing a state of MC excess, are independent risk factors for adverse cardiovascular events, including mortality. It is not the increment in LV mass that accounts for increased risk, but rather an associated structural remodeling, due to fibrosis mediated by primary or secondary increments in these steroid hormones, that impairs myocardial stiffness and leads to electrical dispersion with ventricular arrhythmias.

and occurs in response to mineralocorticoid (MC) excess, relative to sodium intake.[10,11] This fibrosis is seen within the adventitia of intramyocardial coronary and systemic arterioles and their neighboring interstitial spaces and does not require parenchymal cell injury (a *reactive* fibrosis). Elevations in plasma concentrations of the MC hormones ALDO or deoxycorticosterone (DOC), relative to dietary sodium intake, have each been linked to this pathological structural remodeling of not only the myocardium but of systemic organs as well.[11-13] The extracellular accumulation of fibrillar collagen alters the function of any organ, including the myocardium. Clinical and experimental studies alike have identified the functional significance of fibrillar collagen accumulation in raising myocardial stiffness[14,15] and promoting ventricular arrhythmias.[16-18] In addition to this reactive fibrosis, chronic MC excess with enhanced urinary potassium excretion is associated with reduced stores of potassium within the myocardium, myocyte necrosis, and a *reparative* myocardial fibrosis, or microscopic scarring.[19]

The objective of this review is to consider myocardial fibrosis and each of its presentations as they are expressed in association with MC excess, which we define as an elevation in plasma ALDO or DOC relative to dietary sodium intake. We emphasize at the outset that although the myocardium may be particularly vulnerable to electrolyte-induced myocyte necrosis and microscopic scarring, it is not unique relative to the reactive fibrous tissue response. Instead, the perivascular and interstitial fibrosis found in the myocardium is representative of the fibrosis seen in multiple organs in MC excess.

Myocardial Fibrosis in Humans With Mineralocorticoid Excess

Morphological studies have shown that the concentration of collagen is increased in the hypertensive hypertrophied human left ventricle.[20-22] This fibrosis is present in several distinct morphological patterns[20] including: (a) a perivascular fibrosis of intramyocardial coronary arteries, together with an associated interstitial fibrosis of neighboring extracellular spaces (Figure 2), representing a reactive fibrosis (without parenchymal cell loss) seen throughout the myocardium; and (b) microscopic scars, or a reparative (replacement) fibrosis, that follows cardiac myocyte necrosis and can favor the endomyocardium.

These postmortem studies did not include a profiling of the RAAS. Therefore, the relationship between myocardial fibrosis and

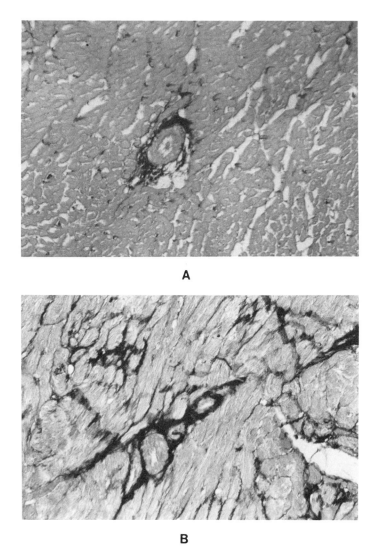

Fig. 2. (A) A normal intramyocardial coronary artery of the rat with fibrillar collagen in its adventitia and interstitial spaces. (B) Perivascular fibrosis of intramyocardial coronary arteries in the rat with extensions of fibrillar collagen into neighboring interstitial spaces to create an interstitial fibrosis. This reactive fibrosis is distinguished from the reparative fibrosis, or scarring, that replaces necrotic myocytes. (Picrosirius red ×40.)

abnormal elevations in plasma A II or ALDO in humans is uncertain. This gap in our knowledge needs to be addressed through a greater use of endomyocardial biopsies, especially in patients with diastolic dysfunction. Postmortem studies in patients having primary or secondary MC excess, however, suggest that such a relationship exists (see below).

Myocardial fibrosis was found at autopsy in a young normotensive woman with Bartter's syndrome (secondary hyperaldosteronism with hypokalemia), who died suddenly; her epicardial coronary arteries at autopsy were anatomically normal in appearance.[23] The observed microscopic scarring was therefore thought to be secondary to chronic hypokalemia with associated myocyte necrosis.

Following the sudden cardiac death of a young weight lifter who had been taking parenteral anabolic steroids, a marked reactive and reparative fibrosis of the right and left ventricles, as well as the atria, was found postmortem.[24,25] Myocardial fibrosis, as well as a perivascular and interstitial fibrosis of intramural arteries in systemic organs, has likewise been observed in the rat administered anabolic steroids or testosterone over weeks.[26,27] Administration of 17 α-methyl-androstenediol causes an inhibition of 11β- and 18-hydroxylation of steroid hormone synthesis and, as a result, there is an increased secretion of DOC.[28] This secondary MC excess state that occurs with chronic androgen administration can be prevented by adrenalectomy.[29]

Campbell et al.[30] have observed a marked perivascular and interstitial fibrosis, as well as microscopic scarring of the myocardium, in patients with autopsy-proven adrenal adenoma. This abnormal reactive fibrous tissue response was evident in systemic organs as well and may explain the increased incidence of cardiovascular complications that have been recognized in patients with primary hyperaldosteronism.[31]

These postmortem findings do not permit a clear distinction to be made regarding the relative importance of hemodynamic versus hormonal components of the RAAS in mediating the abnormal fibrous tissue response in the myocardium. For this purpose, experimental studies can be used to advantage.

Myocardial Fibrosis in Experimental Animals With Mineralocorticoid Excess

Chronic elevations in plasma ALDO or DOC are inappropriate when dietary sodium intake is normal or enhanced. Under these circumstances, MC excess is associated with arterial hypertension, provided cardiac output and intravascular volume are normal or near normal. On the other hand, when MC excess occurs in the presence of myocardial failure with reduced cardiac output, arterial hypertension is absent.

Myocardial Fibrosis in Mineralocorticoid Excess with Hypertension

Various models of arterial hypertension have been used to examine LVH and the structural remodeling of the myocardium that accompany the hypertrophic process. Often, however, raising left-ventricular systolic pressure was the primary objective, and little attention was paid to whether or not the RAAS was also activated or whether there was associated MC excess. For example, reducing renal perfusion by placing a constrictive band around either the ascending aorta, thoracic aorta, or the abdominal aorta above the renal arteries each represents models of left-ventricular pressure overload associated with secondary hyperaldosteronism. Arterial hypertension that accompanies surgically-induced unilateral renal ischemia is an obvious example of secondary hyperaldosteronism. Primary MC excess accompanies the chronic administration of mineralocorticoids (d-aldosterone or deoxycorticosterone acetate, DOCA). In each of these various models of arterial hypertension, with associated primary or secondary MC excess, collagen concentration is increased in the hypertrophied left ventricle and, when measured, in the nonhypertrophied right ventricle.[11,32] A rise in mRNA expression for type I and type III fibrillar collagens[33] and increased collagen synthesis[34] is known to precede fibrosis in unilateral and bilateral renal ischemia. Fibroblast proliferation has also been observed with renal ischemia in the right and left ventricles[35,36] and suggests the importance of a circulating (vis-à-vis hemodynamic) factor.

To distinguish more clearly between the importance of ventricular loading and hormonal factors in mediating reactive myocardial fibrosis, Brilla et al.[32] examined collagen concentration by both morphometric and biochemical techniques, in the normotensive right ventricle and in the hypertensive left ventricle, in various models of arterial hypertension. Models that provide a diverse profile of the RAAS were selected: unilateral renal ischemia, with elevated plasma A II and ALDO; infrarenal aorta banding with normal RAAS; uninephrectomized rats receiving ALDO and elevated dietary sodium, where only plasma ALDO is elevated; and uninephrec-tomized animals receiving increased dietary sodium without ALDO administration, where the RAAS is not activated. Comparable arterial hypertension and LVH were found with renal ischemia, infrarenal banding, and chronic ALDO administration, whereas the right ventricle was not hypertrophied in any of these models. A reactive myocardial fibrosis was found in both ventricles, but only with unilateral renal ischemia and primary hyperaldosteronism. Fibrosis was not found with infrarenal banding or sodium loading alone (that is, an uninephrectomy and a high sodium diet). These in vivo studies demonstrated that cardiac myocyte hypertrophy was most closely related to ventricular systolic pressure, whereas the fibrous tissue response was governed by hormonal factors. Additional studies, using various pharmacological probes, were needed to address the relative importance of A II and ALDO.

Brilla and Weber[37] found that right and left ventricular fibrosis could be prevented in the rat with either unilateral renal ischemia or hyperaldosteronism by the ALDO receptor-antagonist spironolactone. This was true whether arterial hypertension and LVH were or were not prevented by using a large or small dose of spironolactone, respectively. Angiotensin-converting enzyme (ACE) inhibition with captopril was only effective in preventing fibrosis in unilateral renal ischemia; not unexpectedly, it did not prove cardioprotective in hyperaldosteronism. Thus, the evidence implicating MC excess in mediating the perivascular and interstitial fibrosis of the myocardium is compelling. Selye[12] emphasized this concept years ago when he found a similar fibrous tissue response in multiple organs, including the heart, with chronic DOCA administration. A similar structural remodeling of systemic organs and the heart has been observed with MC excess induced by the chronic administration of d-aldosterone,[13] 17 α-methyl androstenediol,[26] and testosterone.[27]

A reparative fibrosis specific to the heart accompanies chronic (greater than 4 weeks) MC administration and can be prevented by enhanced dietary potassium supplementation[19] or the potassium-conserving agents spironolactone or amiloride.[38,39] This scarring follows cardiac myocyte necrosis in response to reduced myocardial stores of potassium and is not evident in skeletal muscle.

Myocardial Fibrosis in Mineralocorticoid Excess Without Hypertension

A perivascular and interstitial fibrosis of the canine myocardium has been observed after chronic ventricular pacing.[40] In this model of myocardial failure with low cardiac output and ventricular dilatation the RAAS is activated. Unlike the secondary hyperaldosteronism that occurs with rapid pacing, the ventricular dilatation and high cardiac output seen early after aortacaval fistula in either the dog or rat is not associated with MC excess, and myocardial fibrosis has not been observed.[40,41] In other models of volume overload in which an activation of the RAAS does not occur, such as an atrial septal defect or chronic anemia, ventricular collagen concentration remains normal.[42,43]

Banding of the pulmonary artery is associated with ascites and pleural effusions. In this model of MC excess due to RAAS activation, collagen concentration is increased in the pressure-overloaded, hypertrophied right ventricle and the normotensive, nonhypertrophied left ventricle.[44]

Genetic Hypertension

Myocardial fibrosis is also seen in the rat with a genetic predisposition to hypertension. In these rats with spontaneously appearing hypertension (SHR), myocardial collagen concentration rises progressively with age.[45] Early in life, and before hypertension and LVH appear, an unexplained rise in collagen synthesis has been observed.[46]

The mechanism responsible for the fibrous tissue response is not clear. Abnormal elevations in the plasma concentration of various components of the RAAS have not been observed in SHR. On the other hand, the fact that the plasma renin activity of SHR is in the expected "normal" range and is not suppressed does raise the possibility that an abnormality of the RAAS, whether in the circulation or intrinsic to vascular tissue, may be operative. In treating fetal SHR with an ACE inhibitor and then continuing the treatment for an additional 14 weeks, it was possible to prevent myocardial fibrosis, as well as hypertension and LVH.[47] In contrast, 32 weeks of hydralazine administration introduced at 4 weeks of age was effective in preventing hypertension and LVH, but not the appearance of myocardial fibrosis.[48]

Mineralocorticoids and Fibroblasts

Cultured fibroblasts, obtained from the rat aorta, have high-affinity, low-capacity corticoid receptors.[49] Their contribution to altered collagen metabolism (synthesis and degradation) and fibroblast growth has not been addressed.

In preliminary studies using quiescent, cultured adult rat cardiac fibroblasts studied at confluence, Brilla et al.[50] found that aldosterone enhances collagen synthesis. The increment in ^{3}H proline incorporation was found for concentrations of ALDO that corresponded to plasma levels seen in experimental models of primary and secondary hyperaldosteronism.[32] Angiotensin II also increased cardiac fibroblast collagen synthesis, but only at nonphysiological concentrations.[51] A similar concentration-dependent response to A II-mediated collagen synthesis has been observed in cultured cardiac fibroblasts obtained from adult SHR, as well as in their genetic controls (WKY). However, fibroblasts from SHR were more sensitive to A II.[52]

Future Directions

Experimental evidence regarding the cardioprotective and cardioreparative properties of ACE inhibition and anti-ALDO therapy relative to myocardial fibrosis has been reported.[37–39,47,53,54] In recognizing that MC excess can mediate a structural remodeling of the myocardium and cardiovascular system, expressed as a pathological accumulation of fibrillar collagen, it should be possible to develop therapeutic strategies that can prevent or even reverse the structural remodeling responsible for ventricular dysfunction and arrhythmias in humans. Experimental evidence regarding the cardioprotective and cardioreparative properties of ACE inhibition and anti-ALDO therapy relative to myocardial fibrosis has been reported.[37–39,47,53,54]

Acknowledgements

This work was supported in part by NIH grant R01-31701.

Summary

Left-ventricular hypertrophy (LVH) is the major risk factor associated with adverse cardiovascular outcomes, including symptomatic heart failure. At the same time and independent of the influence of LVH, patients with elevated plasma renin activity and plasma aldosterone concentration are thought to be at increased risk for adverse cardiovascular events. These seemingly unrelated risk factors may indeed be interrelated when one considers the adverse structural remodeling of the myocardium and cardiovascular system that accompanies primary or secondary mineralocorticoid excess, relative to dietary sodium intake. Clinical and experimental evidence is presented in support of this hypothesis, with a particular emphasis directed toward the pathological accumulation of fibrillar collagen that appears in the myocardium and systemic organs on either a reactive or reparative basis under circumstances of chronic mineralocorticoid excess.

References

1. Kannel WB. Epidemiological aspects of heart failure. Cardiol Clin 1989; 7:1–9.
2. Levy D, Garrison RJ, Savage DD, Kannel WB, Castelli WP. Prognostic implications of echocardiographically determined left-ventricular mass in the Framingham Heart Study. N Engl J Med 1990; 322:1561–1566.
3. Casale PN, Devereux RB, Milner M, Zullo G, Harshfield GA, Pickering TG, et al. Value of echocardiographic measurement of left ventricular mass in predicting cardiovascular morbid events in hypertensive men. Ann Intern Med 1986; 105:173–178.
4. Koren MJ, Devereux RB, Casale PN, Savage DD, Laragh JH. Relation of left ventricular mass and geometry to morbidity and mortality in uncomplicated essential hypertension. Ann Intern Med 1990; 115: 345–352.
5. Cooper RS, Simmons BE, Castaner A, Santhanam V, Ghali J, Mar M. Left ventricular hypertrophy is associated with worse survival independent of ventricular function and number of coronary arteries severely narrowed. Am J Cardiol 1990; 65:441–445.
6. Ghali JK, Kadakia S, Cooper RS, Liao Y. Impact of left ventricular hypertrophy on ventricular arrhythmias in the absence of coronary artery disease. J Am Coll Cardiol 1991; 17:1277–1282.
7. Brunner HR, Laragh JH, Baer L, Newton MA, Goodwin FT, Krakoff LR, et al. Essential hypertension: renin and aldosterone, heart attack and stroke. N Engl J Med 1972; 286:441–449.
8. Alderman MH, Madhaven S, Ooi WL, Cohen H, Sealey JE, Laragh JH. Association of the renin-sodium profile with the risk of myocardial infarction in patients with hypertension. N Engl J Med 1991; 324: 1098–1104.
9. Swedberg K, Eneroth P, Kjekshus J, Wilhelmsen L. Hormones regulating cardiovascular function in patients with severe congestive heart failure and their relation to mortality. CONSENSUS Trial Study Group. Circulation 1990; 82:1730–1736.
10. Weber KT. Cardiac interstitium in health and disease: the fibrillar collagen network. J Am Coll Cardiol 1989; 13:1637–1652.
11. Weber KT, Brilla CG. Pathological hypertrophy and cardiac intersti-

tium: fibrosis and renin-angiotensin-aldosterone system. Circulation 1991; 83:1849–1865.

12. Selye H. The general adaptation syndrome and the diseases of adaptation. J Clin Endocrinol 1946; 6:117–230.

13. Hall CE, Hall O. Hypertension and hypersalimentation. I. aldosterone hypertension. Lab Invest 1965; 14:285–294.

14. Weber KT, Brilla CG, Janicki JS. Structural remodeling of myocardial collagen in systemic hypertension: functional consequences and potential therapy. Heart Failure 1990; 6:129–137.

15. Weber KT, Janicki JS, Shroff SG, Pick R, Abrahams C, Chen RM, et al. Collagen compartment remodeling in the pressure overloaded left ventricle. J Appl Cardiol 1988; 3:37–46.

16. Spach MS, Miller WT III, Dolber PC, Kootsey JM, Sommer JR, Mosher CE Jr. The functional role of structural complexities in the propogation of depolarization in the atrium of the dog. Circ Res 1982; 50:175–191.

17. Strain JE, Grose RM, Factor SM, Fisher JD. Results of endomyocardial biopsy in patients with spontaneous ventricular tachycardia but without apparent structural heart disease. Circulation 1983;68:1171–1181.

18. Sugrue DD, Holmes DR, Gersh BJ, Edwards WD, McLaran CJ, Wood DL, et al. Cardiac histologic findings in patients with life-threatening ventricular arrhythmias of unknown origin. J Am Coll Cardiol 1984; 4:952–957.

19. Darrow DC, Miller HC. The production of cardiac lesions by repeated injections of desoxycorticosterone acetate. J Clin Invest 1942; 21:601–611.

20. Anderson KR, St. John Sutton MG, Lie JT. Histopathological types of cardiac fibrosis in myocardial disease. J Pathol 1979; 128:79–85.

21. Pearlman ES, Weber KT, Janicki JS, Pietra G, Fishman AP. Muscle fiber orientation and connective tissue content in the hypertrophied human heart. Lab Invest 1982; 46:158–164.

22. Huysman JAN, Vliegen HW, VanderLaarse A, Eulderink F. Changes in nonmyocyte tissue composition associated with pressure overload of hypertrophic human hearts. Pathol Res Pract 1989; 184:577–581.

23. Potts JL, Dalakos TG, Streeten DHP, Jones D. Cardiomyopathy in an adult with Bartter's syndrome: hemodynamic, angiographic, and metabolic studies. Am J Cardiol 1977; 40:995–999.

24. Luke JL, Farb A, Virmani R, Sample RHB. Sudden cardiac death during exercise in a weight lifter using anabolic androgenic steroids: pathological and toxicological findings. J Forensic Sci 1990; 35:1441–1447.

25. Campbell SE, Farb A, Weber KT. Pathologic remodeling of the myocardium in a weightlifter taking anabolic steroids. Case report. Blood Pressure 1993; 2:213–216.

26. Skelton FR. The production of hypertension, nephrosclerosis and cardiac lesions by methylandrostenediol treatment in the rat. Endocrinology 1953; 53:492–505.

27. Colby HD, Skelton FR, Brownie AC. Testosterone-induced hypertension in the rat. Endocrinology 1970; 86:1093–1101.

28. Fink CS, Gallant S, Brownie AC. Peripheral serum corticosteroid concentrations in relation to the rat adrenal cortical circadian rhythm in androgen-induced hypertension. Hypertension 1980; 2:617–622.

29. Salgado E, Selye H. The role of the adrenals in the production of cardio-

vascular and renal changes by methylandrostenediol. Arch Int Physiol 1954; 62:352–358.

30. Campbell SE, Diaz-Arias AA, Weber KT. Fibrosis of the human heart and systemic organs in adrenal adenoma. Blood Pressure 1992; 1: 149–156.

31. Shionoiri H, Young SC, Takasaki I, Kihara M, Ishii M. Hypertensive vascular complications in patients with primary aldosteronism [abstract]. In: 17th International Aldosterone Conference. Evansville, Ind.: Meetings and Events Communications, 1991:48.

32. Brilla CG, Pick R, Tan LB, Janicki JS, Weber KT. Remodeling of the rat right and left ventricle in experimental hypertension. Circ Res 1990; 67:1355–1364.

33. Chapman D, Weber KT, Eghbali M. Regulation of fibrillar collagen types I and III and basement membrane type IV collagen gene expression in pressure overloaded rat myocardium. Circ Res 1990; 67:787–794.

34. Lindy S, Turto H, Uitto J. Protocollagen proline hydroxylase activity in rat heart during experimental cardiac hypertrophy. Circ Res 1972; 30:205–209.

35. Morkin E, Ashford TP. Myocardial DNA synthesis in experimental cardiac hypertrophy. Am J Physiol 1968; 215:1409–1413.

36. Moore RD, Schoenberg MD, Koletsky S. Cardiac lesions in experimental hypertension. Arch Pathol 1963; 75:28–44.

37. Brilla CG, Matsubara LS, Weber KT. Anti-aldosterone treatment and the prevention of myocardial fibrosis in primary and secondary hyperaldosteronism. J Mol Cell Cardiol 1993; 25:563–575.

38. Brilla CG, Weber KT. Reactive and reparative myocardial fibrosis in arterial hypertension. Cardiovasc Res 1992; 26:671–677.

39. Campbell SE, Janicki JS, Matsubara BB, Weber KT. Myocardial fibrosis in the rat with mineralocorticoid excess: prevention of microscopic scarring by amiloride. Am J. Hypertens 1993: 6:487–495.

40. Weber KT, Pick R, Silver MA, Moe GW, Janicki JS, Zucker IH, et al. Fibrillar collagen and the remodeling of the dilated canine left ventricle. Circulation 1990; 82:1387–1401.

41. Michel JB, Salzmann JL, Ossondo Nlom M, Bruneval P, Barres D, Camilleri JP. Morphometric analysis of collagen network and plasma perfused capillary bed in the myocardium of rats during evolution of cardiac hypertrophy. Basic Res Cardiol 1986; 81:142–154.

42. Marino TA, Kent RL, Uboh CE, Fernandez E, Thompson EW, Cooper G. Structural analysis of pressure versus volume overload hypertrophy of cat right ventricle. Am J Physiol 1985; 18:H371–H379.

43. Bartosova D, Chvapil M, Korecky B, Poupa O, Rakusan K, Turek Z, et al. The growth of the muscular and collagenous parts of the rat heart in various forms of cardiomegaly. J Physiol 1969; 200:285–295.

44. Buccino RA, Harris E, Spann JF, Sonnenblick EH. Response of myocardial connective tissue to development of experimental hypertrophy. Am J Physiol 1969; 216:425–428.

45. Pfeffer JM, Pfeffer MA, Fishbein MC, Froehlich ED. Cardiac function and morphology with aging in spontaneously hypertensive rat. Am J Physiol 1979; 6:H461–H468.

46. Sen S, Bumpus FM. Collagen synthesis in development and reversal of cardiac hypertrophy in spontaneously hypertensive rats. Am J Cardiol 1979; 44:954–958.

47. Brilla CG, Weber KT. Prevention of myocardial fibrosis and medial thickening of coronary resistance vessels in SHR [abstract]. Circulation 1991; 84:II-738.
48. Narayan S, Janicki JS, Shroff SG, Pick R, Weber KT. Myocardial collagen and mechanics after preventing hypertrophy in hypertensive rats. Am J Hypertens 1989; 2:675–682.
49. Meyer WJ III, Nichols NR. Mineralocorticoid binding in cultured smooth muscle cells and fibroblasts from rat aorta. J Steroid Biochem 1981; 14:1157–1168.
50. Brilla CG, Zhou G, Matsubara L, Weber KT. Collagen metabolism in cultured adult cardiac fibroblasts: response to angiotensin and aldosterone. J Mol Cell Cardiol 1993 (in press).
51. Zhou G, Matsubara L, Brilla CG, Tyagi SC, Weber KT. Angiotensin II and aldosterone regulate collagen turnover in cultured adult rat cardiac fibroblasts [abstract]. J Mol Cell Cardiol 1993; 25(suppl. III):S40.
52. Sano H, Okada H, Kawaguchi H, Yasuda H. Increased angiotensin II-stimulated collagen synthesis in cultured cardiac fibroblasts from spontaneously hypertensive rats [abstract]. Circulation 1991; 84:II-48.
53. Brilla CG, Janicki JS, Weber KT. Cardioreparative effects of lisinopril in rats with genetic hypertension and left ventricular hypertrophy. Circulation 1991; 83:1771–1779.
54. Brilla CG, Janicki JS, Weber KT. Impaired diastolic function and coronary reserve in genetic hypertension: role of interstitial fibrosis and medial thickening of intramyocardial coronary arteries. Circ Res 1991; 69:107–115.

10

Role of the Cardiac Renin-Angiotensin System in Left-Ventricular Hypertrophy

Masahiro Nagano and Toshio Ogihara

Mechanisms of Left-Ventricular Hypertrophy

In patients with hypertension, left-ventricular hypertrophy (LVH) is a common complication and an independent risk factor for morbidity and mortality.[1] An increase of afterload to the left ventricle by the elevation of systemic blood pressure is a major determinant of left-ventricular mass. Casual and ambulatory blood pressures have been reported to correlate with left-ventricular mass assessed by echocardiography.[2,3] However, these correlations were relatively weak,[3] suggesting that elevated blood pressure cannot solely explain the development of LVH. Frohlich[4] discussed two cases of hypertension in patients of the same age and race, similar level and course of high blood pressure, and a similar occupation and family history, but with very different cardiac complications: one patient developed obvious LVH and the other had a normal heart. On the basis of this evidence and his cumulative data, Frohlich proposed a multifactorial model for the development of LVH similar to "Page's mosaic of hypertension".[4] There is much data to support the hypothesis that several factors other than elevated blood pressure contribute to cardiac hypertrophy.[5,6]

Lindpaintner K and Ganten D (editors): *The Cardiac-Renin Angiotensin System,* © Futura Publishing Co., Inc., Armonk, NY, 1994.

The Renin-Angiotensin System and Cardiac Hypertrophy

The renin-angiotensin system (RAS) has been suggested as one of the possible factors contributing to cardiac hypertrophy.[7] In addition to the major physiological role of the RAS in vasoconstriction and stimulation of aldosterone production, recent data have demonstrated that A II stimulates cell proliferation in vascular smooth muscle cells (VSMC).[8] The binding site for A II was demonstrated in the nucleus of myocytes.[9] Infusion of A II analogues increased left-ventricular weight without blood pressure elevation.[10] In the chick heart, A II has been shown to stimulate protein synthesis and cardiac growth directly.[11]

Recently, the extrarenal RAS has been demonstrated in the heart, and its possible role in cardiac hypertrophy was proposed.[12,13] Experimental data from in vivo studies support this hypothesis. Cardiac angiotensinogen mRNA was significantly increased in the left ventricle by pressure overload.[14] Also, mRNA expression and cardiac ACE activity were increased in aortic stenosis.[15] These results suggest that the cardiac RAS is important in cardiac adaptations to pressure overload.

Regression of Cardiac Hypertrophy by ACE Inhibitors

In considering the mechanism of LVH, other lines of research have been directed to examining the role of the RAS in the regression of LVH. Reduction of afterload by antihypertensive drugs may be one of the mechanisms of regression of cardiac hypertrophy, and control of high blood pressure by antihypertensive drugs has been shown to cause reduction of left-ventricular weight. However, even if a similar decrease in blood pressure is achieved, antihypertensive drugs do not cause equal reduction of cardiac mass.[16,17] Therefore, factors other than blood pressure reduction are implicated in the mechanism of regression of LVH.

Regression of cardiac hypertrophy by treatment with ACE inhibitors has been widely demonstrated in humans[18,19] and in animal hypertension models.[20,21] Dahlöf et al.[17] reviewed the 109 studies evaluating the effect of various antihypertensive drugs on LVH in a total of 2,357 patients. This meta-analysis showed that the ratio of left-ventricular mass reduction to blood pressure reduction differed depending on whether the treatments were ACE inhibitors, β-blockers, calcium antagonists, or diuretics, and showed that ACE inhibitors were the most effective.[17] The inhibitory action of ACE inhibitors on the RAS has been suggested as a possible mechanism for their regression of LVH. Kromer and Riegger[22] reported that cardiac hypertrophy induced by coarctation of the ascending aorta was prevented by quinapril. Because pressure overload to the heart persisted during treatment, other factors were strongly suggested as the mechanisms of the regression of hypertrophy. Linz et al.[23] also demonstrated that a subdepressor dose of ramipril caused regression of hypertrophy induced by ligation of the abdominal aorta. Thus, these results indicate that ACE inhibitors have a cardioprotective effect, possibly through the inhibition of the RAS, in addition to their hypotensive activity.

ACE inhibitors suppress cardiac tissue ACE activity.[24,25] We therefore hypothesized that inhibition of the cardiac RAS may account for the regression of hypertrophy by ACE inhibitors. To clarify the direct relation of the cardiac RAS to regression of LVH, we measured tissue A II in the hypertrophied heart of SHR.[26] Chronic oral treatment with either enalapril or trandolapril decreased left-ventricular weight with a parallel reduction of left-ventricular tissue A II (Figure 1). Plasma A II, by contrast, was increased by ACE inhibitors. It has also been demonstrated that long-term treatment with enalapril increased plasma A II, and it has been suggested that

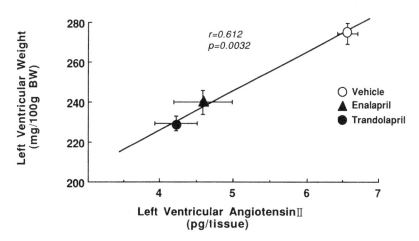

Fig. 1. Relationship between left-ventricular weight and left-ventricular angiotensin II in hearts obtained from SHR treated with ACE inhibitors. Significant positive correlation was observed between their parameters. Mean $\pm$ SE; n = 7 in each group.

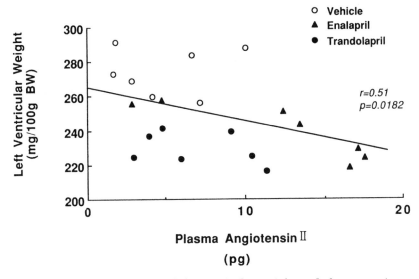

Fig. 2. Relationship between left-ventricular weight and plasma angiotensin II in SHR treated with ACE inhibitors. Left-ventricular weight was inversely correlated with plasma angiotensin II. N = 7 in each group.

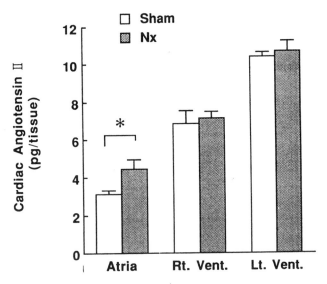

Fig. 3. Cardiac tissue angiotensin II in rats that received sham operation or bilateral nephrectomy. Rt. Vent. = right ventricle; Lt. Vent. = left ventricle; Sham = sham operation; Nx = bilateral nephrectomy; * $p < 0.05$ by unpaired t-test; mean ± SEM; n = 4 in each group.

the actions of ACE inhibitors are independent of their blockade of plasma A II formation.[27] Unexpectedly, plasma A II was inversely correlated with left-ventricular weight after treatment with ACE inhibitors (Figure 2). These results indicate that regression of LVH by ACE inhibitors cannot be explained by their effects on circulating A II. We obtained similar results in SHR treated with spirapril.[28] In SHR, bilateral nephrectomy did not decrease cardiac A II (Figure 3).[28] These results suggest that the cardiac RAS is regulated independently of the RAS in the plasma, and it may be one of the factors accounting for the regression of LVH by ACE inhibitors in SHR.

Isoproterenol–Induced Left–Ventricular Hypertrophy

In another model of cardiac hypertrophy, we investigated the role of cardiac A II in the development and prevention of hypertrophy.[29] Infusion of isoproterenol has been shown to induce cardiac hypertrophy.[30,31] Since isoproterenol does not increase blood pressure, this model of hypertrophy is not mediated by afterload change. In Wistar rats, subcutaneous infusion of isoproterenol (4.2 mg/kg/day) for 7 days increased left-ventricular weight and left-ventricular A II, whereas α-adrenergic stimulation by phenylephrine (3.2 mg/kg/day) did not change either parameters (Figure 4A). In cultured myocytes from the neonatal rat heart, norepinephrine increased protein synthesis, whereas isoproterenol did not.[32] Differences in materials (whether the cultured cells were from the neonate or the in vivo adult heart) may have been the cause of this discrepancy. Xenophontos et al.[33] reported that the elevation of cyclic AMP, the second messenger of the β-adrenoceptor, by forskolin or IBMX (1-methyl-3-isobutylxanthine) stimulated protein synthesis in the adult rat heart. Therefore, it is possible that the α-adrenoceptor has a significant role in cell growth of neonatal myocytes, whereas the β-receptor is more important in the hypertrophy of adult cardiac myocytes. Dzau[34] reported that isoproterenol increased expression of renin mRNA in cardiac myocytes. Therefore, the increase in cardiac tissue A II by β-adrenergic system stimulation may be mediated by renin.

Isoproterenol stimulates renin release from the kidney.[35] Subcutaneous infusion of isoproterenol increased plasma renin activity and A II concentration (Figure 4B). In addition, production of vascular A II was shown to be increased by isoproterenol.[36] Therefore, it is possible that cardiac A II measured in isoproterenol-infused rats originated from the plasma or the vascular tissue in the heart. To

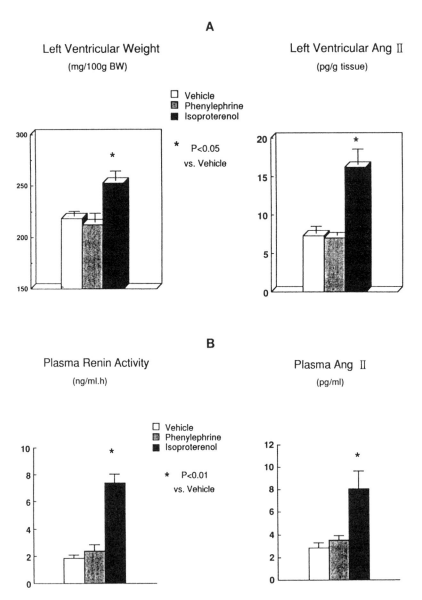

Fig. 4. Effects of subcutaneous infusion of either vehicle (0.9% saline), phenylephrine (3.2 mg/kg/day), or isoproterenol (4.2 mg/kg /day) for 7 days on left-ventricular weight, left-ventricular angiotensin II, plasma renin activity, and plasma angiotensin II. Mean ± SE; n = 6 in each group.

examine this possibility, isoproterenol was infused after bilateral nephrectomy. Plasma renin activity and A II were significantly decreased by nephrectomy (Figure 5A). Isoproterenol did not increase these parameters in anephric rats. In contrast, nephrectomy per se did not decrease cardiac A II (Figure 5B). Isoproterenol increased left-ventricular weight and left-ventricular A II concentration even

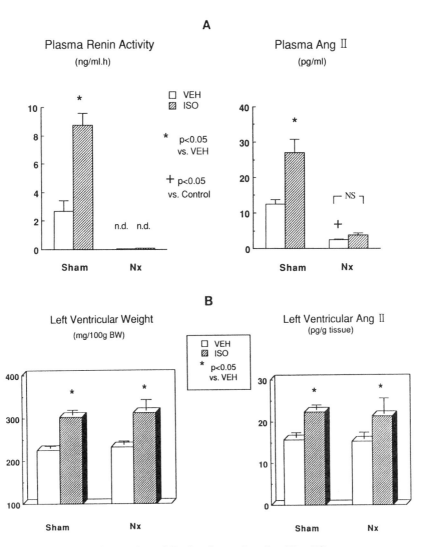

Fig. 5. A and B. See legend under Fig. 5C.

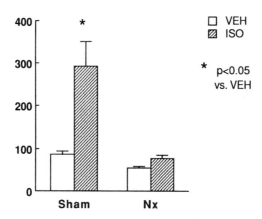

Fig. 5. Effects of bilateral nephrectomy on isoproterenol-induced changes in plasma renin activity, plasma angiotensin II concentration, left-ventricular weight, left-ventricular angiotensin II, and aortic angiotensin II. VEH = vehicle; ISO = isoproterenol; Sham = sham operation; Nx = bilateral nephrectomy; n.d. = not detected; mean ± SE; n = 6 in each group.

in nephrectomized rats, similar to its effects in sham-operated rats (Fig. 5B). In the absence of kidneys, aortic A II concentration was not increased by isoproterenol (Figure 5C). Therefore, these results suggest that (1) circulating and vascular A II are derived from renal renin, (2) synthesis of cardiac A II does not require renal renin, and (3) cardiac A II accounts for the LVH induced by isoproterenol.

Tissue A II levels in the right ventricle and atria were also increased by infusion of isoproterenol but not by phenylephrine (Figure 6). Interestingly, these elevations were not associated with weight changes (Fig. 6). Therefore, the role of tissue A II in the right ventricle and atria may be different from that in the left ventricle. Further research assessing the significance of tissue A II in the right ventricle and atria may demonstrate an alternative pathophysiological role of the cardiac RAS.

The mechanism for the prevention of cardiac hypertrophy by ACE inhibitors was also investigated in chronically isoproterenol-infused rats.[29] Concomitant oral administration of trandolapril itself

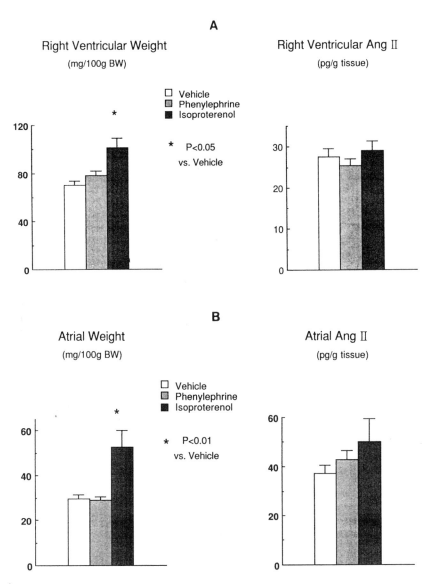

Fig. 6. Weights and angiotensin II concentrations of the right ventricle and atria from Wistar rats treated with either vehicle, phenylephrine, or isoproterenol. Mean ± SE; n = 6 in each group.

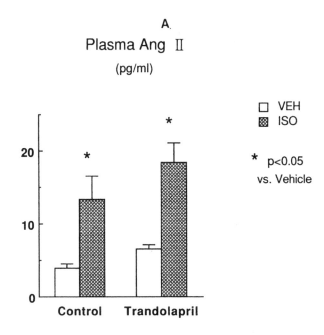

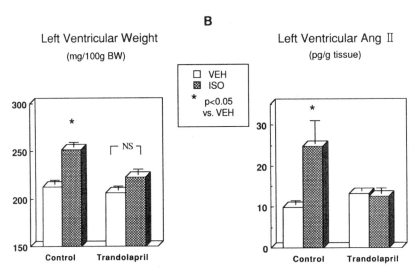

Fig. 7. A and B. See legend under Fig. 7C.

did not affect plasma A II in either vehicle or isoproterenol-infused rats (Figure 7A). However, trandolapril prevented cardiac A II and left-ventricular weight increases by isoproterenol (Figure 7B). These results suggest that trandolapril prevented LVH by suppressing the tissue A II increase by isoproterenol.

Blood pressure was not changed by isoproterenol; however, it was decreased by concomitant administration of trandolapril (Figure 7C). This hypotensive activity may also explain the preventive effect of trandolapril. However, this is unlikely because the addition of hydralazine to isoproterenol decreased blood pressure similarly (Figure 8A) but failed to suppress the increases in left-ventricular weight and cardiac A II by isoproterenol (Figure 8B). From these results, it was concluded that the cardiac tissue RAS partly accounts for the induction of LVH by isoproterenol and its prevention by ACE inhibitors.

We do not think that all types of LVH are explained by the cardiac RAS. We evaluated cardiac A II in LVH of volume-dependent, low-renin hypertensive rats.[37] Five-sixth renal ablation (uninephrectomy plus ablation of the remaining kidney by the upper and lower poles, thus leaving five-sixths of the original renal mass) and sodium load induced hypertension and LVH with low concentrations

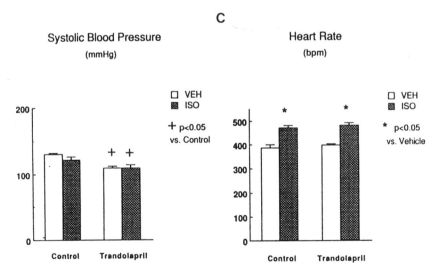

Fig. 7. Effects of concomitant oral administration of trandolapril (3 mg/kg/day) on isoproterenol-induced changes in plasma angiotensin II, left-ventricular weight, left-ventricular angiotensin II, systolic blood pressure, and heart rate. VEH = vehicle; ISO = isoproterenol; mean ± SE; n = 12 in each group.

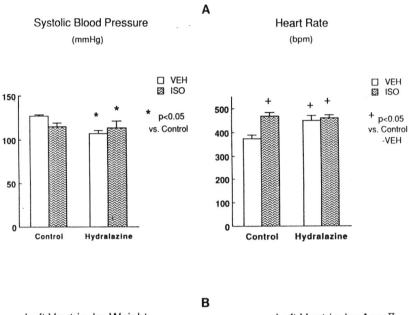

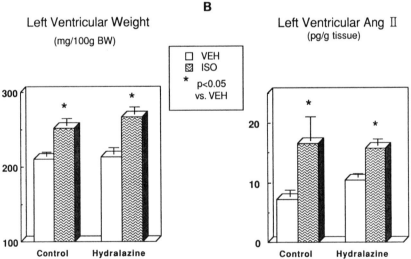

Fig. 8. Effects of concomitant oral administration of hydralazine (8 mg/kg/day) on isoproterenol-induced changes in systolic blood pressure, heart rate, left-ventricular weight, and left-ventricular angiotensin II. VEH = vehicle; ISO = isoproterenol; Mean ± SE; n = 6 in each group.

of A II in plasma and cardiac tissue. Treatment with ACE inhibitors did not decrease blood pressure but prevented LVH. Plasma and left-ventricular A II were not altered by concomitant administration of ACE inhibitors. Therefore, the mechanisms of the progression and the regression of LVH are multifactorial. The cardiac RAS may be one of the factors comprising the "mosaic of left ventricular hypertrophy."[4]

Summary

Several lines of study have provided evidence that the tissue RAS exists in the heart. Angiotensin II (A II), a biologically active peptide of the RAS, has been reported to stimulate protein synthesis in cardiac myocytes, suggesting that cardiac tissue A II plays a significant role in left-ventricular hypertrophy (LVH). To examine this hypothesis, cardiac A II has been measured during the development and regression of hypertrophy. In spontaneously hypertensive rats (SHR), cardiac weight was decreased by administration of angiotensin-converting enzyme (ACE) inhibitors, with a parallel reduction of tissue A II. Bilateral nephrectomy decreased plasma A II but had no effect on cardiac A II. In adult Wistar rats, continuous infusion of isoproterenol resulted in increases of LVH weight and A II concentrations of both plasma and cardiac tissue. Angiotensin II in plasma was significantly decreased by bilateral nephrectomy, whereas A II in tissue was not. In anephric rats, isoproterenol increased left-ventricular weight and tissue A II, similar to the changes in sham-operated rats. In contrast, plasma A II was decreased by nephrectomy, whereas isoproterenol failed to increase plasma A II in nephrectomized rats. Concomitant oral administration of ACE inhibitors prevented the increases in left-ventricular A II and weight by isoproterenol but not the increase by isoproterenol in plasma A II. Hydralazine, on the other hand, did not prevent an A II increase and LVH, despite blood pressure reduction similar to that caused by ACE inhibitors.

Thus, these parallel changes of cardiac weight and tissue A II suggest that the cardiac RAS accounts for the mechanism of development and regression of LVH.

References

1. Levy D, Garrison RJ, Savage DD, Kannel WB, Castelli WP. Prognostic implications of echocardiographically determined left ventricular mass

in the Framingham Heart Study. New Engl J Med 1990; 322: 1561–1566.

2. Drayer JIM, Weber MA, De Young JL. Blood pressure as a determinant of cardiac left ventricular muscle mass. Arch Intern Med 1983; 143: 90–92.

3. Devereux RB, Pickering TG, Harshfield GA, et al. Left ventricular hypertrophy in patients with hypertension: importance of blood pressure response to regularly recurring stress. Circulation 1983; 68:470–476.

4. Frohlich ED. The heart in hypertension: a 1991 overview. Hypertension 1991; 18[suppl III]:III-62–III-68.

5. Frohlich ED, Tarazi RC. Is arterial pressure the sole factor responsible for hypertensive cardiac hypertrophy? Am J Cardiol 1979; 44:959–963.

6. Dahlöf B. Factors involved in the pathogenesis of hypertensive cardiovascular hypertrophy. Drugs 1988; 35(suppl 5):6–26.

7. Devereux RB, Pickering TG, Cody RJ, Laragh JH. Relation of renin-angiotensin system activity to left ventricular hypertrophy and function in experimental and human hypertension. J Clin Hypertens 1987; 3: 87–103.

8. Geisterfer AAT, Peach MJ, Owens GK. Angiotensin II induces hypertrophy, not hyperplasia, of cultured rat aortic smooth muscle cells. Circ Res 1988; 62:749–756.

9. Robertson Jr AL, Khairallah PA. Angiotensin II: rapid localization in nuclei of smooth and cardiac muscle. Science 1971; 172:1138–1139.

10. Sen S, Tarazi C, Bumpus FM. Cardiac effects of angiotensin antagonists in normotensive rats. Clin Sci 1979; 56:439–443.

11. Kato Y, Komoro I, Shibasaki Y, Yamaguchi H, Yazaki Y. Angiotensin II induced hypertrophy and oncogene expression in cultured rat heart myocyte. (abstract) Circulation 1989; 80(suppl II):II-450.

12. Dzau VJ. Cardiac renin-angiotensin system. Am J Med 1988; 84(suppl 3A):22–27.

13. Lindpaintner K, Ganten D. The cardiac renin-angiotensin system. Circ Res 1991; 68:905–921.

14. Baker KM, Chernin MI, Wixson SK, Aceto JF. Renin-angiotensin system involvement in pressure-overload cardiac hypertrophy in rats. Am J Physiol 1990; 259:H324–H332.

15. Schunkert H, Dzau VM, Tang SS, Hirsch A, Apstein CS, Lorell BH. Increased rat cardiac angiotensin converting enzyme activity and mRNA expression in pressure overload left ventricular hypertrophy. J Clin Invest 1990; 86:1913–1920.

16. Balogum MO, Dunn FG. Regression of left ventricular hypertrophy in patients with hypertension. J Human Hypertens 1990; 4(suppl 4): 29–34.

17. Dahlöf B, Pennert K, Hansson L. Reversal of left ventricular hypertrophy in hypertensive patients. A metaanalysis of 109 treatment studies. Am J Hypertens 1992; 5:95–110.

18. Nakashima Y, Fouad FM, Tarazi RC. Regression of left ventricular hypertrophy from systemic hypertension. Am J Cardiol 1984; 53: 1044–1049.

19. Nagano N, Iwatsubo H, Hata T, Mikami H, Ogihara T. Effects of antihypertensive treatment on cardiac hypertrophy and cardiac function in elderly hypertensive patients. J Cardiovasc Pharmacol 1991; 17(suppl 2):S163–S165.

20. Sen S, Bumpus FM. Collagen synthesis in development and reversal of cardiac hypertrophy in spontaneously hypertensive rats. Am J Cardiol 1979; 44:954–958.

21. Sen S, Tarazi RC, Bumpus FM. Effect of converting enzyme inhibitor (SQ 14,225) on myocardial hypertrophy in spontaneously hypertensive rats. Hypertension 1980; 2:169–176.

22. Kromer EP, Riegger GAJ. Effects of long-term angiotensin converting enzyme inhibition on myocardial hypertrophy in experimental aortic stenosis in the rat. Am J Cardiol 1988; 62:161–163.

23. Linz W, Scholkens BA, Ganten D. Converting enzyme inhibition specifically prevents the development and induces regression of cardiac hypertrophy in rats. Clin Exp Hypertens [A] 1989; A11:1325–1350.

24. Chevillard C, Brown NL, Mathieu M-N, Laliberte F, Worcel M. Differential effects of oral trandolapril and enalapril on rat tissue angiotensin-converting enzyme. Eur J Pharmacol 1988; 147:23–28.

25. Chevillard C, Brown NL, Jouquey S, Mathieu M-N, Laliberte F, Hamon G. Cardiovascular actions and tissue-converting enzyme inhibitory effects of chronic enalapril and trandolapril treatment of spontaneously hypertensive rats. J Cardiovasc Pharmacol 1989; 14:297–301.

26. Nagano M, Higaki J, Mikami H, et al. Converting enzyme inhibitors regressed cardiac hypertrophy and reduced tissue angiotensin II in spontaneously hypertensive rats. J Hypertens 1991; 9:595–599.

27. Mento PF, Wilkes BM. Plasma angiotensins and blood pressure during converting enzyme inhibition. Hypertension 1987; 9[suppl III]:III-42–III-48.

28. Nagano M, Higaki J, Ogihara T, et al. Role of cardiac angiotensin II in left ventricular hypertrophy in spontaneously hypertensive rats. J Vasc Med Biol 1993; 4:64–70.

29. Nagano M, Higaki J, Nakamura F, et al. Role of cardiac angiotensin II in isoproterenol-induced left ventricular hypertrophy. Hypertension 1992; 19:708–712.

30. Stanton HC, Brenner G, Mayfield ED. Studies on isoproterenol-induced cardiomegaly in rats. Am Heart J 1969; 7:72–80.

31. Pagano VT, Inchiosa Jr MA. Cardiomegaly produced by chronic beta-adrenergic stimulation in the rat: comparison with alpha-adrenergic effects. Life Sci 1977; 21:619–624.

32. Simpson P. Norepinephrine-stimulated hypertrophy of cultured rat myocardial cells is an alpha adrenergic response. J Clin Invest 1983; 72:732–738.

33. Xenophontos XP, Watson PA, Chua BHL, Haneda T, Morgan HE. Increased cyclic AMP content accelerates protein synthesis in rat heart. Circ Res 1989; 65:647–656.

34. Dzau VJ. Cardiac renin-angiotensin system: molecular and functional aspects. Am J Med 1988; 84(suppl 3A): 22–27.

35. Ganong WF. Sympathetic effects on renin secretion: mechanism and physiological role. In: Control of Renin Secretion. New York: Plenum Press, 1972, 17–32.

36. Nakamaru M, Jackson EK, Inagami T. β-adrenoceptor-mediated release of angiotensin II from mesenteric arteries. Am J Physiol 1986; 250:H144–H148.

37. Nakamura F, Nagano M, Higaki J, et al. Regression of left ventricular hypertrophy by angiotensin-converting enzyme inhibitor in reduced renal mass hypertensive rats. J Hypertens 1991; 9(suppl 6):S398–S399.

11

Induction of the Cardiac Angiotensin-Converting Enzyme in Pressure-Overload Hypertrophy: Implications for Diastolic Function

Beverly H. Lorell and Heribert Schunkert

Introduction

Pressure-overload hypertrophy is the biological response to increased load imposed on cardiac muscle cells. The hypertrophic process is initiated by induction of early intermediate genes such as proto-oncogenes and stimulation of protein synthesis in the cardiac myocyte. Macroscopically, this adaptation is characterized by left-ventricular remodeling in which concentric thickening of the left-ventricular walls develops with minimal cavity dilatation. Pressure-overload hypertrophy is also characterized by coordinated changes in gene expression that recapitulate fetal gene programming and appear to promote a slower rate of systolic myofiber shortening at an efficient myocardial economy.[1-3] However, pressure-overload hypertrophy is also associated with impaired diastolic function characterized by the slowing of left-ventricular relaxation and a decrease in left-ventricular chamber distensibility.[4,5] Diastolic dysfunction in advanced cardiac hypertrophy may be due, in part, to changes in

Lindpaintner K and Ganten D (editors): *The Cardiac-Renin Angiotensin System,* © Futura Publishing Co., Inc., Armonk, NY, 1994.

gene expression that modify and prolong the availability of intracellular calcium to the myofibers for crossbridge cycling.[6-8] In addition, gene reprogramming in cardiac hypertrophy may result in increased cardiac ACE activity and local synthesis of A II. The aim of this chapter is to review recent experiments that examine the physiological role of local cardiac A II and its inhibition by ACE on diastolic dysfunction in the hypertrophied heart.[9-13]

Cardiac ACE and Cardiac Physiology

ACE is a peptidase that is intimately involved in the metabolism of a whole group of peptides and substances regulating cardiac and vascular function.[14] First, ACE facilitates the cleavage of A I to generate the active metabolite A II, which acts as a regulator of cardiovascular homeostasis. In addition, A II controls the activity of the RAS by feedback regulation[15] and mediates norepinephrine release.[16] However, ACE is also involved in the metabolism of bradykinin that, in part, acts through formation of prostacyclin and nitric oxide (EDRF).[17] The enzyme is identical with kininase II, which is involved in bradykinin metabolism by liberating the C-terminal dipeptide phenylalanyl-arginine.[14]

Recent experiments support the existence of a tissue RAS in the heart. ACE, angiotensinogen, renin, and A II receptors have been localized in cardiac tissue using techniques of protein biochemistry and molecular biology.[18,19] Furthermore, A II receptors[20,21] and at least two receptor subtypes have been identified and are currently being characterized in myocardial tissue. The intracardiac conversion of A I to A II has also been shown in isolated perfused hearts.[9,22] The physiological actions of cardiac A II activation are still not understood and may include the modulation of excitation-contraction-relaxation coupling as well as cardiac myocyte and vascular cell growth.[1,22,23]

Material and Methods

To study the role of the cardiac RAS in adaptive LVH, we employed the experimental model of chronic aortic stenosis by banding of the ascending aorta in weanling male Wistar rats.[9]

The hearts of the LVH and sham groups were studied with molecular biological techniques for the analysis of cardiac ACE mRNA.

Cardiac RNA was extracted and further purified for polyadenylate (poly A)$_1$ sequenced by oligo (Dt)-cellulose columns. RNA was then run on an agarose gel, transblotted, and hybridized with a human ACE cDNA. For measurement of ACE activity, biochemical studies were performed using a synthetic ACE substrate and a fluorimetric assay first described by Cushman and Cheung.[24]

To analyze the functional implications of the cardiac RAS, another subgroup of hearts was studied in a buffer-perfused isovolumic heart apparatus under normothermic conditions. To assess left-ventricular contractility and relaxation, a collapsed latex balloon, slightly larger than the left-ventricular chamber, was inserted into the left ventricle via a left-atrial incision. The balloon was filled with bubble-free saline and attached to a fluid-filled pressure transducer or to a micromanometer. Coronary perfusion pressure was measured via a Y-shaped connector attached to the aortic infusion cannula. In this preparation, changes in left-ventricular diastolic pressure relative to constant balloon volume are a measure of left-ventricular diastolic chamber distensibility, whereas isovolumic relaxation is assessed by -dp/dt and the time constant, τ, of left-ventricular pressure decay.[25,26]

The intracardiac conversion of A I to A II was studied by quantification of the peptides in the coronary effluent after perfusion of the isolated heart with A I. The perfusates were subjected to high-performance liquid chromatography (HPLC) and radioimmunoassay (RIA). The conversion rate was calculated as A II/A II + II [M] × 100 = %.

Induction of Cardiac ACE and Implications for Cardiac Function

Eight weeks after surgical intervention, banding of the ascending aorta resulted in slightly lower body weights at sacrifice as compared with sham-operated controls (218 g vs. 243 g; $p < 0.16$). The ratio of left-ventricular weight to body weight was significantly higher in aortic-banded animals (LVH) as compared with shams (3.6 vs. 2.6 g/kg; $p < 0.005$).

Using a fluorimetric assay, cardiac ACE activity was significantly higher in tissue obtained from several regions of the left ventricle, whereas there was no difference in tissue ACE activity of the nonhypertrophied right ventricle between the aortic-banded and control groups.[9] Thus, the amplified left-ventricular ACE activity did not appear to be related to the altered activity of the systemic

RAS but was related to the magnitude and site of pressure-overload stress. Northern blot analyses showed the presence of ACE mRNA in left-ventricular tissue from both the aortic banded and control groups. However, there was induction of cardiac ACE mRNA expression in the aortic-banded group, which was increased fourfold in comparison with the control group (Figure 1).

The effects of the amplified cardiac conversion of A I to A II on cardiac function were also studied. Coronary flow was adjusted to achieve similar levels of flow per gram in the aortic-banded and control hearts, and left-ventricular balloon volume was adjusted to achieve a level of left-ventricular end-diastolic pressure (LVEDP) of

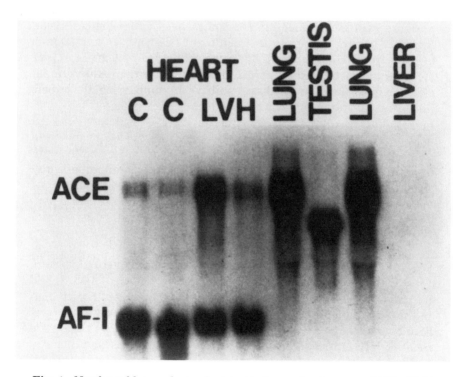

Fig. 1. Northern blot analysis of rat testicular and pulmonary ACE mRNA and cardiac mRNA from left-ventricular tissue obtained from the LVH and control groups. The blot was hybridized with an oligolabeled human ACE cDNA. Using 25 mg poly(A)$^+$ RNA, all hearts gave a clear signal. This demonstrates the local expression of ACE mRNA in the rat heart. Furthermore, the signal from tissues of the LVH group hearts is increased relative to the controls. Anglerfish insulin mRNA (AF-1) served as a recovery marker. (from Schunkert H, et al.[9]).

10 mm Hg in both groups and then held constant. At this operational point on the diastolic pressure-volume relation of these animals, left-ventricular volumes were similar in both groups. In the hearts of aortic-banded rats that were studied at a stage of compensatory hypertrophy, left-ventricular systolic-developed pressure per unit of left-ventricular mass and $+dP/dt$ were not depressed and were actually higher in the hypertrophy group compared with the control group. In the isolated perfused hearts, A I was infused to measure the intracardiac fractional conversion of A I to A II and its effects on left-ventricular function. In the isolated beating hypertrophied hearts, the intracardiac fractional conversion to A II was significantly higher in the hypertrophied hearts ($17.3 \pm 4.1\%$ vs. $6.8 \pm 1.3\%$; $p < 0.01$). The intracardiac activation of A II caused a similar dose-dependent increase in coronary vascular tone in both groups. Angiotensin II activation had no significant effect on indices of systolic contractility in either group in these hearts that were studied at a physiological heart rate and perfusate calcium concentration.

In the control hearts, intracardiac A II activation had minimal effect on diastolic chamber distensibility.[9] In comparison, the hypertrophied hearts showed a dose-dependent depression of left-ventricular diastolic relaxation and a decrease in diastolic chamber distensibility during A I infusion (Figure 2). Angiotensin I infusion caused a similar dose-related increase in coronary vascular tone in both groups, whereas the deleterious effect of A I infusion on both diastolic relaxation and diastolic chamber distensibility was observed only in the hypertrophied hearts. Preliminary studies of A II receptor affinity and density in hypertrophied left-ventricular tissue from rats with aortic banding have demonstrated a lower receptor density and no change in affinity compared with sham-operated control hearts.[9] An alternate explanation for the differential response of coronary reactivity and diastolic properties in the hypertrophied and normal hearts may be that the major site of increased A II activation in the hypertrophied heart is at the location of the cardiac myocytes rather than the cardiac microvasculature. Further study is needed regarding the cellular sites of cardiac angiotensin activation.

In this experiment, it was not resolved whether the effects of A II activation on diastolic function in hypertrophied hearts were simply related to a higher local availability of A II or to a differing functional response to A II in comparison with control hearts. Recent preliminary studies from our laboratory have examined the direct effects of equivalent doses of A II in this model of hypertrophied and control rat hearts.[27] The hypertrophied and control hearts were studied under baseline conditions of similar coronary flow per gram

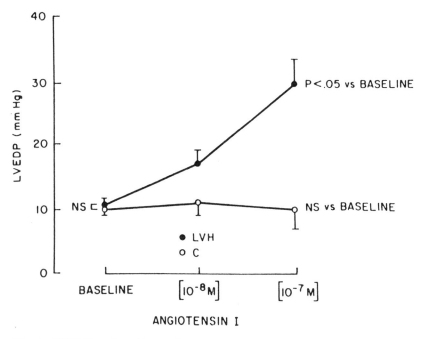

Fig. 2. LVEDP at baseline and in response to angiotensin I infusion in the LVH and control groups. There was no change in LVEDP in the control group in response to angiotenesin I infusion. However, in response to angiotensin I infusion and its intracardiac activation to angiotensin II, there was a marked dose-related increase in isovolumic LVEDP in the LVH group. (from Schunkert H, et al.[9]).

and an identical level of isovolumic LVEDP. The infusion of 10^{-8}M A II caused a mild increase of coronary vascular tone (20% increase relative to baseline) with no significant effect on left-ventricular developed pressure, myocardial adenosine triphosphate (ATP) levels, or aerobic metabolism in the hypertrophied and control hearts. The equivalent concentration of A II altered diastolic function in both groups. However, the rise in isovolumic LVEDP was significantly higher in the hypertrophied versus the control hearts. Isovolumic LVEDP was also more marked when normalized for left-ventricular mass and was associated with a greater slowing of relaxation in comparison with the control hearts. Thus, these data suggest that rat hearts with pressure-overload hypertrophy develop more severe diastolic dysfunction in response to A II, in addition to an enhanced capacity for induction of cardiac ACE and increased local conversion of A II.

Does ACE Mediate the Cardiac Generation of Angiotensin II in the Hypertrophied Heart?

The activity of cardiac ACE appears to be increased in other experimental models of cardiac remodeling and hypertrophy as well. Hirsch and coworkers[28] and Jackson and coworkers[29] have recently studied tissue-specific activation of the cardiac RAS in an experimental model of hypertrophy and heart failure due to late cardiac remodeling following myocardial infarction in male rats. Drexler and coworkers have previously shown that the rat model of myocardial infarction is associated with a transient increase in the expression of cardiac angiotensinogen soon after experimental infarction that normalizes later in the chronic failure state.[30]. Hirsch and coworkers studied hearts in the state of compensated heart failure approximately 85 days after experimental coronary ligation.[28] In this model of postinfarct hypertrophy and heart failure, plasma renin concentrations and serum ACE activities were not different between experimental failure and control animals. However, the animals with chronic failure due to postinfarction remodeling were characterized by increased cardiac ACE activity and the expression of ACE messenger RNA compared with sham-operated control animals. These investigations as well as our studies suggest that ACE may be the critical enzyme for cardiac A II generation. In a recent study of cardiac membrane preparation from human hearts, a non-ACE chymase peptidase has been shown to catalyze A II generation in an in vitro preparation.[31] This non-ACE peptidase is not inhibited by specific ACE inhibitors and could possibly catalyze the local activation of A I to A II in the aortic-banded rat model.

To address this, we have performed studies to determine the relative role of ACE on the enhanced A II activation and its effects on cardiac function in the aortic-banded rat heart.[12] In vitro autoradiography experiments showed increased ACE density in the myocardium of hypertrophied versus control hearts. In addition, the isolated beating aortic-banded and control hearts were perfused with A I in the presence of parallel infusion of enalaprilat. In this preliminary report,[12] the intracardiac fractional conversion of A I to A II was higher in the hypertrophied hearts than in the control hearts. Furthermore, the coinfusion of enalaprilat and A I inhibited A I to A II conversion in the hypertrophied hearts by about 70%. These experimental data lend support to the idea that the major pathway for the intracardiac conversion of A I to A II in this hypertrophy rat model is via the A II-converting enzyme (ACE).

In this study, the coinfusion of A I and enalaprilat prevented the increase in coronary vascular tone induced in hearts treated with A I alone. This experiment confirmed the earlier finding that A I infusion impaired diastolic function in the hypertrophied hearts. However, hypertrophied hearts perfused with both enalaprilat and A I showed no adverse change in diastolic function. These observations support the hypothesis that specific ACE inhibition decreases the exaggerated intracardiac activation of A II and prevents its detrimental actions on diastolic function in the hypertrophied rat heart. Further work is needed to clarify the angiotensin receptor subtypes that mediate the actions of A II on coronary vasomotor tone as well as on excitation-contraction-relaxation coupling in hypertrophied hearts. Tests using experimental AT_1 and AT_2 receptor subtype blockers to look at this question are in progress.

Angiotensin and Ischemic Diastolic Dysfunction in Hypertrophied Hearts

Enhanced local A II generation in the hypertrophied heart may also modify the response of the hypertrophied heart to ischemia and reperfusion. Previous clinical studies from our laboratory[32] and experiments in hypertrophied hearts[13,25,26,33] and myocytes[34] have shown that the hypertrophied heart has an impaired capacity to maintain normal diastolic relaxation in response to both constant flow hypoxia, low-flow ischemia, and metabolic inhibition. The susceptibility of the hypertrophied heart to develop ischemic diastolic dysfunction has been reported by others.[35,36]

Mochizuki and coworkers in our laboratory have shown that A II exacerbates ischemic diastolic dysfunction in isovolumic red cell-perfused rabbit hearts.[37] Low-flow ischemia was induced by reducing coronary perfusion pressure to 15 mm Hg, and hearts were studied in the presence and absence of perfusion with A II at baseline and during the period of low-flow ischemia. Whereas the level of ischemic coronary flow was comparable in both groups at the onset of ischemia, the A II-treated hearts showed a further progressive reduction of coronary flow during ischemia. Thus, an increased local cardiac availability of A II may adversely affect coronary vasomotor regulation during an ischemic insult. In additional hearts, the direct actions of A II on left-ventricular contractility and relaxation were studied under conditions of matched levels of reduced coronary flow per gram during the 30-minute period of low-flow ischemia. Under the condition of matched levels of ischemic flow in the angiotensin-treated and no-drug groups, the ischemic depression of left-ventricular developed pressure, reduction of myocardial ATP, and aerobic lactate production were comparable. In contrast, the ischemic depression of myocardial relaxation and the rise in isovolumic LVEDP was significantly greater in the angiotensin-treated hearts, and recovery of normal diastolic function during reperfusion was incomplete in the angiotensin group. These recent experiments suggest the concept that A II directly impairs left-ventricular diastolic function during the imposition of transient low-flow ischemia and limits recovery during reperfusion.

The finding of adverse actions of A II on ischemic diastolic dysfunction in normal hearts raised the issue of whether the exaggerated ischemic diastolic dysfunction, which is characteristic of hypertrophied hearts, can be influenced by local cardiac ACE inhibition. A recent study by Eberli and coworkers showed that specific ACE inhibition selectively modifies ischemic diastolic dysfunction in hypertrophied hearts.[33] Isolated isovolumic red-cell-perfused control and hypertrophied rat hearts were subjected to 30 minutes of low-flow ischemia and 30 minutes of reperfusion. Subsets of hypertrophied and control hearts received enalaprilat perfusion at baseline and during the low-flow ischemia and reperfusion periods. By experimental design, coronary flow per gram was comparable in the hypertrophy and control groups at baseline and during ischemia and reperfusion. Cardiac ACE inhibition with enalaprilat had no effect on systolic function during ischemia or reperfusion. Consistent with prior observations, the ischemic depression of diastolic distensibility during low-flow ischemia was more severe in the hypertrophied versus control hearts in the absence of ACE inhibition. Enalaprilat infusion had no effect on ischemic diastolic function or its recovery in the normal hearts. However, enalaprilat prevented the exaggerated ischemic diastolic dysfunction in the hypertrophied hearts (Figure 3). This effect was not attributed to differing ischemic lactate production and washout, myocardial ATP depletion, or tissue-glycogen levels, which were similar in all groups. These observations support the hypothesis that cardiac ACE inhibition has a favorable effect on ischemic diastolic failure in hypertrophied hearts.

A beneficial effect of ACE inhibition on ischemia-reperfusion injury has been seen by others.[38-41] In these experiments, the beneficial actions of ACE inhibition during ischemia and reperfusion could

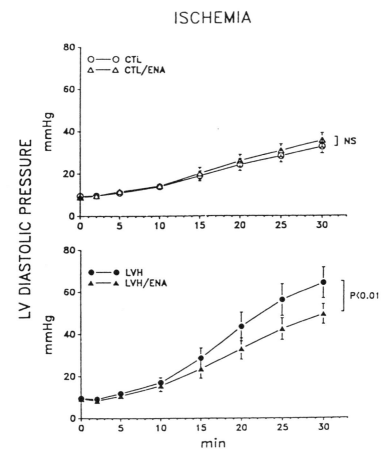

Fig. 3. Graphs showing LVEDP for untreated and enalaprilat- treated, non-hypertrophied age-matched control hearts (CTL and CTL/ENA) in the upper panel and untreated and enalaprilat-treated hypertrophied hearts (LVH and LVH/ENA) in the lower panel. LVEDP increased to a significant higher level in hypertrophied hearts than in nonhypertrophied hearts in either untreated hearts (LVH versus CTL; $p < 0.01$) or enalaprilat-treated hearts (LVH/ENA versus CTL/ENA; $p < 0.01$). Enalaprilat had no effect in nonhypertrophied hearts, but it attenuated the greater increase in LVEDP in hypertrophied hearts ($p < 0.01$) (from Eberli FR, et al.[33]).

be related to multiple factors such as reduced bradykinin degradation, the inhibition of angiotensin-induced norepinephrine release, induction of prostaglandin synthesis, and antifree radical effect of the specific ACE inhibitor that was used. Taken together, these studies suggest that ACE inhibition may protect against ischemia-reperfusion arrhythmias, whereas the untreated hearts showed longer episodes of ventricular fibrillation. In these studies, any favorable effect of ACE inhibition on postischemic recovery of cardiac function may have been confounded by the indirect effect of limiting energy-costly fibrillation and arrhythmias rather than a direct myocardial effect. Eberli's study[33] avoided the confounding influence of fibrillation on myocardial metabolism and function by eliminating hearts with ventricular fibrillation from the study.

Possible Mechanisms

Advanced cardiac hypertrophy is characterized by prolongation of the calcium transient and slowed diastolic myofilament calcium-sensitive force inactivation.[42,43] This disturbance of calcium regulation appears to be related in part to a reduced density of calcium ATPase pumps and the slowed reuptake of calcium by the sarcoplasmic reticulum.[2,6–8] The alteration in myocardial calcium homeostasis may be a compensatory adaptation under basal, well-oxygenated conditions, which would promote a longer duration and magnitude of systolic force development in the presence of an increased load. However, this adaptation also results in a very fragile calcium homeostasis in the hypertrophied heart since the lusitropic reserve for maintaining normal calcium uptake and relaxation is impaired during the imposition of ischemia, which further blunts calcium reuptake and elevates diastolic calcium levels.[44,45]

The deleterious actions of A II on diastolic function in hypertrophied hearts may be mediated by the interplay of angiotensin's effects on myocardial calcium handling and the intrinsic changes in calcium regulation in hypertrophied myocytes. The subcellular signaling of A II appears to be partially mediated by the activation of phosphoinositide second messengers.[46,47] The actions of A II on excitation-contraction-relaxation in neonatal rat heart myocytes can be simulated by phorbol ester activation of protein kinase C.[48] Angiotensin II-induced phosphoinositide hydrolysis stimulates the production of two metabolites. Inositol triphosphate may promote calcium release from the sarcoplasmic reticulum,[49] which is reported to be enhanced in hypertrophied hearts.[50] Phosphoinositide hydrolysis also promotes formation of diacylglycerol and protein kinase C. Protein kinase C may depress calcium transport by the sarcoplasmic reticulum and may promote the phosphorylation of the sarcolemmal sodium-proton antiporter causing intracellular alkalinization and enhanced myofilament calcium sensitivity. Recent studies in our laboratory suggest that the effects of A II infusion on contractility and relaxation may be predominantly mediated by intracellular alkalinization and alteration in myofilament calcium responsiveness.[51] The intracellular signaling of A II in the heart appears to be remarkably analogous to endothelin, whose intracellular signaling appears to be mediated by alkalinization induced by protein kinase C activation that alters myofilament calcium sensitivity.[52]

Neyses and coworkers have studied the actions of A II on isolated cardiac myocytes from hypertensive SHR and normotensive WKY rats.[53] They observed that A II caused a shift in the relationship for calcium and contractility, indicating a greater calcium sensitivity in hypertrophied myocytes.[53] Furthermore, studies from our laboratory suggest that the effects of angiotensin on diastolic function in rats with pressure-overload hypertrophy are simulated by protein kinase C activation with phorbol ester and can be attenuated by amiloride, an inhibitor of sodium-proton exchange.[10,11] The actions of A II on intracellular cation regulation and diastolic relaxation are very complex; they may differ between species and may be mediated by multiple signaling pathways. Additional studies are needed to clarify the intracellular signaling pathways that mediate the actions of A II in experimental animal models and in humans with hypertrophy and failure.

Conclusion

ACE appears to be the major enzyme activating A I to A II in the rat experimental model of pressure-overload hypertrophy. The peptide A II has multiple local actions including vasoconstriction and positive inotropy in some species. Furthermore, A II can promote deterioration of diastolic function of the ventricle, in particular when pressure-overload LVH is evident. In addition, cardiac ACE inhibition has a favorable effect on the exaggerated diastolic dysfunction that is characteristic of the hypertrophied heart during ischemic stress. Inhibition of cardiac ACE may attenuate the functional changes seen after intracardiac A I administration. Ongoing clinical studies are testing the efficacy of ACE inhibitors in the treatment of diastolic dysfunction in patients with advanced LVH.[54]

Acknowledgements

   The assistance of Ms. Barbara Zillman in preparation of the manuscript is greatly appreciated.

Summary

Systemic infusion of A II in patients with coronary artery disease or normal control subjects can cause an increase in systolic pressure, or left-ventricular pressure (LVP), and left-ventricular end-diastolic pressure (LVEDP). In this clinical setting, A II produces an increase in both afterload and preload that makes it difficult to discriminate possible local myocardial effects of the peptide. The studies summarized in the present paper were designed to examine the physiological role of local cardiac A II generation and local bradykinin degradation within the heart. Therefore, the effects of A I, A II, bradykinin, and ACE inhibition on cardiac function were studied in the normal and hypertrophied rat heart. Angiotensin I and A II, infused in isolated, well-oxygenated, buffer-perfused normal rat hearts, produced a mild increase in LVEDP with no change in systolic function. In contrast, in isolated perfused hypertrophied rat hearts, A I and A II caused a marked deterioration of diastolic function, evident as an increase in LVEDP at constant volume and a slowing of left-ventricular relaxation. There was no significant difference in metabolism or coronary perfusion rate per gram between the normal and hypertrophied rat hearts, which might account for the effects of angiotensin on LVEDP. Instead, preliminary evidence suggests that A II effects on diastolic function are mediated via a protein kinase C dependent pathway that might involve Na^+-H^+ exchange. When cardiac ACE was blocked by infusion of an ACE inhibitor prior and in parallel to A I infusion, no changes in diastolic function were noted. Bradykinin infusion or prevention of bradykinin breakdown by ACE inhibition, on the other hand, had no effect on diastolic function in isolated normal oxygenated rat or rabbit hearts, despite causing a mild vasodilation. In summary, these studies suggest that cardiac A II activation may promote deterioration of cardiac relaxation in rat hearts with established LVH. ACE inhibition, on the other hand, may improve diastolic function in the setting of ischemia or cardiac hypertrophy in the presence of an activated RAS.

References

1. Morgan HE, Baker KM. Cardiac hypertrophy: mechanical, neural, and endocrine dependence. Circulation 1991; 83:13–25.

2. Schwartz K, Mercardier J-J, Swynghedauw B, Lompre A-M. Modifications in gene expression in cardiac hypertrophy. Heart F 1988; 4: 154–163.
3. Izumo S, Nadal-Ginard B, Mahdavi V. Proto-oncogene induction in reprogramming of cardiac gene expression produced by pressure overload. Proc Natl Acad Sci 1988; 85:339–343.
4. Lorell BH. Significance of diastolic dysfunction of the heart. Ann Rev Med 1991; 42:411–436.
5. Peterson KL, Tsugi J, Johnson A, et al. Diastolic left ventricular pressure-volume and stress-strain relations in patients with valvular aortic stenosis and left ventricular hypertrophy. Circulation 1978; 58:77–90.
6. De la Bastie D, Levitsky DD, Rappaport L, Mercardier JJ, Marotte F, Wisnewsky C, et al. Function of the sarcoplasmic reticulum and expression of its Ca^{2+}-ATPase gene in pressure overload induced cardiac hypertrophy in the rat. Circ Res 1990; 66:554–564.
7. Mercadier J-J, Lompré A-M, Duc P, Boheler KR, Fragsse J-B, Wisnewsky C, et al. Altered sarcoplasmic reticulum Ca^{2+}-ATPase gene expression in the human ventricle during end-stage heart failure. J Clin Invest 1990; 85:305–309.
8. Gwanthmey JK, Copelas L, MacKinnon R, Schoen FJ, Feldman MD, Grossman W, et al. Abnormal intracellular calcium handling in myocardium from patients with end-stage heart failure. Circ Res 1987; 61: 70–76.
9. Schunkert H, Dzau VJ, Tang SS, Hirsch AT, Apstein C, Lorell B. Increased rat cardiac angiotensin-converting enzyme activity and mRNA levels in pressure overload left ventricular hypertrophy: effects on coronary resistance, contractility and relaxation. J Clin Invest 1990; 86: 1913–1920.
10. Mochizuki T, Schunkert H, Ngoy S, Apstein CS, Lorell BH. The effects of angiotensin on pressure-overload hypertrophy are simulated by protein kinase C activation. Circulation 1991; 84 (suppl. II):II-308.
11. Mochizuki T, Weinberg E, Apstein CS, Schunkert H, Lorell BH. Impairment of diastolic function by angiotensin II in pressure overload hypertrophy: evidence for Na^+-H^+ exchange. Circulation 1991; 84 (suppl. II): II-280.
12. Schunkert H, Jackson B, Tang SS, Schoen FJ, Smits, JFM, Apstein CS, et al. Distribution and functional significance of cardiac angiotensin-converting enzyme in hypertrophied rat hearts. Circulation 1993; 87: 1328–1339.
13. Lorell BH, Apstein CS, Cunningham MJ, Schoen FJ, Weinberg E, Peeters GA, et al. Contribution of endothelial cells to calcium dependent fluorescence transient in rabbit hearts loaded with indo 1. Circ Res 1990; 67:415–425.
14. Erdös EG: Angiotensin I converting enzyme and the changes in our concepts through the years. Hypertension 1990; 16:363–370.
15. Schunkert H, Hirsch AT, Pinto Y, Pelletier P, Jacob H, Remme WJ, et al. Feedback regulation of angiotensin converting enzyme mRNA and activity by angiotensin II. Circulation 1990; 82 (suppl. III):III-230.
16. Xiang J, Linz W, Becker H, Ganten D, Lang RE, Schölkens B, et al. Effects of converting enzyme inhibitors: ramipril and enalapril on peptide action and sympathetic neurotransmission in the isolated rat heart. Eur J Pharmacol 1984; 113:215–223.

17. Wiemer G, Schölkens BA, Becker RHA, Busse R. Ramiprilat enhances endothelial autacoid formation by inhibiting breakdown of endothelium derived bradykinin. Hypertension 1991; 18:558–563.
18. Lindpaintner K, Ganten D. The cardiac renin-angiotensin system: an appraisal of present experimental and clinical evidence. Circ Res 1991; 68(4):905–921.
19. Kunapuli SP, Kumar A. Molecular cloning of human angiotensinogen cDNA and evidence for the presence of its mRNA in rat heart. Circ Res 1987; 60:786–790.
20. Baker KM, Campanile CP, Trachte GJ, Peach MJ. Identification and characterization of the rabbit angiotensin II myocardial receptor. Circ Res 1984; 54:286–293.
21. Saito K, Gutkind JS, Saavedra JM. Angiotensin II binding sites in the conduction system of rat hearts. Am J Physiol 1987; 253:H1618–H1622.
22. Lindpaintner K, Jin M, Wilhelm MJ, Suzuki F, Linz W, Schölkens BA, et al. Intracardiac generation of angiotensin and its physiologic role. Circulation 1988; 77 (suppl. 1):18–23.
23. Kromer EP, Riegger GAJ. Effects of long-term ACE inhibition on myocardial hypertrophy in experimental aortic stenosis in the rat. Am J Cardiol 1988; 62:161–163.
24. Cushman DW, Cheung HS. Concentration of angiotensin converting enzyme in tissues of the rat. Biochem Biophys Acta 1971; 250:261–265.
25. Lorell, B.H., et al. The influence of pressure overload left ventricular hypertrophy on diastolic properties during hypoxia in isovolumically contracting rat hearts. Circ Res 1986; 58:653–663.
26. Lorell BH, Grice WN, Apstein CS. Influence of hypertension with minimal hypertrophy on diastolic function during demand ischemia. Hypertension 1989; 13:361–370.
27. Lorell BH, Weinberg E, Ngoy S, Apstein CS. Angiotensin II directly impairs diastolic function in pressure-overload hypertrophy. (abstract) Circ 1986; (III):82:111–112.
28. Hirsch AT, Talsness CE, Schunkert H, Paul M, Dzau VJ. Tissue-specific activation of cardiac angiotensin converting enzyme in experimental heart failure. Circ Res 1991; 69:475–482.
29. Jackson B, Fabris B, Kohzuki M, Mendelsohn FAO, Johnston CI. Angiotensin converting enzyme in the myocardium of rats with heart failure following myocardial infarct. J Hypertens 1990; 8 (suppl.3):S40.
30. Drexler H, Lindpaintner K, Lu W, Schieffer B, Ganten D. Transient increase in the expression of cardiac angiotensinogen in rat model of myocardial infarction and failure. Circ 1989; 80 (suppl.II):II-459.
31. Urata H, Healy B, Stewart RW, Bumpus FM, Husain A. Angiotensin II-forming pathways in normal and failing human hearts. Circ Res 1990; 6: 883–890.
32. Fifer MA, Bourdillon PD, Lorell BH. Altered left ventricular diastolic properties during pacing-induced angina in patients with aortic stenosis. Circ 1986; 74:675–683.
33. Eberli FR, Apstein CS, Ngoy S, Lorell BH. Exacerbation of left ventricular ischemic diastolic dysfunction by pressure-overload hypertrophy: modification by specific inhibition of cardiac angiotensin converting enzyme. Circ Res 1992; 70:931–943.
34. Kagaya Y, Grossman W, Lorell BH. Effects of glycolytic inhibition on

diastolic relaxation and $[Ca^{2+}]$ in hypertrophied myocytes. (abstract) Circulation 1994.

35. Gaasch WH, Zile MR, Hoshino PK, Weinberg EO, Rhodes DR, Apstein CS. Tolerance of the hypertrophic heart to ischemia: studies in compensated and failing dog hearts with pressure overload hypertrophy. Circ 1990; 81:1644–1653.

36. Buser PT, Wikman-Caffelt J, Wu ST, Derugin N, Parmley WW, Higgins CB. Post-ischemic recovery of mechanical performance and energy metabolism in the presence of left ventricular hypertrophy: a ^{31}P-MRS study. Circ Res 1990; 66:735–746.

37. Mochizuki T, Eberli FR, Apstein CS, Lorell BH. Exacerbation of ischemic dysfunction by angiotensin II in red-cell perfused rabbit hearts: effects on coronary flow, contractility, and high energy phosphate metabolism. J Clin Invest 1992; 89:490–498.

38. van Gilst WH, de Graeff PA, Wesseling H, de Langen CDJ. Reduction of reperfusion arrhythmias in the ischemic isolated rat heart by angiotensin converting enzyme inhibitors: a comparison of captopril, enalapril and HOE 498. J Cardiovasc Pharmacol 1986; 8:722–728.

39. Linz W, Schölkens BA, Han Y-F. Beneficial effects of the converting enzyme inhibitor, ramipril, in ischemic rat hearts. J Cardiovasc Pharmacol 1986; 8(suppl.10):S91–S99.

40. Linz W, Schölkens BA. Influence of local converting enzyme inhibition on angiotensin and bradykinin effects in ischemic rat hearts. J Cardiovasc Pharmacol 1987; 10 (suppl.7):S75–S82.

41. Li K, Chen X. Protective effects of captopril and enalapril on myocardial ischemia and reperfusion damage of rat. J Mol Cell Cardiol 1987; 19: 909–915.

42. Gwathmey JK, Morgan JP. Altered calcium handling in experimental pressure-overload hypertrophy in the ferret. Circ Res 1985; 57:836–843.

43. Morgan JP, Morgan KG. Calcium and cardiovascular function: intracellular calcium levels during contraction and relaxation of mammalian cardiac and vascular smooth muscle as detected with aequorin. Am J Med 1984; 77 (suppl. 5A):33–46.

44. Ikenouchi H, Kohmoto O, McMillan M, Barry WH. The contributions of $[Ca^{2+}]_i$ and pH_i to altered diastolic myocyte tone during partial metabolic inhibition. J Clin Invest 1991; 88:55–61.

45. Kihara Y, Grossman W, Morgan JP. Direct measurement of changes in $[Ca^{2+}]_i$ during hypoxia, ischemia, and reperfusion of the intact mammalian heart. Circ Res 1989; 65:1029–1044.

46. Baker KM, Singer HA. Identification and characterization of guinea pig angiotensin II ventricular and atrial receptors: coupling to inositol phosphate production. Circ Res 1988; 62:896–904

47. Baker KM, Aceto JA. Characterization of avian angiotensin II cardiac receptors: coupling to mechanical activity and phosphoinositide metabolism. J Mol Cell Cardiol 1989; 21:375–38.

48. Dosemeci A, Dhallan RS, Cohen NM, Lederer WJ, Rogers TB. Phorbol ester increases calcium current and simulates the effect of angiotensin II on cultured neonatal rat heart myocytes. Circ Res 1988; 62:347–357.

49. Nosek TM, Williams MF, Zeigler ST, Godt RE. Inositol triphosphate enhances calcium release in skinned cardiac and skeletal muscle. Am J Physiol 1986; 250:C807–C811.

50. Kawaguchi H, Shouki M, Yasuda H. Calcium release from microsomes was stimulated by inositol triphosphate in rat heart. (abstract) Circulation 1989; 80 (suppl. II):II-443.

51. Ikenouchi H, Barry WH, Weinberg E, Apstein CA, Bridje JHB, Lorell BH. Effects of angiotensin II on intracellular Ca^{2+} transients and pH: in isolated beating rabbit hearts and myocytes loaded with the indicator Indo 1. J Physiol (London); in press.

52. Kramer BK, Smith TW, Kelly RA. Endothelin and increased contractility in adult rat ventricular myocytes: role of intracellular alkalosis induced by activation of the protein kinase C-dependent Na^+-H^+ exchanger. Circ Res 1991; 68:269–279.

53. Neyses L, Molls M, Vetner H. Altered activation of the myocardium by angiotensin II in early hypertrophy. Circulation 1991; (suppl. II) 84:II-308.

54. Friedrich SP, Lorell BH, Douglas PS, et al. Intracardiac ACE inhibition improves diastolic distensibility in patients with left ventricular hypertrophy due to aortic stenosis. Submitted for publication.

12

The Cardiac Renin-Angiotensin System in Different Ischemic Syndromes of the Heart

Pieter A. de Graeff, Wiek H. van Gilst,
and Harry Wesseling

Introduction

Although renin-like enzymes had been extracted from a variety of organs other than the kidney, including the uterus, placenta, heart, brain, adrenal glands, and submaxillary gland,[1] it was initially thought that these extrarenal sources did not play any physiological role in cardiovascular homeostasis. However, this changed when clinical studies with ACE inhibitors demonstrated that, although the acute blood-pressure lowering effect of ACE inhibitors correlated with initial plasma renin activity, the chronic response showed little relationship to pretreatment plasma hormonal levels.[2] Further circumstantial evidence for the importance of the RAS in tissues other than blood was obtained by other studies which demonstrated that chronic administration of ACE inhibitors also lowered blood pressure when plasma renin activity was not elevated,[3] or even low, as in anephric subjects.[4]

Direct evidence for an inhibition of ACE in various tissues, including the vascular wall, following administration of an ACE inhibitor was subsequently provided in SHR.[5] Furthermore, the prolonged

Lindpaintner K and Ganten D (editors): *The Cardiac-Renin Angiotensin System,* ©
Futura Publishing Co., Inc., Armonk, NY, 1994.

antihypertensive action was unrelated to ACE inhibition in the plasma but was associated with persistent ACE inhibition in the kidney and vascular wall. This led to the hypothesis that the RAS in the vascular wall played an important role in cardiovascular homeostasis.[2] Further studies confirmed this hypothesis. ACE is widespread on endothelial cells, and both renin mRNA and angiotensin mRNA have been detected in the vascular wall, demonstrating beyond doubt that A II can be generated locally in the vasculature.[6] This led to the revised concept that the primary function of the circulating RAS is not systemic delivery of A II to the tissues but rather the delivery of angiotensinogen and prorenin.[7] Thus, a major fraction of both A I and A II may be produced locally rather than in the circulating plasma itself. This hypothesis has recently been confirmed in humans.[8]

Now, what about the heart? As early as in 1973, it was demonstrated in the blood-perfused Langendorff rat heart that A I could be converted into A II when administered into the coronary artery.[9] Several other investigators subsequently confirmed this cardiac generation of A II from A I in guinea pig atria,[10] in the coronary vasculature of the rabbit,[11] and in the isolated perfused rat heart.[12] Further proof of the existence of a cardiac RAS was obtained by biochemical characterization of components of the RAS and the demonstration of renin and angiotensinogen mRNAs in the heart.[13] The marked rise in atrial and ventricular contents of A I after nephrectomy in rats and the presence of functional A II receptors in the heart gave further proof that this cardiac RAS is a functional and locally integrated system.[13]

Pathophysiological Effects of the Cardiac RAS in the Heart During Myocardial Ischemia

A number of functions of locally generated A II, either direct or mediated via activation of cardiac sympathetic neurotransmission, have been demonstrated in various experimental models (Table 1).[13–15] Direct effects on contractility and heart rate increase myocardial oxygen demand, and coronary vasoconstriction reduces myocardial oxygen supply. Detrimental effects on cell membrane integrity enhance myocardial damage and ventricular arrhythmias during ischemia and reperfusion, and stimulation of cardiac myocyte growth ultimately promotes myocardial ischemia. As a consequence,

Table 1
Functional Aspects of the Locally Generated Angiotensin II and
Bradykinin in the Heart

Angiotensin II	*Bradykinin*
Coronary vasoconstriction	Coronary vasodilatation
Increased contractility	Increased contractility*
Positive chronotropy	Positive chronotropy*
Stimulation of cardiac myocyte growth	Reduction of cardiac myocyte growth
Worsening of myocardial metabolism during ischemia and reperfusion	Improvement in myocardial metabolism during ischemia and reperfusion
Increase in myocardial damage during ischemia and reperfusion	Reduction in myocardial damage during ischemia and reperfusion
Increase in ventricular arrhythmias during ischemia and reperfusion	Reduction in ventricular arrhythmias during ischemia and reperfusion

* Variable results have been reported.

a major role for this system in the pathophysiology of myocardial ischemia and its consequences may be postulated, be it the symptomatology of angina pectoris, the myocardial damage following coronary occlusion, or the course of events following reperfusion.

It is therefore remarkable that, as yet, there is no direct and reliable evidence for an activation of the cardiac RAS in ischemia. We do know that the RAS can be activated during myocardial ischemia during coronary occlusion[16–18] and atrial pacing,[17,19] but whether this occurs locally as a result of myocardial ischemia or systemically on the basis of hemodynamic factors remains to be established. Similarly, ventricular angiotensinogen mRNA levels may increase selectively in the heart following myocardial infarction,[20] and a correlation between ACE cardiac mRNA levels and infarct size has been shown,[21] but this may similarly be due to indirect hemodynamic changes and not as a direct consequence of myocardial ischemia. Even the exact site in the heart where the system is activated remains to be established; both the coronary vasculature and the endocardium and the myocardium should be considered. Differences between the atria and the ventricles appear to be present and, so far, the presence of ACE activity has not been conclusively established in the smooth muscle cell of the vascular wall and the myocardium.

In the absence of data that unequivocally show direct patho-physiological effects of intracardially activated RAS in ischemic syndromes, one has to rely on experiments with pharmacological agents that antagonize these effects, especially ACE inhibitors. It is now well recognized that ACE inhibitors exert their principal action at local sites, including the heart and the vasculature.[14,22] Inhibition of cardiac ACE activity and intracardiac A II generation by ACE inhibitors has been demonstrated in vitro and ex vivo.[14,22] Thus, major conclusions with regard to the role of the cardiac RAS in various ischemic syndromes can be drawn from experimental data that have been obtained with these pharmacological agents. In this chapter, we will summarize these data as obtained by us and others and discuss the therapeutic implications.

Effects of ACE Inhibitors on the Heart

Although the majority of data obtained with ACE inhibitors in the experimental setting of ischemia/reperfusion do suggest that the cardiac RAS does play an important pathophysiological role in ischemic heart disease, a number of reservations should be made. First, no in vivo data selectively demonstrating the effects of ACE inhibitors on the cardiac RAS are available, owing to the complexity of the direct and indirect actions of ACE inhibitors on a number of effector systems involved in cardiovascular homeostasis, such as arterial and venous vascular smooth muscle, adrenal cortex, and the central and autonomic systems. Even results in isolated organs and tissue preparations may still be confounded by variable and differential effects of ACE inhibitors on selective anatomic and cellular components present in such experimental systems.

Second, one should realize that the heart is an endocrine organ, and changes in cardiac RAS will be counteracted by other locally effective systems. This applies especially to the kinin-kallikrein system because the angiotensin-converting enzyme, or kininase II, is also responsible for the breakdown of bradykinin. Since there is increasing evidence that the heart and vascular tissue contain a local kallikrein-kinin pathway,[23] ACE inhibition will not only result in a reduction of local A II but also in an increase in local kinin concentrations. This is important because many of the effects of bradykinin on the heart are opposite to those of A II, as will be discussed by us and others in this volume (Table 1). It induces coronary vasodilatation, it reduces myocardial damage due to hypoxia, and it has an antiproliferative effect following endothelial injury. Thus, the underlying mechanism of direct cardiac effects of ACE inhibitors in ischemic heart disease may also be due to local stimulation of the bradykinin.

Finally, sulfhydryl(SH)-containing ACE inhibitors, like captopril and zofenopril, may exert cardiac effects due to the presence of the thiol moiety, independent of their ACE inhibiting property. SH-containing agents may act as scavengers of free radicals and/or as antioxidant agents that may play an important role in reperfusion-induced depression of contractility and reperfusion arrhythmias.[24–26] Furthermore, SH groups are involved in the vascular smooth muscle response to endogenous and exogenous nitrovasodilators, and SH-containing agents may induce coronary vasodilation on their own.[27] Figure 1 summarizes all the mechanisms of action, which must be taken into account when the cardioprotective effects

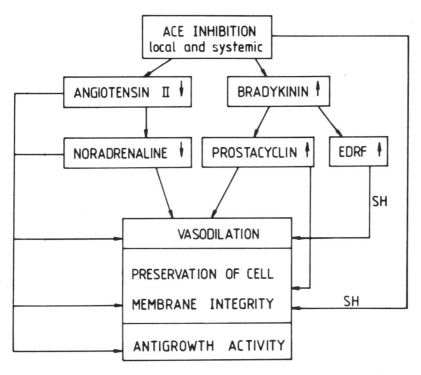

Fig. 1. Tentative scheme explaining the mechanisms of action of ACE inhibitors in ischemic heart disease. EDRF: endothelium-derived relaxing factor; SH: sulfhydryl group.

of these agents in ischemic disease and their underlying mechanisms are discussed.

ACE Inhibitors and Ischemia Reperfusion–Induced Myocardial Injury

On the basis of the concept that A II might be detrimental to the ischemic heart, a number of animal experiments with ACE inhibitors on ventricular performance and infarct size after coronary occlusion have been performed to study their potentially beneficial effects. All studies in intact animals with acute left-ventricular failure following coronary occlusion showed an improvement in global ventricular performance, irrespective of which ACE inhibitor was applied.[16,28-30] This beneficial effect was attributed primarily to the reduction of preload and afterload and not to a direct cardioprotective effect.

In the first study that was published on the effect of ACE inhibitors on infarct size (see also Table 2), it was shown that, following myocardial infarction, ACE inhibitors do not only beneficially influence the hemodynamic changes as a consequence of left-ventricular dysfunction but also the amount of myocardial damage.[31] Captopril treatment reduced both the myocardial area at risk and the size of the myocardial damage following 6 hours of coronary occlusion in anesthetized dogs.[31] In contrast, two subsequent studies with captopril, also in dogs, showed no limitation of infarct size 24 hours after coronary occlusion.[32,33] A conclusive explanation for these negative results could not be found, although differences in anesthesia and duration of ischemia were postulated to be of importance. Further evidence of a beneficial effect of ACE inhibitors in the setting of acute myocardial infarction was obtained by studies with enalapril, which showed reduction in infarct size following permanent acute left-coronary artery ligation after 48 hours in the rat and after 5 hours in the cat.[34,35] At the time of publication of these experiments, the underlying mechanism was primarily attributed to a reduction of systemic A II, although the involvement of kinin-mediated mechanisms was also suggested.[35] Reduction in microcirculatory damage was suggested when it was also shown in the rat that administration of enalapril in conjunction with reperfusion produced a significant preservation of CK activity to 88% of the sham MI rats following 10 minutes of ischemia.[35]

More evidence for a direct effect on the heart was obtained when we described for the first time that captopril, administered in a high

Table 2
In Vivo Animal Studies on the Effect of ACE Inhibitors During Myocardial Ischemia and Reperfusion

Investigator	ACE Inhibitor	Species	Ischemia	Reperfusion	Results
Ertl[31]	Captopril	Dog	6 hrs	—	↓ Infarct size
Liang[32]	Teprotide/Captopril	Dog	24 hrs	—	No effect infarct size
Daniell[33]	Captopril	Dog	24 hrs	—	No effect infarct size
Lefer[34]	Enalapril	Cat	5 hrs	—	↓ Myocardial CK activity
Hock[35]	Enalapril	Rat	48 hrs	+	↓ CK activity
	Enalapril	Rat	10 min	+	↓ CK activity
Elfellah[51]	Captopril	Dog	30 min	+	↓ Occlusion arrhythmias
	Enalapril				↓ Occlusion + reperfusion arrhythmias
Li[40]	Enalapril*	Rat	8 hrs	—	↓ CK and myocardial ischemia
Rochette[52]	Captopril	Rat	30 min	—	↓ VF ↓ mortality
	Perindopril				Idem
de Graeff[37,50]	Captopril	Pig	60 min	+	↓ CK activity and catecholamines upon reperfusion
					↓ Inducibility arrhythmias after 2 weeks
Westlin[53]	Captopril	Dog	15 min	+	↓ Reperfusion arrhythmias ↑ myocardial segmental function
Tio[54]	Enalaprilat				↓ Reperfusion arrhythmias
	Zofenopril**	Pig	45 min	+	↓ Purine overflow and catecholamines upon reperfusion
					↓ Inducibility arrhythmias and late potentials after 2 weeks
Martorana[59]	Ramiprilat	Dog	6 hrs	—	↓ Infarct size
Przyklenk[26,55]	Zofenopril***	Dog	15 min	+	↑ Myocardial segmental function
	Captopril***				↑ Myocardial segmental function
	Enalaprilat***				↑ Myocardial segmental function
van Wijngaarden[57]	Perindoprilat	Pig	45 min	+	No effect CK and purine overflow
Tobé[56]					↓ Mortality after 2 weeks
Muller[58]	Perindoprilat	Pig	20 min	—	↑ VF threshold ↓ cyclic AMP ischemic zone

CK = creatine kinase; VF = ventricular fibrillation.
* Intraperitoneal pretreatment; ** Oral pretreatment; *** Given only during reperfusion.

concentration (80 μg/ml), improved contractility and reduced myocardial ATP breakdown and reperfusion arrhythmias after reversible 15 minutes ligation of the left-coronary artery in the isolated rat heart.[36] An extension of these experiments showed that these cardioprotective effects were dose dependent and already present at a therapeutic concentration.[37] This cardioprotective effect was, among others, demonstrated by a concentration-dependent reduction of the incidence and duration of ventricular fibrillation upon reperfusion (Figure 2). Subsequently, a number of in vitro studies have been performed in the isolated rat heart on the effect of ACE inhibitors on ischemia/reperfusion-induced myocardial damage (Table 3). Although the type of ACE inhibitor and dosage, the duration and extent of ischemia, and the size of beneficial effect varied among the different studies, in all studies at least some favorable

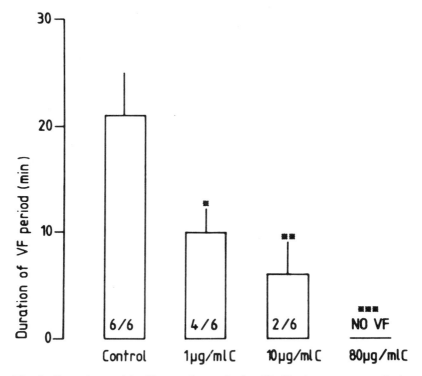

Fig. 2. Duration and incidence of ventricular fibrillation upon reperfusion in control hearts and captopril-treated hearts. The values in the vertical bars represent the total number of hearts that fibrillated upon reperfusion in each group (n = 6); (from de Graeff PA, et al.[37]). $*p < 0.05$; $**p < 0.02$; $***p < 0.001$, compared with the control group.

Table 3

Effects of ACE Inhibitors on Ischemia/Reperfusion-Induced Myocardial Damage in Vitro

Investigator	ACE Inhibitor	Dose*	Duration	Type Ischemia	Results
van Gilst[36]	Captopril	80 μg/ml	15 min	Regional	↓ Reperfusion arrhythmias ↓ Purine overflow ↑ Myocardial function
de Graeff[37,42] van Gilst[38]	Captopril Ramiprilat Ramipril Enalaprilat	1–80 μg/ml 15 μg/ml 15 μg/ml 8 μg/ml	15 min	Regional	Captopril idem, concentration dependent Ramiprilat idem but less No effect Enalaprilat only ↓ purine overflow
Linz[39,44,45]	Ramipril	1 mg/kg**	15 min	Regional	↓ Reperfusion arrhythmias ↑ energy stores ↓ lactate
	Ramiprilat Enalapril Captopril	10 μg/ml 10 mg/kg** 50 mg/kg**			Idem Idem No effect reperfusion arrhythmias
Rochette[52]	Captopril Perindopril	$5 \cdot 10^{-5}$M $5 \cdot 10^{-5}$M	10 min	Regional	↓ Reperfusion arrhythmias Idem
Li[40]	Enalapril	2.5 mg/kg***	20 min	Global	→ Reperfusion arrhythmias ↓ function
	Captopril	10^{-5} M	20 min	Regional	↑ CK release ↑ contractility
Rahusen[41]	Captopril	80 μg/ml	15 min	Global	↑ Recovery ATP after normo- and hypothermic ischemia
Bagchi[43]	Captopril	50 μM	60 min	Global	↓ CK release ↓ LDH ↑ high energy Phosphates
Fleetwood[46]	Enalaprilat	70 nM	40 min	Global	→ Reperfusion arrhythmias No effect CK release No effect LVP
Grover[47]	Captopril Enalaprilat Zofenopril Fosinoprilat Ramiprilat	400 μM 0.03–400 μM 0.03–400 μM 100 μM 0.03–400 μM	25 min	Global	↑ Contractile function ↓ LDH release No effects ↑ Contractile function ↓ LDH No effects No effects
Arad[48]	Captopril	80 μg/ml	5–30 min	Global	↓ Duration VF ↓ CK release
Menasché[49]	Captopril Enalapril	75 mg**** 7.5 mg****	90 min	Global Global	↓ Contractility Idem, but less

CK = creatine kinase; VF = ventricular filbrillation; LVP = left-ventricular pressure; LDH = lactic dehydrogenase.
* Concentration in perfusion fluid; ** Oral pretreatment; *** Intraperitoneal pretreatment; **** Total dose administered subcutaneously in 48 hours.

effect of the ACE inhibitor on ischemia/reperfusion damage occurred.[36–49]

These beneficial effects on ischemia and reperfusion damage in vitro were subsequently confirmed in vivo in different animal species as summarized in Table 2.[26,35,40,42,50–59] Pretreatment with an ACE inhibitor reduced enzymatic infarct size,[35,40,42,50] showed antiarrhythmic action,[42,51–54,58] and improved segmental function.[53] In studies with perindopril, even a reduction in mortality was found.[56,57] The effect appeared to be more consistent in ischemia plus reperfusion than in ischemia alone, although in a recent study ramipril significantly reduced infarct size after 6 hours of coronary occlusion.[59] This study suggests that ACE inhibitors do not only affect myocardial damage as result of ischemia but also reperfusion. Early reperfusion may represent a "double-edged sword," that is, that it paradoxically may sometimes cause additional myocardial injury.[60] Several mechanisms may be involved, among others catecholamine efflux, generation of free radicals, and activation of neutrophils. These are all affected by ACE inhibition and may explain why these agents appear to have a specific cardioprotective effect on reperfusion damage. This is further shown by in vitro and in vivo experiments in which the ACE inhibitor was given during, or even at the end of, the ischemic period, which still showed beneficial effects on reperfusion phenomena, although in some experiments to a lesser extent.[26,44–46,53,55]

The in vivo studies on reperfusion phenomena again showed variable results between the different ACE inhibitors. These differences can partly be explained by differences in species, and especially duration of ischemia, which varied from 10 to 60 minutes (Table 2). This influences the extent of myocardial damage and type of reperfusion arrhythmia.[61] Another explanation may be differences in degree of ACE inhibition. In the heart, where ACE inhibitors may prevent ischemic damage to the myocardium, single oral doses of captopril, fosinopril, and particularly zofenopril produced striking and long-lasting inhibition, whereas equivalent doses of ramipril and enalapril only induced minimal inhibition.[62] However, this selective inhibition, which was attributed to the degree of lipophilicity, was not found by others.[63] Other factors must be involved, related to underlying mechanisms of the ischemia/reperfusion damage and its interference by ACE inhibitors. This will be discussed more in detail.

The Role of the Cardiac ACE in Ischemia/Reperfusion Injury

As shown by the use of ACE inhibitors, enzymatic activity of ACE in the myocardium, coronary vasculature, and blood may influence the effects of A II and bradykinin on the heart. These effects appear to be antagonistic (Table 1).

Large doses of A II cause tissue necrosis in rabbits.[64] Both administration of A I and A II in the coronary effluent of isolated rat hearts induced coronary vasoconstriction, increased the incidence and duration of reperfusion arrhythmias, and worsened metabolic conditions.[12,39,44,45] Infusion of A II causes inducible ventricular tachycardias 2 weeks after myocardial infarction in pigs.[65] Conversely, administration of an A II antagonist or a renin inhibitor produced protective effects on reperfusion arrhythmias similar to those of enalaprilat.[46] Angiotensin II may exert these deleterious effects both by impairment of coronary perfusion and by facilitation of sympathetic neurotransmission. A marked outflow of norepinephrine has been reported upon reperfusion in vitro and in vivo, and reduction of this outflow may beneficially influence the chain of events leading to irreversible cell damage.[37,50,52,54,66]

Administration of bradykinin salvages myocardial tissue following coronary occlusion[59] and reperfusion.[67] It has been shown experimentally that bradykinin is stimulated during ischemia and reperfusion, and this effect can be potentiated by captopril.[68] Addition of bradykinin to the perfusate of isolated rat hearts reduces the occurrence of reperfusion arrhythmias and improves cardiac and metabolic events similar to the effect of ACE inhibitors.[39,44,45] Bradykinin, administered during ischemia and reperfusion, also reduces ischemia-induced arrhythmias in anesthetized dogs[69] and inducibility of ventricular tachycardia 2 weeks after myocardial infarction.[70] Conversely, the cardioprotective effects of bradykinin and ACE inhibitors can be abolished completely by concomitant administration of a specific bradykinin antagonist.[44,45,59]

These bradykinin-mediated beneficial effects may be mediated in large part to the release of prostaglandins, most notably PGI_2. Administration of captopril in the isolated rat heart during ischemia and reperfusion stimulated prostacyclin production progressively during reperfusion.[43] Coadministration of the cyclo-oxygenase inhibitor indomethacin attenuated the effects of bradykinin[44] and those of ACE inhibitors.[26,38,40,44] Several mechanisms for the cardioprotective effects of prostacyclin have been proposed, such as the inhibition of myocardial catecholamine release, preservation of free radical scavenging systems, inhibition of neutrophil activation, and inhibition of intracellular lysosome disruption.[71] Other bradykinin activities may also contribute to the cardioprotective effects, especially bradykinin's capacity to increase glucose uptake in the heart and to release EDRF, which may induce further protection of the cardiac and coronary endothelium.[45]

In conclusion, the RAS, locally and systemically, appears closely linked with the kinin-kallikrein system with the ACE as the primary regulating enzyme. Changes in one system will be contraregulated by the other. ACE inhibitors will favorably influence this balance, and this explains why ACE inhibitors in general are beneficial in acute myocardial infarction plus reperfusion.

As shown in Tables 2 and 3, in most comparative studies, the SH-containing ACE inhibitors were more effective than the non-SH-containing ACE inhibitors,[38,47,49,53] although not in all.[26,45,51] This may be related to the aforementioned antioxidant properties of the sulfhydryl moiety, which may influence free radical-induced myocardial injury.[24] This is further demonstrated by the fact that in a number of studies stereoisomers or inactive prodrugs of the SH-containing captopril and zofenopril also demonstrated beneficial effects.[26,47,53] However, as indicated above, a number of studies have indicated beneficial effects of non-SH-containing ACE inhibitors (Tables 2 and 3), and these effects could only be obtained when the active ACE-inhibiting form was given.[38] It should also be taken into account that ACE inhibitors may also affect free radical injury by indirect ACE-dependent mechanisms like activation of prostacyclin and/or EDRF.[25,26,43,49]

Effects of Converting-Enzyme Inhibitors on Coronary Flow and Myocardial Ischemia

The regulation of coronary hemodynamics is a complex process. It depends on three interrelated factors: myocardial oxygen consumption, coronary vasomotor tone, and perfusion pressure. Coronary vasoconstrictive effects of A II, either directly or via facilitation of sympathetic tone, may be counteracted in vivo by other mechanisms, and this may mask its effects. More information about local effects can be derived from studies in vitro because perfusion pressure can be controlled, and there is no influence of changes in preload and afterload on myocardial oxygen consumption.

When an ACE inhibitor was added to the perfusate in rat Langendorff preparations, coronary flow clearly increased (Figure 3).[12,39,45,49,72,73] Pretreatment in vivo, both with captopril and other ACE inhibitors, resulted in flow increase in vitro throughout the experiments.[12,39,73] A more complex picture emerged from in vivo animal experiments. When captopril was given via either the intravenous or intracoronary routes to anaesthetized dogs under normoxic conditions, it did not produce a marked change in coronary

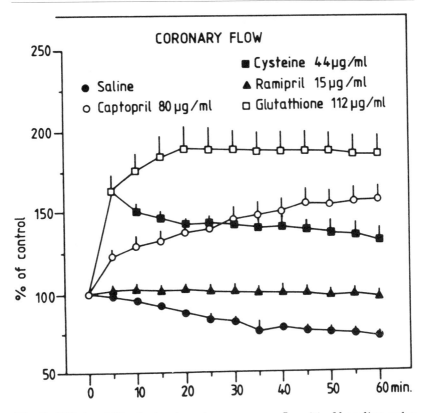

Fig. 3. Effects of 60 min treatment on coronary flow (% of baseline value at t = 0) in the isolated rat heart. Values are the mean ± SEM (from van Gilst WH, et al.[73]).

blood flow.[74] However, the proportional contribution changed during myocardial ischemia or other conditions in which the RAS was stimulated.[16,29,74] Converting-enzyme inhibition may thus cause redistribution of regional blood flow in favor of the brain, heart, and kidney, especially in conditions when the RAS is stimulated.

This finding may be of special importance in ischemic heart disease. Several studies have shown that myocardial ischemia induces renin release.[16,75] In various models of myocardial ischemia, saralasin and captopril acted as coronary vasodilators.[76] However, other investigators found no increase in myocardial blood flow with ACE inhibition; this lack of effect was presumably due to metabolic autoregulation and a drop in coronary perfusion pressure.[32,77] Nevertheless, when systemic vasodilatory effects were excluded, saralasin completely prevented further decreases in coronary blood flow during atrial pacing.[76]

Clinical studies on the effects of ACE inhibitors on coronary blood flow suggest that these theoretical considerations and experimental findings may also be relevant in humans. In patients with heart failure and hypertension, a reduction in coronary blood flow was observed as part of the acute effects of ACE inhibitors corresponding to a reduction in myocardial oxygen consumption due primarily to a reduction in the rate pressure product.[78–80] Variable effects were observed in patients without CHF. Captopril increased coronary blood flow in both healthy subjects[79] and patients with hypertension and no evidence of coronary artery disease,[81] despite the fact that captropril did not change the rate-pressure product; however this increase only occurred in the presence of an activated RAS. Further evidence of a coronary vasodilating effect was shown in a study by Foult et al., which showed that intracoronary administration of enalaprilat produced coronary vasodilation independent of its systemic effects.[82] In 1989, Remme et al. confirmed that ACE inhibitors preferentially dilate the coronary vasculature, and thereby improve coronary flow, in patients with coronary artery disease in the absence of heart failure.[83] This improvement in cororary blood flow was also demonstrated by studies with ACE inhibitors during incremental atrial pacing in patients with coronary artery disease,[84,85] and during the cold pressor and diving test when the sympathetic nervous system is activated.[86]

The Role of the Cardiac ACE in Coronary Blood Flow

All these results suggest that, in contrast to basic conditions, under conditions of neurohumoral activation, ACE activity does play a role in the regulation of coronary vasoconstrictive tone. It regulates the balance between the vasoconstrictive properties of A II and the vasodilating properties of bradykinin.

Regulation of locally generated A II may affect coronary vascular tone both by a direct vasoconstrictive effect or indirectly by facilitation of sympathetic activity. It has been demonstrated in the isolated rat heart that both A I and A II were able to induce coronary vasoconstriction, corroborating both the vasoconstrictive properties of A II and the presence of a local converting enzyme in the endothelium of the coronary vasculature.[12] In vivo, coronary extraction of renin occurs during experimental coronary occlusion, which also suggests local generation of A II during myocardial ischemia.[17] As is also shown by experiments with ACE inhibitors, local regulation of A II may contribute to coronary vascular tone but only under stimulated conditions.

Bradykinin is an endothelium-dependent vasodilator, stimulating local production of prostacyclin and EDRF, which is identical to nitric oxide (NO). Interest in the role of locally generated bradykinin on coronary flow increased markedly when selective bradykinin antagonists became available. Subsequently, it was shown that the increase in coronary flow by enalaprilat and ramiprilat, given in vitro and ex vivo, was completely abolished by these antagonists.[45,68] Similarly, in vivo, in rat experiments using a microsphere technique, the presence of a bradykinin antagonist reduced the increase in local conductance in the heart as induced by enalaprilat.[87] However, a more puzzling picture arose when captopril and zofenoprilat were studied in these models. These SH-containing ACE inhibitors induced a much more pronounced effect than the non-SH-containing ACE inhibitors enalaprilat and ramiprilat.[72,73] Evidence that this effect was due to the presence of a SH group was obtained by other experiments with the inactive (R,S)-isomer of captopril and other SH-containing agents, like cysteine and glutathione, which also demonstrated an increase in coronary flow under similar conditions (Figure 3).[72,73] We also knew from studies with nitrates, which as exogenous nitrovasodilators act by the formation of intermediate metabolites, NO among them, that their effects can be enhanced by SH-containing agents.[88] Apparently, more than one mechanism was involved (Figure 4).

Subsequently, we performed a number of experiments to prove this hypothesis. First, we concentrated on the effects of prostacyclin synthesis. Although we could measure a slow increase in 6-keto-PGF1α, the stable metabolite of prostacyclin, in the coronary effluent following administration of high dosages of bradykinin[68] or ACE inhibitors,[72,73] coadministration of cyclooxygenase inhibitors like indomethacin and acetylsalicylic did not demonstrate any effect on these coronary vasodilating effects,[68,72,89] despite effective blockage of the outflow of prostacyclin.[89] All these results suggested that under stable, normoxic conditions the role of a bradykinin-mediated effect on prostacyclin, potentiated by ACE inhibitors, is limited. However, this may change under ischemic conditions as has been shown in patients with coronary artery disease, in whom indomethacin significantly reduced coronary sinus blood flow.[90] Notwithstanding, other underlying mechanisms must be involved in the regulation of coronary flow by bradykinin, and attention has recently concentrated on the release of EDRF.

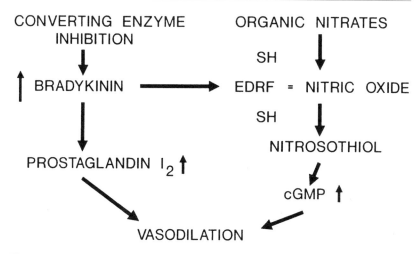

Fig. 4. Postulated mechanisms whereby SH-containing ACE inhibitors may interact with organic nitrates. cGMP: cycline guanosine monophosphate; SH: sulfhydryl group.

The importance of this mechanism was shown in vitro by complete inhibition of nitric oxide release when bradykinin was administered in the presence of a bradykinin antagonist.[91] Further evidence of a contribution of bradykinin-mediated release of EDRF to coronary flow was demonstrated in vivo in the canine coronary circulation by attenuation of the effects of bradykinin by concomitant administration of inhibitors of EDRF, especially L-N^G-monomethylarginine (L-N-MMA).[92] The effects of ACE inhibitors on the release of EDRF may mimic those of bradykinin, suggesting a contribution of locally generated kinins in the vascular wall, and subsequent release of EDRF, to the vasodilatory effects of these drugs. Studies in cultured bovine and human endothelial cells with ramiprilat and enalaprilat have shown that ACE inhibitors are able to unmask a release of bradykinin with a subsequent increase in EDRF.[91,93] In vivo studies in SHR have shown that coadministration of L-N-MMA attenuated the hypotensive effect of several ACE inhibitors.[94]

We studied the effects of captopril both in the presence of L-arginine, the "true" precursor of EDRF, and L-N-MMA, the "false" precursor of EDRF (Figure 5).[27] L-arginine increased the effect of captopril, whereas L-N-MMA showed a competitive antagonism for the effect of captopril on coronary flow in the isolated rat heart. These results strongly suggest that a bradykinin-mediated release

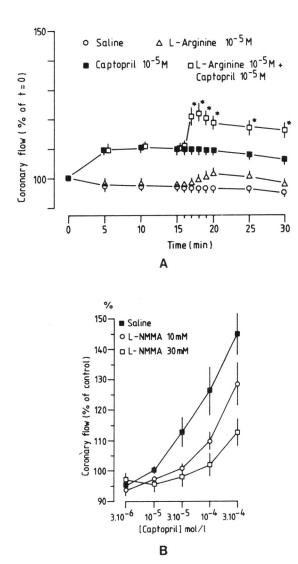

Fig. 5. (A) Effect of captopril, arginine, and the combination of both compounds on coronary flow in the isolated rat heart. (B) Effect of L-N-monomethylarginine (L-N-MMA) on the cumulative dose-response curve of captopril (from van Gilst WH, et al.[27]).*$p < 0.05$

of EDRF indeed plays a role in the coronary vasodilating effects of ACE inhibitors. Since both the "true" and the "false" precursors affected coronary flow even in the absence of the ACE inhibitor, it has been suggested that EDRF is produced under normal conditions and participates in the regulation of coronary flow.

The bradykinin-induced release of prostaglandins and EDRF is a transient response that does not persist in the continuous presence of bradykinin or during repeated administration of the compound.[95] This tachyphylaxis occurs at the receptor level and is due to a homologous downregulation of the kinin receptors, occurring in vitro within a few minutes. However, another mechanism may also be involved. Already in 1967, potentiation of the effect of bradykinin by SH-containing compounds was observed.[96] We know from studies with organic nitrates that tissue SH groups in vascular smooth muscle are involved in their mechanism of action, supposedly by activation of guanylate cyclase through the formation S-nitrosothiols from intermediate metabolites, among which is NO.[97] It has been shown repeatedly that administration of SH-containing agents like acetylcysteine enhances nitrate vascular effects.[88] Furthermore, EDRF is destroyed by free oxygen radicals that may be scavenged by SH-containing agents, including the ACE inhibitor captopril, thus leading to a potentiation of its effect.[98]

The interaction of SH-containing agents on the effect of bradykinin on coronary flow was a subject of study in a number of experiments in the isolated rat heart under normoxic conditions.[27] The effect of 5 minutes of bradykinin infusion showed a biphasic pattern with a maximum after 1 to 2 minutes followed by a complete loss of its effect, suggesting the development of tolerance. Concomitant treatment with the SH donor 10 μM of cysteine increased and prolonged this effect. This effect was also reflected by a potentiation of the dose-response curves of bradykinin on coronary flow in the presence of different concentrations of SH-containing ACE inhibitors, and, to lesser extent, other SH-containing agents like cysteine.[27] Further proof was obtained by another set of experiments showing a reduced response of bradykinin and an unchanged response to captopril on coronary flow when endogenous SH depletion was evoked by pretreatment with high dosages of nitrates (Figure 6). Similarly, in our in vitro heart model, captopril potentiated the coronary vascular response to isosorbide dinitrate, comparable to cysteine, whereas ramiprilat, lacking a SH-moiety, had no significant effect.[99]

Apparently, thiol-groups are important for the vasorelaxing action of EDRF. One should be cautious, however, to extrapolate our

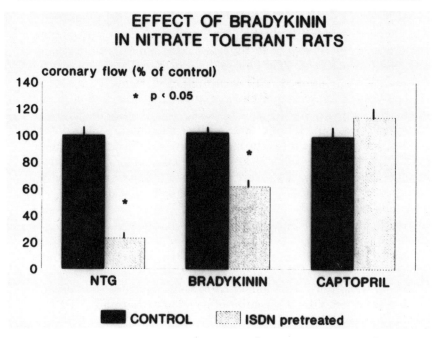

Fig. 6. Effects of nitroglycerin (NTG; 10^{-5}M), bradykinin (10^{-8}M), and captopril (10^{-8}M) on coronary flow in control hearts and in hearts pretreated with isosorbide dinitrate (15 mg daily) for 2 weeks. All responses are related to responses of a separate, nontreated group of control rats (n = 16) (from van Gilst WH, et al.[27]). $*p < 0.05$

findings to the in vivo situation because high levels of free radicals under basic conditions are only found in vitro and not in vivo. Furthermore, the in vivo capacity of SH-containing agents to interact with locally generated EDRF needs to be studied further. Some clinical data are already available on the interaction with exogenous nitrovasodilators, as will be discussed below.

Therapeutic Implications

Acute Myocardial Infarction

After acute coronary occlusion in the clinical setting, there are various factors to consider at different times that may influence the development of ventricular dilatation and the subsequent occurrence of heart failure. The evolution of transmural infarction may lead to early infarct expansion.[100] Despite healing, infarct expansion may be accompanied by compensatory hypertrophy in the noninfarcted region and progressive global dilatation, the major stimulus being wall stress. It has been shown repeatedly that ACE inhibitors may interfere with this process of remodeling, and this may result in a reduction of cardiovascular morbidity and mortality.[101] Whether these effects are a result of the reduction of wall stress or whether local effects also contribute remain to be established.

A major question that remains to be solved is the optimal timing of the treatment with ACE inhibitors. Remodeling is a process that starts within a few hours after myocardial infarction, and it has been shown that treatment within 24 to 28 hours after the onset of symptoms may already influence the process of hypertrophy and dilatation.[102,103] ACE inhibitors may block compensatory mechanisms necessary to maintain cardiac performance, and a recent study with enalaprilat, which started within hours of myocardial infarction, did not show any clinical benefit on the clinical outcome.[104]

Another approach may be the reduction of myocardial damage in the acute phase, similar to the animal experiments. In the clinical setting, thrombolytic treatment is given in patients with coronary occlusion to achieve reperfusion and to salvage myocardial tissue. However, the introduction of oxygen and cellular elements into the ischemic zone may initiate a deleterious cascade of events that limits myocardial salvage after reperfusion.[60] Clearly, despite the benefits of thrombolytic therapy, the use of adjuvant therapies to reduce this reperfusion damage must be explored.

ACE inhibitors appear to be a particularly attractive choice. In the acute phase, they may scavenge free radicals, blunt the catecholamine response, elicit coronary vasodilation, and increase prostacyclin and bradykinin levels. In the subacute and chronic phase, remodeling may be attenuated. In a pilot study with captopril, given within 30 minutes after the start of streptokinase infusion, a significant reduction in norepinephrine levels was found. Safety appeared acceptable.[105] Currently, two controlled studies are being carried out to study the effects of early intervention with ACE inhibitors after thrombolytic treatment, followed by maintenance treatment.[105,106] These studies will hopefully confirm the beneficial effects on myocardial damage, ventricular arrhythmias, and myocardial function as shown by the experimental studies.

Angina Pectoris

Despite the aforementioned role of the ACE, controlled trials have failed to demonstrate a significant effect of ACE inhibitors on exercise tolerance.[107] Although in some studies some therapeutic effect has been suggested, this effect appears to be inferior to that of β-adrenergic blocking agents and calcium antagonists. Even worsening of anginal complaints may occur, as was reported recently in a placebo-controlled study in patients with severe heart failure.[108] In this study, the risk of adverse effects was directly related to the magnitude of the drug's hypotensive effects. Indeed, part of the conflicting results of the clinical trials on ACE inhibitors in angina may be due to the high dosage, augmenting the likelihood of producing a reduction in coronary perfusion pressure. Thus, further studies should employ cardioselective ACE inhibitors, starting with a low dose and continuing for a longer period.

More benefit may be obtained in the presence of hypertension and early heart failure, especially following myocardial infarction. Left-ventricular pressure or volume overload leads to LVH, which may be accompanied by an impairment of coronary vasodilator reserve.[97] ACE inhibitors have been shown to reduce left-ventricular mass in these patients and to correct vascular structure abnormalities. These properties, together with the vasodilating effects of ACE inhibitors, make these drugs especially suitable for the treatment of angina in patients with hypertension, as well as in patients with left-ventricular dysfunction with no or only mild to moderate symptoms of CHF. This is confirmed by a recent study in patients with hypertension and angina, which showed that captopril has both antianginal as well as anti-ischemic effects on exercise-induced ST segment shift on the ECG when these conditions coexist.[109] Furthermore, recent results (in part unpublished) of two large controlled trials in patients with left-ventricular dysfunction and no symptoms, the SAVE trial and the SOLVD trial, indicate that part of the beneficial effects of ACE inhibitors on cardiovascular morbidity and mortality is based on a reduction of the number of ischemic events (unstable angina and/or recurrent myocardial infarction).[98,110] Thus, under certain circumstances, ACE inhibitors can be beneficial in the situation of myocardial ischemia with or without symptoms by an interplay between their vascular and tissue effects on a local and on a systemic level.

Our experimental studies have shown that especially SH-containing ACE inhibitors may potentiate the action of nitrate therapy. This is important because nitrates are frequently used in angina pectoris, and the effect of continuous nitrate therapy decreases in time due to the development of tolerance. This was confirmed by us in a clinical study in which a single dose of captopril significantly improved the therapeutic effect of long-term treatment with isosorbide dinitrate.[27] However, conflicting results have been obtained by other investigators, and this interaction needs further confirmation, especially with regard to the clinical importance of the thiol moiety.[107]

Finally, main emphasis has been put on the effects of exercise-induced ischemia. In contrast, pacing-induced ischemia in patients at rest is clearly improved by ACE inhibition.[83–85] This may be due to the fact that ischemia-induced neurohumoral activation is probably of less importance in exercise-induced than in pacing-induced ischemia.[111] It may be anticipated in patients with myocardial ischemia at rest, that is, with unstable angina, that a similar or even more pronounced neuroendocrine activation will be observed. Reduction of this activation may be beneficial. First results are hopeful,[112] but caution is warranted, especially in the light of the hypotensive effect.

Conclusion

An impressive body of evidence has been generated to support both the existence and functional importance of a local, intracardiac RAS system. On the basis of the physiological effects of A II, a major role of this system in the pathophysiology of myocardial ischemia and its consequences may be postulated. However, in vivo it is very difficult, if not impossible, to differentiate between local (autocrine/paracrine) and circulating (endocrine) effects of A II. The effects may also be influenced by other regulatory systems like the autonomous nervous system and the kinin-kallikrein system, which also may be activated in ischemic syndromes.

In the absence of conclusive evidence, one has to rely on studies with specific antagonists of components of the RAS to prove its role in myocardial infarction and angina pectoris. A number of experimental studies with ACE inhibitors, both in vitro and in vivo, do suggest that cardiac ACE activity does indeed play some role during ischemia and reperfusion, regulating both the synthesis of A II and the breakdown of bradykinin. However, clinical studies with these agents so far have failed to show a major benefit of these agents in symptomatic ischemic heart disease, although the reduction in occurrence of reinfarction and symptomatic angina pectoris following treatment after myocardial infarction is promising.

More studies are needed to demonstrate the activation of the cardiac RAS during various settings of myocardial ischemia and to elucidate its physiological significance. They should include experimental studies focusing on biochemical and molecular biological techniques, functional studies with more specific antagonists of the different components of the RAS, and clinical studies with ACE inhibitors, using very low dosages in order to achieve specific tissue effects and to obviate interfering effects on preload and afterload. We think that these studies will confirm the hypothesis that the cardiac RAS does play a major role in myocardial ischemia, influencing the course of events leading to irreversible cell damage.

Summary

Evidence for a functional and locally integrated RAS both in myocardial tissue and in the coronary vasculature has been established by using biochemical and molecular biological techniques. Despite the well-known physiological effects of A II on coronary blood flow, contractility, and heart rate, its growth-stimulating potential and its potentially cardiotoxic effects, there is no direct evidence that this system does indeed play a role in the course of events that occur during myocardial ischemia and lead to cardiovascular morbidity and mortality. More proof can be obtained by studies with ACE inhibitors, which can interfere with tissue ACE and thereby block the cardiac RAS.

We and others performed a number of experimental studies both in vitro and in vivo to study the effects of ACE inhibitors on ischemia-reperfusion-induced myocardial injury. Decrease in infarct size, better metabolical conditions, reduction in ventricular arrhythmias, and improvement in myocardial function were found, all indicating a potentially beneficial effect. At least part of the effect appeared related to the ACE-inhibitory properties in the heart itself. This strongly suggests that the cardiac RAS is involved in the process of myocardial ischemia, leading to irreversible cell damage. However, other mechanisms may also be involved, especially a reduction in bradykinin breakdown, and SH-containing ACE inhibitors may exert additional effects due to their antioxidant and/or free-radical scavenging properties.

The cardiac RAS also plays a role in the regulation of coronary blood flow, at least under ischemic conditions. ACE inhibitors have been shown to increase coronary blood flow under stimulated conditions but, as we have shown, this was not only due to the inhibition of locally generated A II. Reduction in the breakdown of bradykinin may lead to the release of prostacyclin and EDRF in the coronary vasculature, and the latter effect may be potentiated by the presence of SH groups.

Thus, although conclusive evidence is lacking, the cardiac RAS does appear to play a role in certain ischemic syndromes. Potentially beneficial effects of ACE inhibitors may, at least partly, be explained by an inhibition of this cardiac RAS. However, there appears to be a close interaction with other locally active neurohumoral systems, which may also be affected. More studies are needed to differentiate both the separate effects on these systems and the local versus systemic effects.

References

1. Ganten D, Schelling P, Vecsei P, Ganten U. Iso-renin of extrarenal origin: the tissue angiotensinogenase systems. Am J Med 1976; 60: 760–772.
2. Dzau VJ. Significance of the vascular renin-angiotensin pathway. Hypertension 1986; 8:553–559.
3. Gavras H, Brunner HR, Turini GA, et al. Antihypertensive effect of the oral angiotensin converting-enzyme inhibitor SQ 14225 in man. N Engl J Med 1978; 298: 991–995.
4. Man in 't Veld AJ, Schicht IM, Derkx FHM, de Bruyn JHB, Schalekamp MADH. Effects of an angiotensin-converting enzyme inhibitor (captopril) on blood pressure in anephric subjects. Br Med J 1980; 280: 288–290.
5. Cohen ML, Kurz KD. Angiotensin converting enzyme inhibition in tissues from spontaneously hypertensive rats after treatment with captopril or MK-421. J Pharmacol Exp Ther 1982; 220:63–69.
6. Dzau VJ. Possible prorenin activating mechanisms in the blood vessel wall. J Hypertens 1987; 5 (suppl 2):S15–S18.
7. Campbell DJ. Tissue renin-angiotensin system: sites of angiotensin formation. J Cardiovasc Pharmacol 1987; 10 (suppl 7): S1–S8.
8. Admiraal PJJ, Derkx FHM, Danser AHJ, Pieterman H, Schalekamp MADH. Intrarenal de novo production of angiotensin I in subjects with renal artery stenosis. Hypertension 1990; 16:555–563.
9. Gerlings ED, Gilmore P. Evidence for myocardial conversion of angiotensin I. Basic Res Cardiol 1973; 69:222.
10. Ziogas J, Story DF, Rand MJ. Effects of locally generated angiotensin II on noradrenergic transmission in guinea-isolated atria. Eur J Pharmacol 1984; 106:11–18.
11. Needleman P, Marshall GR, Sobel BE. Hormone interactions in the isolated rabbit heart: synthesis and coronary vasomotor effects of prostaglandins, angiotensin, and bradykinin. Circ Res 1975; 37:802–808.
12. Xiang JZ, Linz W, Becker H, et al. Effects of converting enzyme inhibitors: ramipril and enalapril on peptide action and sympathetic neurotransmission in the isolated rat heart. Eur J Pharmacol 1985; 113: 215–223.
13. Lindpaintner K, Ganten D. The cardiac renin-angiotensin system. An

appraisal of present experimental and clinical evidence. Circ Res 1991; 68:905–921.

14. Dzau VJ. Cardiac renin-angiotensin system: molecular and functional aspects. Am J Med 1988; 84 (suppl 3A): 22–27.

15. Grinstead WC, Young JB. The myocardial renin angiotensin system: existence, importance, and clinical implications. Am Heart J 1991; 123:1039–1045.

16. Liang C, Gavras H. Renin-angiotensin system inhibition in conscious dogs during acute hypoxemia: effects on systemic hemodynamics, regional blood flows and tissue metabolism. J Clin Invest 1978; 62: 961–970.

17. Ertl G, Meesman M, Kochsiek K. On the mechanism of renin release during experimental myocardial ischemia. Eur J Clin Invest 1985; 15: 375–381.

18. Santos RAS, Brum JM, Brosnihan KB, Ferrario CM. The renin-angiotensin system during acute myocardial ischemia in dogs. Hypertension 1990; 15 (suppl I): I-121–I-127.

19. Remme WJ, de Leeuw PW, Bootsma M, Look M, Kruijssen DACM. Systemic neurohumoral activation and vasoconstriction during pacing-induced acute myocardial ischemia in patients with stable angina pectoris. Am J Cardiol 1991; 68:181–186.

20. Drexler H, Lindpaintner K, Lu W, Schieffer B, Ganten D. Transient rise in the expression of cardiac angiotensinogen in a rat model of myocardial infarction and failure (abstract). Circulation 1989; 80:II-459.

21. Hirsch AT, Talsness CE, Schunkert H, Paul M, Dzau VJ. Tissue specific activation of cardiac angiotensin converting enzyme in experimental heart failure. Circ Res 1991; 69:475–482.

22. Unger T, Gohlke P. Tissue renin-angiotensin systems in the heart and vasculature: possible involvement in the cardiovascular actions of converting enzyme inhibitors. Am J Cardiol 1990; 65: 3I–10I.

23. Scicli AG, Farhy R, Scicli G, Nolly H. The kinin-kallikrein system in heart and vascular tissue. In: Bönner G, Schölkens BA, Scicli AG, eds. The Role of Bradykinin in the Cardiovascular Action of the Converting Enzyme Inhibitor Ramipril. Sussex, United Kingdom: Media Medica, 1992:17–28.

24. Chopra M, Scott N, McMurray J, et al. Captopril: a free radical scavenger. Br J Clin Pharmacol 1989; 27:396–399.

25. Pi X, Chen X. Captopril and ramiprilat protect against free radical injury in isolated working rat hearts. J Mol Cell Cardiol 1989; 21: 1261–1271.

26. Przyklenk K, Kloner RA. Angiotensin converting enzyme inhibitors improve contractile function of stunned myocardium by different mechanisms of action. Am Heart J 1991; 121:1319–1330.

27. van Gilst WH, de Graeff PA, de Leeuw MJ, Scholtens E, Wesseling H. Converting enzyme inhibitors and the role of the sulfhydryl group in the potentiation of exo- and endogenous nitrovasodilators. J Cardiovasc Pharmacol 1991; 18:429–436.

28. Sweet CS, Ludden CT, Frederick CM, Bush LR, Ribeiro LGT. Comparative hemodynamic effects of MK-422, a converting enzyme inhibitor, and a renin inhibitor in dogs with acute left ventricular failure. J Cardiovasc Pharmacol 1984; 6:1067–1075.

29. Drexler H, Depenbusch JW, Truog AG, Zelis R, Flaim SF. Acute regional vascular effects of intravenous captopril in a rat model of myocardial function and failure. J Pharmacol Exp Ther 1987; 241:13–19.

30. Shionoiri H, Jinno Y, Kobayashi H, et al. Cardiovascular effects of the converting enzyme inhibitors captopril, enalaprilate, or ramiprilate in anesthetized dogs with acute ischemic heart. Curr Ther Res 1987; 42:988–994.

31. Ertl G, Kloner RA, Alexander RW, Braunwald E. Limitation of experimental infarct size by an angiotensin converting enzyme inhibitor. Circulation 1982; 65:40–48.

32. Liang C, Gavras H, Black J, Sherman LG, Hood WB. Renin-angiotensin system inhibition in acute myocardial infarction in dogs. Circulation 1982; 66:1249–1255.

33. Daniell HB, Carson RR, Ballard KD, Thomas GR, Privitera PJ. Effects of captopril on limiting infarct size in conscious dogs. J Cardiovasc Pharmacol 1984; 6:1043–1047.

34. Lefer AM, Peck RC. Cardioprotective effects of enalapril in acute myocardial ischemia. Pharmacology 1984; 29:61–69.

35. Hock CE, Ribeiro LGT, Lefer AM. Preservation of ischemic myocardium by a new converting enzyme inhibitor, enalaprilic acid, in acute myocardial infarction. Am Heart J 1985; 109:222–228.

36. van Gilst WH, de Graeff PA, Kingma JH, Wesseling H, de Langen CDJ. Captopril reduces purine loss and reperfusion arrhythmias in the rat heart after coronary occlusion. Eur J Pharmacol 1984; 100: 113–117.

37. de Graeff PA, van Gilst WH, de Langen CDJ, Kingma JH, Wesseling H. Concentration-dependent protection by captopril against ischemia-reperfusion injury in the isolated rat heart. Arch Int Pharmacodyn Ther 1986; 280:181–193.

38. van Gilst WH, de Graeff PA, Wesseling H, de Langen CDJ. Reduction of reperfusion arrhythmias in the ischemic isolated rat heart by angiotensin converting enzyme inhibitors: a comparison of captopril, enalapril, and HOE 498. J Cardiovasc Pharmacol 1986; 8:722–778.

39. Linz W, Schölkens BA, Han YF. Beneficial effects of the converting enzyme inhibitor ramipril in ischemic rat hearts. J Cardiovasc Pharmacol 1986; 8(suppl 10):S91–S99.

40. Li K, Chen X. Protective effects of captopril and enalapril on myocardial ischemia and reperfusion damage of rat. J Mol Cell Cardiol 1987; 19:909–915.

41. Rahusen FD, va Gilst WH, Robillard GT, Dijkstra K, Wildevuur CRH. Captopril improves recovery of adenosine triphosphate during reperfusion of the ischemic isolated rat heart: a 31-phosphorus-nuclear magnetic resonance study. Basic Res Cardiol 1988; 83:540–549.

42. de Graeff PA, de Langen CDJ, van Gilst WH, et al. Protective effects of captopril against ischemia/reperfusion-induced ventricular arrhythmias in vitro and in vivo. Am J Med 1988; 84(suppl 3A):67–74.

43. Bagchi D, Iyengar J, Stockwell P, Das DK. Enhanced prostaglandin production in the ischemic-reperfused myocardium by captopril linked with its free radical scavenging action. Prostaglandins Leukot Essent Fatty Acids 1989; 38:145–150.

44. Linz W, Schölkens BA, Kaiser J, et al. Cardiac arrhythmias are ame-

liorated by local inhibition of angiotensin formation and bradykinin degradation with the converting-enzyme inhibitor ramipril. Cardiovasc Drugs Ther 1989; 3:873–882.

45. Linz W, Martorana PA, Grötsch H, Bei-Yin Q, Schölkens BA. Antagonizing bradykinin (BK) obliterates the cardioprotective effects of bradykinin and angiotensin-converting enzyme (ACE) inhibitors in ischemic hearts. Drug Dev Res 1990; 19:393–408.

46. Fleetwood G, Boutinet S, Meier M, Wood JM. Involvement of the renin-angiotensin system in ischemic damage and reperfusion arrhythmias in the isolated perfused rat heart. J Cardiovasc Pharmacol 1991; 17: 351–356.

47. Grover GJ, Sleph PG, Dzwonczyk S, et al. Effects of different angiotensin-converting enzyme (ACE) inhibitors on ischemic isolated rat hearts: relationship between cardiac ACE inhibition and cardioprotection. J Pharmacol Exp Ther 1991; 257:919–929.

48. Arad M, Shotan A, Horowitz L, Klein R, Rabinowitz B. Effects of captopril on metabolic and hemodynamic alterations in global ischemia and reperfusion in the isolated working rat heart. J Cardiovasc Pharmacol 1992; 19:319–323.

49. Menasché P, Grousset G, Peynet J, Mouas C, Loch G, Piwnica A. Pretreatment with captopril improves myocardial recovery after cardioplegic arrest. J Cardiovasc Pharmacol 1992; 19:402–407.

50. de Graeff PA, van Gilst WH, Bel K, de Langen CDJ, Kingma JH, Wesseling H. Concentration-dependent protection by captopril against myocardial damage during ischemia and reperfusion in a closed-chest pig model. J Cardiovasc Pharmacol 1987; 9(suppl 2):S37–S42.

51. Elfallah MS, Ogilvie RI. Effect of vasodilator drugs on coronary occlusion and reperfusion arrhythmias in anesthetized dogs. J Cardiovasc Pharmacol 1985; 7:826–832.

52. Rochette L, Ribuot C, Belichard P, Bril A, Devissaguet M. Protective effect of angiotensin converting enzyme inhibitors (CEI): captopril and perindopril on vulnerability to ventricular fibrillation during myocardial ischemia and reperfusion in rat. Clin Exp Hypertens 1987; A9: 365–368.

53. Westlin W, Mullane K. Does captopril attenuate reperfusion-induced myocardial dysfunction by scavenging free radicals? Circulation 1988; 77 (suppl I):I30–I39.

54. Tio RA, de Langen CDJ, de Graeff PA, et al. The effects of oral pretreatment with zofenopril, an angiotensin converting enzyme inhibitor on early reperfusion and subsequent electrophysiologic stability in the pig. Cardiovasc Drug Ther 1990; 4:695–704.

55. Przyklenk K, Kloner RA. Acute effects of hydralazine and enalapril on contractile function of postischemic myocardium. Am J Cardiol 1987; 60:934–936.

56. Tobé TJM, de Langen CDJ, Weersink EGL, et al. The angiotensin converting enzyme inhibitor perindopril improves survival after experimental myocardial infarction in pigs. J Cardiovasc Pharmacol 1992; 19:732–740.

57. van Wijngaarden J, Tobé TJM, Weersink EGL, et al. Effects of early angiotensin-converting enzyme inhibition in a pig model of myocardial ischemia and reperfusion. J Cardiovasc Pharmacol 1992; 19:408–416.

58. Muller CA, Opie LH, Peisach M, Pineda CA. Antiarrhythmic effects of angiotensin converting enzyme inhibitor perindoprilat in a pig model of acute regional myocardial ischemia. J Cardiovasc Pharmacol 1992; 19:748–754.

59. Martorana PA, Kettenbach B, Breipohl G, Linz W, Schölkens BA. Reduction of infarct size by local angiotensin-converting enzyme inhibition is abolished by a bradykinin-antagonist. Eur J Pharmacol 1990; 182:395–396.

60. Forman MB, Puett DW, Virmani R. Endothelial and myocardial injury during ischaemia and reperfusion: pathogenesis and therapeutic implications. J Am Coll Cardiol 1989; 13:450–459.

61. Manning AS, Hearse DJ. Reperfusion-induced arrhythmias: mechanisms and prevention. J Mol Cell Cardiol 1984; 16: 497–518.

62. Cushman DW, Wang FL, Fung WC, Harvey CM, DeForrest JM. Differentiation of angiotensin-converting enzyme (ACE) inhibitors by their selective inhibition of ACE in physiologically important target organs. Am J Hypertens 1989; 2:294–306.

63. Frohlich ED, Horinaka S. Cardiac and aortic effects of angiotensin converting enzyme inhibitors. Hypertension 1991; 18(suppl II): II-2–II-7.

64. Gavras H, Kremer D, Brown JJ, et al. Angiotensin- and norepinephrine-induced myocardial lesions: experimental and clinical studies in rabbits and man. Am Heart J 1974; 89: 321–332.

65. de Langen CDJ, de Graeff PA, van Gilst WH, Bel K, Kingma JH. Effects of angiotensin II and captopril in inducible ventricular tachycardias two weeks after myocardial infarction in the pig. J Cardiovasc Pharmacol 1989; 13:186–191.

66. Carlsson L, Abrahamsson T. Ramiprilat attenuates the local release of noradrenaline in the ischemic myocardium. Eur J Pharmacol 1989; 166:7–64.

67. Tio RA, Tobé TJM, Bel KJ, de Langen CDJ, van Gilst WH, Wesseling H. Beneficial effects of bradykinin on porcine ischemic myocardium. Basic Res Cardiol 1991; 86:107–116.

68. Tio RA, van Gilst WH, Rett K, Wolters K, Dietze GJ, Wesseling H. The effects of bradykinin and the ischemic isolated rat heart. Horm Metab Res 1990; 22: 85–89.

69. Vegh A, Szekeres L, Paratt JR. Local intracoronary infusions of bradykinin profoundly reduce the severity of ischemia-induced arrhythmias in anaesthetized dogs. Br J Pharmacol 1991; 104: 294–295.

70. Tobé T, de Langen CDJ, Tio RA, Bel KJ, Mook PH, Wesseling H. In vivo effect of bradykinin during ischemia and reperfusion: improved electrical stability two weeks after myocardial infarction in the pig. J Cardiovasc Pharmacol 1991; 17:600–607.

71. Schrör K. Actions of prostaglandins on the heart. In: Gryglewski RJ, Stock G, eds. Prostacyclin and Its Stable Analogue Iloprost. Berlin: Springer Verlag, 1987:159–178.

72. van Gilst WH, van Wijngaarden J, Scholtens E, de Graeff PA, de Langen CDJ, Wesseling H. Captopril-induced increase in coronary flow: an SH-dependent effect on arachidonic acid metabolism? J Cardiovasc Pharmacol 1987; 9(suppl 2):S31–S36.

73. van Gilst WH, Scholtens E, de Graeff PA, de Langen CDJ, Wesseling

H. Differential influences of angiotensin converting-enzyme inhibitors on the coronary circulation. Circulation 1988; 77(suppl I):I-24–I-29.

74. Noguchi K, Kato T, Ito H, Aniya Y, Sakanashi M. Effect of intracoronary captopril on coronary blood flow and regional myocardial function in dogs. Eur J Pharmacol 1985; 110:11–19.

75. Ertl G, Alexander RW, Kloner RA. Interactions between coronary occlusion and the renin-angiotensin system in the dog. Basic Res Cardiol 1983; 78:518–533.

76. Ertl G. Coronary vasoconstriction in experimental myocardial ischemia. J Cardiovasc Pharmacol 1987; 9(suppl 2):S9–S17.

77. Berdeaux A, Bonhenry C, Giudicelly JF. Effects of four angiotensin I converting enzyme inhibitors on regional myocardial blood flow and ischemic injury during coronary occlusion in dogs. Fund Clin Pharmacol 1987; 1:201–212.

78. Halperin, JL, Faxon DP, Creager MA, et al. Coronary hemodynamic effects of angiotensin inhibition by captopril and teprotide in patients with congestive heart failure. Am J Cardiol 1982; 50:967–972.

79. Faxon DP, Creager MA, Halperin JL, Sussman HA, Gavras H, Ryan TJ. The effect of angiotensin converting enzyme inhibition on coronary blood flow and hemodynamics in patients without coronary artery disease. Int J Cardiol 1982; 2:251–262.

80. Daly P, Mettauer B, Rouleau J-L, Cousineau D, Burgess JH. Acute effects of captorpil on the coronary circulation of patients with hypertension and angina. Am J Med 1984; 76(suppl 3B): 111–119.

81. Magrini F, Shimizu M, Roberts N, Fouad FM, Tarazi RC, Zanchetti A. Converting-enzyme inhibition and coronary flow. Circulation 1987; 75(suppl I):I-168–I-174.

82. Foult JM, Tavolaro O, Antony I, Nitenberg A. Direct myocardial and coronary effects of enalaprilat in patients with dilated cardiomyopathy: assessment by a bilateral intracoronary infusion technique. Circulation 1988; 77:337–344.

83. Remme WJ, Look MP, Bootsma M. Enalaprilat improves coronary flow without affecting hemodynamics: a local tissue effect? Circulation 1989; 80(suppl II):II-558.

84. Karsh KR, Voelker W, Mauser M. Myocardial and coronary vascular effects of captopril in stable angina pectoris. Eur Heart J 1990; 11 (suppl B):157–161.

85. Ikram H, Low CJS, Shirlaw T, Webb CM, Richards AM, Crozier IG. Antianginal, hemodynamic and coronary vascular effects of captopril in stable angina pectoris. Am J Cardiol 1990; 66: 164–167.

86. Perondi R, Saino A, Tio RA, et al. ACE inhibition attenuates sympathetic coronary vasoconstriction in patients with coronary artery disease. Circulation 1992; 85:2004–2013.

87. Tio RA, Heiligers J, de Langen CDJ, Saxena PR, Wesseling H. Systemic and regional effects of the ACE-inhibitors zofenoprilat and enalaprilat in the rat, with and without treatment with a bradykinin antagonist. PhD Thesis. University of Groningen, Groningen, The Netherlands, 1990:119–132.

88. Abrams J. A reappraisal of nitrate therapy. JAMA 1988; 259:396–401.

89. van Wijngaarden J, van Tio RA, van Gilst WH, de Graeff PA, de Langen CDJ, Wesseling H. Coronary vasodilation induced by captopril

and zofenoprilat: evidence for a prostaglandin-independent mechanism. Naunyn-Schmiedeberg's Arch Pharmacol 1991; 343:491–495.

90. Friedman PL, Brown EJ, Gunther S, et al. Coronary vasoconstrictor effect of indomethacin in patients with coronary artery disease. N Engl J Med 1981; 305:1171–1175.

91. Wiemer G, Schölkens BA, Becker RHA, Busse R. Ramiprilat enhances endothelial autacoid formation by inhibiting breakdown of endothelium-derived bradykinin. Hypertension 1991; 18: 558–563.

92. Pelc LR, Gross GJ, Warltier DC. Mechanism of coronary vasodilation produced by bradykinin. Circulation 1991; 83: 2048–2056.

93. Alhenc-Galas F, Tsai SJ, Callahan KS, Campbell WB, Johnson AR. Stimulation of prostaglandin formation by vasoactive mediators in cultured human endothelial cells. Prostaglandins 1982; 24:723–742.

94. Cachofeiro V, Sakakibara T, Nasjletti A. Kinins, nitric oxide, and the hypotensive effect of captopril and ramiprilat in hypertension. Hypertension 1992; 19:138–145.

95. Schrör K. Converting enzyme inhibitors and the interaction between kinins and eicosanoids. J Cardiovasc Pharmacol 1990; 15(suppl 6): S60–S68.

96. Auerswald W, Doleschel W. On the potentiation of kinins by sulfhydrylic compounds. Arch Int Pharmacodyn 1967; 168: 188–197.

97. Ignarro LJ, Lippton H, Edwards JC, et al. Mechanisms of vascular smooth muscle relaxation by organic nitrates, nitrites, nitroprusside and nitric oxide: evidence for the involvement of S-nitrosothiols as active intermediates. J Pharmacol Ther 1981; 218: 739–749.

98. Goldschmidt JE, Tallarida RJ. Pharmacological evidence that captopril possesses an endothelium-mediated component of vasodilation: effect of sulfhydryl groups on endothelium-derived relaxing factor. J Pharmacol Exp Ther 1991; 257:1136–1145.

99. van Gilst WH, de Graeff PA, Scholtens E, de Langen CDJ, Wesseling H. Potentiation of isosorbide dinitrate-induced coronary dilatation by captopril. J Cardiovasc Pharmacol 1987; 9:254–255.

100. Weber KT, Anversa P, Amstrong PW, et al. Remodeling and reparation of the cardiovascular system. J Am Coll Cardiol 1992; 20:3–16.

101. Pfeffer MA, Braunwald E, Moyé LA, et al. Effect of captopril on mortality and morbidity in patients with left ventricular dysfunction after myocardial infarction. New Engl J Med 1992; 327:669–677.

102. Sharpe N, Smith H, Murphy J, Greaves S, Hart H, Gamble G. Early prevention of left ventricular dysfunction after myocardial with angiotensin-converting enzyme inhibition. Lancet 1991; 337: 872–876.

103. Nabel EG, Topol EJ, Galeana A, et al. A randomized placebo-controlled trial of combined early intravenous captopril and recombinant tissue-type plasminogen activator therapy in acute myocardial infarction. J Am Coll Cardiol 1991; 17:467–473.

104. The CONSENSUS II Study Group. Effects of the early administration of enalapril on mortality in patients with acute myocardial infarction. New Engl J Med 1992; 327:678–684.

105. Kingma JH, van Gilst WH, van Peels CH, on behalf of the CATS investigators group. Angiotensin-converting enzyme inhibition during thrombolytic therapy in acute myocardial infarction: the captopril and thrombolysis study. J Cardiovasc Pharmacol 1992; 19(suppl 4): S18–S24.

106. Hochman JS, Hahn RT, LeJementel TH, Zielonka JS, Sonnenblick EH. Concomitant angiotensin-converting enzyme inhibition and thrombolysis in acute anterior myocardial infarction. J Cardiovasc Pharmacol 1992; 19(suppl 4):S25–S29.
107. de Graeff PA, van Gilst WH. Role of angiotensin-converting enzyme inhibition in angina pectoris. J Cardiovasc Pharmacol 1992; 19(suppl 4):S30–S37.
108. Cleland JGF, Henderson E, McLenachan J, Findlay IN, Dargie HJ. Effect of captopril, an angiotensin-converting enzyme inhibitor, in patients with angina pectoris and heart failure. J Am Coll Cardiol 1991; 17:733–739.
109. Ahkras F, Jackson G. The role of captopril as single therapy in hypertension and angina pectoris. Int J Cardiol 1991; 33: 259–266.
110. The SOLVD Investigators. Effect of enalapril on mortality and the development of heart failure in asymptomatic patients with reduced left ventricular ejection fractions. New Engl J Med 1992; 327:685–691.
111. Remme WJ, Look MP, Bootsma M, et al. Neurohumoral activation during acute myocardial ischemia: effects of ACE inhibition. Eur Heart J 1990; 11(suppl B):162–171.
112. Haude M, Erbel R, Tschollar W, Meyer J. Sublingual captopril in patients with unstable angina (abstract). Eur Heart J 1989; 10(suppl): 83.

13

The Contribution of Tissue Renin-Angiotensin Systems to Disease Progression in Experimental Heart Failure

Alan T. Hirsch, Michael R. Muellerleile, and Victor J. Dzau

Cardiovascular Homeostasis: The Classic Role of the Renin-Angiotensin System

The circulating renin-angiotensin system (RAS) is activated during states of sodium restriction, hemorrhage, or intravascular volume contraction, during an increased adrenergic state, or as a consequence of acute cardiac decompensation. The effects of this endocrine system are mediated by the peptide hormone A II, which elicits tissue-specific responses at many target organs, including the blood vessels and kidney, heart, brain, and adrenal tissues. Angiotensin receptors in target tissues mediate systemic vasoconstriction, adrenal aldosterone release, hypophyseal vasopressin secretion, and renal sodium reabsorption. The circulating RAS, as a classic hormonal system, is subject to feedback regulation and serves to maintain acute cardiovascular homeostasis.

Abundant investigation over the past 15 years has demonstrated that an endogenous RAS exists in most target tissues that contribute to acute and chronic cardiovascular regulation. The evi-

Lindpaintner K and Ganten D (editors): *The Cardiac-Renin Angiotensin System,* © Futura Publishing Co., Inc., Armonk, NY, 1994.

dence for the presence of tissue RASs has been reviewed extensively elsewhere.[1,2] We have speculated that these tissue RASs might contribute to local A II production, thereby contributing to disease pathophysiology, and serve as logical targets for pharmacological therapeutic interventions. A number of experimental observations now demonstrate that cardiovascular diseases are associated with tissue-specific regulation of these RASs (in the blood vessels and cardiac and renal tissues). We shall review the evidence documenting the presence of these tissue RASs that suggests that tissue RASs are functional systems contributing to the production of A II in target tissues and that demonstrates a possible role for these tissue RASs in the pathophysiology of heart failure.

Potential Contributions of the Circulating and Tissue Renin-Angiotensin Systems in Heart Failure

It is well documented that a reduction in cardiac output elicits compensatory homeostatic responses that are mediated by neurohormonal mechanisms. Activation of the sympathetic nervous system results in systemic vasoconstriction, decreases in renal blood flow and glomerular filtration rate, and an increase in tubular reabsorption of sodium. Activation of the RAS further contributes to the increases in vascular tone and sodium avidity. Vasopression secretion may also be increased during marked reductions in cardiac output, which contributes signficantly to the antidiuretic state of heart failure. The temporal activation of circulating neurohormonal mechanisms was well illustrated in the study by Watkins et al.[3] of the experimental canine model of cardiac decompensation. In this model, reductions in cardiac output and filling pressure result in elevations of plasma renin activity, A II, and aldosterone levels, with associated vasoconstriction and sodium retention. However, these circulating neurohormonal mechanisms return to normal during the compensated stage of heart failure as plasma volume and cardiac stroke volume increase. Additionally, in other animal models of compensated heart failure, such as the coronary-ligated rat or subacute stage of canine rapid ventricular pacing, normal or near-normal plasma renin activity and A II levels have been demonstrated.[4-6] Thus, in experimental heart failure, circulating neurohormonal mechanisms exhibit a time-dependent response, with acute activa-

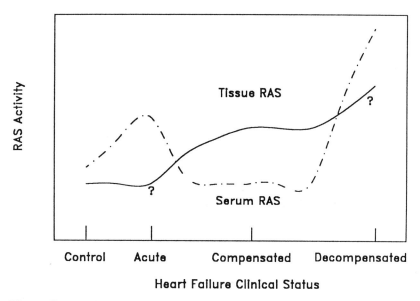

Fig. 1. Proposed contributions of the circulating and tissue RASs during the natural history of heart failure. It is known that the circulating RAS is activated in states of acute cardiac decompensation; subsequent normalization of circulating RAS activity is common despite persistent left ventricular dysfunction during the compensated heart failure state. Episodes of heart failure decompensation again activate the plasma RAS. Present data support a more progressive activation of cardiac and renal RAS activities during compensated heart failure (from Hirsch AT and Dzau VJ[58]).

tion during cardiovascular decompensation and subsequent normalization during the chronic, compensated phase (Figure 1).

A similar pattern of activation of plasma neurohormones has been observed in patients after acute myocardial infarction[7] or during heart failure.[8,9] Patients with mild heart failure or stable disease usually demonstrate normal plasma renin activity, catecholamines, and vasopressin levels at rest. Nevertheless, long-term ACE inhibition elicits salutary responses from both patients and animals with stable cardiac dysfunction. Overall morbidity is decreased, and survival may be prolonged.[10–15] We hypothesize that during the compensated phase, the tissue RAS may contribute to the pathophysiology of heart failure. Examination of the role of the tissue RAS in this disease state may also provide insights into the mechanisms mediating these beneficial therapeutic responses to ACE inhibition. Our data, as well as that of other investigators, demonstrate that tissue RASs indeed are activated during the compensated phase of heart failure. In this review we will focus on cardiac and renal RASs since these are well-studied systems in heart failure.

The Cardiac Renin–Angiotensin System in Heart Failure

The contribution of cardiac RAS activity in pathophysiological states has recently been investigated. We have recently studied cardiac ACE activity in rats with left-ventricular hypertrophy induced by aortic banding[16] and found a marked rise in cardiac ACE activity and ACE mRNA expression and an associated increase in the cardiac conversion rate of A I to A II. This evidence is reviewed in more detail in chapter 11.

Inasmuch as left-ventricular hypertrophy is a prominent and ominous risk factor for the progression of myocardial failure, we have examined the role of the circulating and tissue RASs in a relevant small animal model of chronic heart failure. Rats with heart failure induced by anterior coronary artery ligation mimic the natural history of clinical heart failure via the development of left-ventricular systolic dysfunction, progressive left-ventricular dilatation, regional blood flow redistribution, renal sodium retention, and increased mortality. Administration of ACE inhibitors has been demonstrated to blunt the magnitude of left-ventricular dysfunction as well as to prolong survival. However, the mechanisms underlying these beneficial effects of ACE inhibitors remain incompletely elucidated.

We, therefore, examined the relative activation of the circulating and tissue RASs in heart-failure rats in the chronic, compensated state compared to nonoperated and sham-operated control rats. These investigations have demonstrated[4] that cardiac ACE is significantly elevated in the chronic, compensated state of experimental heart failure in these animals (Figure 2). The ACE activity is increased in the right ventricle and interventricular septum and correlates with the extent of the infarct and the degree of cardiac dilatation (Figure 3). As in stable human disease, circulating renin and ACE activities are not elevated during the chronic, compensated phase in this animal model. In order to determine that the biochemical evidence of increased ACE activity was a result of local cardiac RAS activation, and not a consequence of uptake of ACE from the plasma compartment, we also evaluated the ACE mRNA level in hypertrophied, noninfarcted right-ventricular myocardial tissue. Application of polymerase chain reaction (PCR) techniques permitted the determination that the increase in right-ventricular and in-

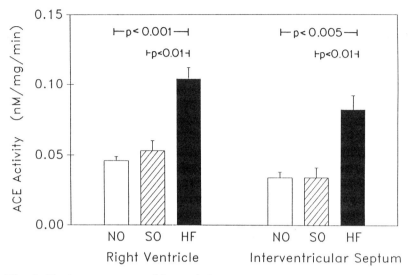

Fig. 2. During compensated heart failure in rats, the interventricular and right-ventricular myocardium demonstrate a twofold increase in ACE activities in the heart failure (HF) animals, as compared to both nonoperated (NO) and sham-operated (SO) control rats.

terventricular septal ACE activities in rats with experimental heart failure was due to a concomitant twofold increase in ACE mRNA expression with increased local enzyme synthesis. Such an induction of myocardial ACE activity has now been demonstrated in the collagenous structures (including the scar) of rats subjected to anterior myocardial infarction,[17] as well as in the myocardial tissue of rats with heart failure induced by rapid cardiac pacing.[18] No studies to date have clarified the exact stimulus responsible for the induction of cardiac ACE. In this model of heart failure, the remodeled myocardium has been demonstrated to express activities for other neurohormonal components. For example, Drexler et al.[19,20] have also demonstrated induction of the expression of both angiotensinogen and the atrial natriuretic factor in the ventricular myocardium in proportion to the extent of myocardial infarction. It is plausible that increased wall stress, increased inflammatory cell or fibroblast migration into the healing myocardium, or increased myocardial neurosympathetic activity may be responsible for the induction of cardiac RAS expression.

The increase in cardiac ACE activity in the hypertrophied or failing myocardium may have important pathophysiological impli-

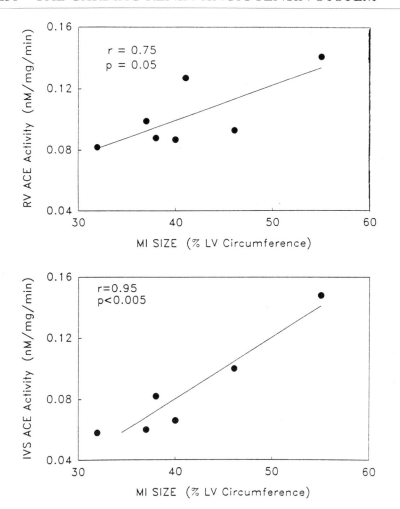

Fig. 3. Both right-ventricular (RV) and interventricular septal (IVS) ACE activities are increased in direct proportion to the magnitude of left-ventricular dysfunction, as denoted by the histopathologic size of the myocardial infarction (MI) of the left ventricle (LV).

cations. Functional A II receptors have been demonstrated in the myocytes of normal and failing human hearts.[21,22] As noted earlier, A II may elicit intense coronary artery vasoconstriction. Indeed, the coronary vasodilatory effect of ACE inhibitors, independent of circulating A II, has been demonstrated in the isolated perfused heart by both Linz et al.[23] and van Gilst et al.[24] Locally synthesized cardiac A II may also directly influence the cardiac inotropic state [25-27] or indirectly augment cardiac systolic function via facilitation of norepinephrine release from sympathetic nerve terminals.[28,29] Whereas these effects might not be prominent in the normal state, we have hypothesized that these hemodynamic effects of A II may be especially important in the failing myocardium.

This possibility has been examined by Foult et al.[30] who evaluated the effects of intracoronary infusion of enalaprilat and the presumed withdrawal of A II on indices of systolic performance in human heart failure. The simultaneous infusion of enalaprilat into the right and left coronary arteries of these patients caused a significant decline in indices of systolic function. The ejection fraction and the cardiac index declined and the end-systolic stress and end-systolic volume ratio diminished in those patients with idiopathic dilated cardiomyopathy. Despite decreased cardiac work, calculated coronary vascular resistance also decreased, suggesting that basal tissue A II concentrations subserved both inotropic and coronary vasoconstrictive responses. Other non-ACE biochemical pathways for A I to A II conversion (chymase) have been demonstrated to exist in the human, but not the rat, heart.[31] Therefore, in humans it is possible that cardiac tissue A II generation might still occur despite administration of systemic ACE inhibitors. Thus, we surmise that tissue A II synthesis could potentially provide positive inotropic effects despite systemic ACE inhibition. As reviewed in chapter 11, the investigations of Lorell et al. have demonstrated that the intracoronary administration of A II may cause severe diastolic dysfunction in models of left-ventricular hypertrophy. In the hypertrophied rat myocardium studied as a Langendorff preparation, infusion of A I induces a dose-dependent increase in left-ventricular end-diastolic pressure.[16] Similar findings have also been reported in patients with left-ventricular hypertrophy due to aortic stenosis.[32] Chronic heart failure is usually characterized by both systolic and diastolic dysfunction; to date, the magnitude of diastolic dysfunction in chronic heart failure that might be attributed to increased cardiac RAS activity has not been determined.

Cardiac angiotensin may also participate directly in ventricular hypertrophy and remodeling via its growth-promoting effects.[33,34] Angiotensin II has been shown to stimulate cardiac myocyte growth. In addition, the enhanced angiotensin-induced norepinephrine release may also promote cardiac hypertrophy. These observations may underlie the ability of ACE inhibitors to produce regression of cardiac hypertrophy secondary to chronic hypertension or aortic banding.[35–37] Thus, the increased cardiac ACE activity and locally synthesized A II may also participate in the ventricular remodeling that is ultimately responsible for cardiac dilation after myocardial infarction or in volume-overload conditions.

Enhanced cardiac A II generation may also contribute to the increased ventricular dysrhythmias that are characteristic of advanced cardiac dysfunction. Linz et al. have demonstrated in the isolated perfused rat heart that both A I and A II perfusion aggravated the arrhythmias induced by transient ischemia.[23] The dysrhythmias induced by A I administration were abolished by pretreatment with the ACE inhibitor ramipril. It is not known whether the dysrhythmias associated with impaired left-ventricular function are due to either subendocardial ischemia, altered adrenergic state, or direct effects of angiotensin on the conduction systems. Indeed, a high density of A II binding sites has been detected in the conduction system.[38] The clinical trials of ACE inhibition in patients with heart failure have noted disparate effects of these agents on the incidence of sudden death, which is presumably a marker of high-grade dysrhythmias.[14,15]

Renal Renin–Angiotensin System in Heart Failure

The progression of heart failure is modulated by the magnitude of renal sodium and fluid retention.[39] Angiotensin II may elicit such sodium retentive responses via the multiple mechanisms previously discussed. Inhibition of A II production via administration of converting-enzyme inhibitors may alter renal function, however, even in states in which the circulating RAS is not activated.[40,41] These data have suggested that the beneficial natriuretic and diuretic effects of ACE inhibition might be mediated via an intrarenal mechanism. Evidence for such a mechanism has been suggested by our recent observations of the effect of experimental heart failure on the activity of the intrarenal RAS.[42] These studies by Schunkert et al. have demonstrated tissue-specific activation of the intrarenal RAS in the chronic, compensated state after experimental myocardial infarction in the rat. In these animals, the renal angiotensinogen mRNA level was increased by 46%, compared with sham-operated controls.[42] The experimental animals were stratified by the histopathologic severity of heart failure into three groups. In those animals with small infarcts (10%–25% of the left-ventricular circumference), the renal angiotensinogen mRNA level was increased slightly (by 31%), though this increase was not statistically different from sham-operated control rats. Animals with medium-sized myocardial infarctions (26%–40%) demonstrated a larger increase (46%,

$p<0.05$). Those rats with the largest infarcts (41%–55%) demonstrated the greatest increase in renal angiotensinogen mRNA level (66%, $p<0.05$), compared to the sham-operated control rats. Additionally, there was a significant correlation between myocardial infarct size and the magnitude of increase of the renal angiotensinogen level ($r = 0.51$, $p = 0.001$). This direct relationship between the magnitude of increase and the histopathologic size of the myocardial infarction implies a possible causal relation to the degree of ventricular dysfunction.

This activation of the intrarenal RAS by heart failure was selective for this single component of the RAS (Figure 4). There were no differences in the liver angiotensinogen mRNA levels, circulating angiotensinogen concentrations, plasma renin concentrations, kidney renin content, renal renin mRNA levels, nor in serum or renal ACE activities in sham and stable heart-failure rats (Figure 5). Thus, these data raised the possibility that the selective increase in the renal angiotensinogen level might alter intrarenal A II concentrations. In order to examine this possibility, renal tissue A II concentration was determined in an additional cohort of sham-operated and heart-failure rats. In these animals, the renal angiotensinogen mRNA levels were 1.8-fold higher in the heart-failure animals, and there was an associated 2.4-fold increase in renal tissue A II concentrations. The concentrations of renal angiotensinogen mRNA and renal A II peptide concentrations exhibited a positive correlation ($r = 0.89$, $p<0.001$).

There are several potential mechanisms that may contribute to the increased renal angiotensinogen mRNA expression observed in this model of experimental heart failure. Increased renal sympathetic activity, hemodynamic effects, and positive feedback effect of renal A II levels on angiotensinogen expression may underlie this phenomenon. The additional finding that intrarenal renin mRNA levels and renal renin concentration were not different from control animals is consistent with the observation that the circulating RAS (e.g., plasma renin activity) is not activated in this compensated disease state.

We subsequently evaluated the effects of treatment with the ACE inhibitors enalapril and captopril in this heart failure model.[43] Most prior investigations of ACE inhibition in this model have examined relatively short treatment periods (1–7 days). In order to evaluate the more clinically relevant effects of prolonged ACE-inhibitor administration, both normal and heart-failure rats were studied during treatment with either vehicle (tap water) or these ACE inhibitors for 7 weeks. Chronic oral treatment with both captopril and

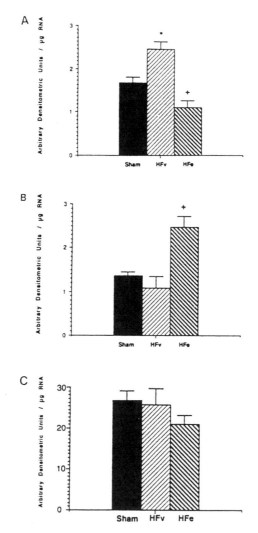

Fig. 4. Quantitative slot-blot analysis demonstrates that experimental heart failure elicits a tissue-specific increase in renal angiotensinogen expression (panel A) but does not alter renal renin (panel B) or hepatic angiotensinogen mRNA levels (panel C). Chronic treatment with oral enalapril caused both a normalization of the renal angiotensinogen mRNA level as well as concomitant increases in the renal renin mRNA level.

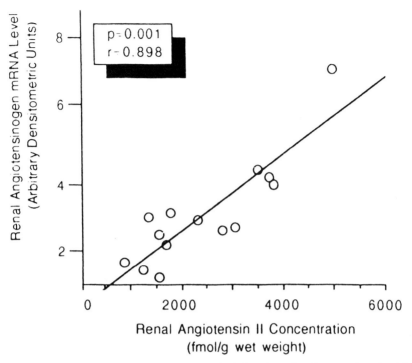

Fig. 5. The renal angiotensinogen mRNA level is closely correlated with the renal concentration of A II.

enalapril caused comparable falls in blood pressure (12–18 mm Hg) in both sham and heart-failure rats. Both ACE inhibitors also caused a comparable inhibition of renal ACE activity. In this study, there was no change in either daily urine volume or sodium excretion in the vehicle- or captopril-treated rats over this prolonged treatment period. In contrast, enalapril-treated animals demonstrated 83% and 10% increases in daily urine volume and sodium excretion, respectively, compared to the control and captopril-treated heart-failure rats. Neither drug treatment caused any significant change in blood urea nitrogen or serum creatinine concentrations. Enalapril, but not captopril, normalized the renal angiotensinogen expression, and the magnitude of this effect correlated with the increase in daily urinary sodium excretion ($r = -0.43, p < 0.005$) (Figure 6). The physiological consequences of intrarenal RAS activation in heart failure may thus be cautiously extrapolated from these findings. Inasmuch as renal perfusion pressure (blood pressure) and renal ACE activities were not different between the two drug treatment groups, we have specu-

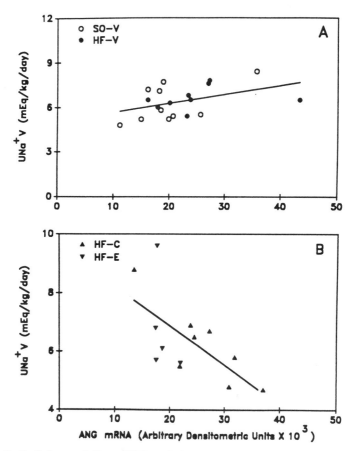

Fig. 6. Both heart failure (HF) and sham-operated (SO) rats treated with vehicle (V) demonstrate variable angiotensinogen mRNA levels and normal urinary sodium excretion (UNa$^+$V). In these rats (panel A), multiple mechanisms preserve normal salt and water homeostasis. Chronic oral treatment with either captopril (C) or enalapril (E) causes a comparable fall in blood pressure (renal perfusion pressure) and decline in renal ACE activity. However, the daily urinary sodium excretion during ACE inhibition in experimental heart failure (panel B) was best predicted by the renal angiotensinogen mRNA level (and thus by intrarenal concentrations of A II).

lated that an intrarenal mechanism must differentiate the disparate diuretic, natriuretic, and renal angiotensinogen mRNA responses. In these ACE-inhibitor-treated animals, renin was undoubtedly present in excess. It is plausible that during chronic ACE inhibition, the intrarenal angiotensinogen level may, therefore, determine the rate of intrarenal A II synthesis. These differing renal physiological effects of these two ACE inhibitors suggest that intrarenal A II levels may cause positive feedback regulation of angiotensinogen expression in the kidney. More sustained inhibition of renal ACE by enalapril, compared to captopril, and consequent decreased intrarenal A II levels would be responsible for both normalization of intrarenal angiotensinogen mRNA levels and natriuresis. Thus, oral administration of ACE inhibitors may differentially block both systemic and intrarenal A II formation. These data may explain why treatment with ACE inhibitors may elicit significant renal vasodilation and natriuresis despite normal activity of the circulating RAS.[40,44]

Stage-Dependent Activation of Tissue Renin-Angiotensin Systems—A Hypothesis in Evolution

It has been demonstrated that activation of circulating neurohormones (e.g., plasma renin activity, norepinephrine, and the atrial natriuretic factor) is predictive of worsened survival in human heart failure.[45,46] However, multiple investigations have also demonstrated that progressive left-ventricular dilation and renal sodium retention occur despite near-normal activity of these circulating hormones in patients with stable, compensated disease. Thus, we hypothesized that the primary role of the plasma RAS was to aid in the preservation of cardiovascular homeostasis during acute cardiac decompensation, whereas changes in tissue RAS might contribute to homeostatic responses during chronic, sustained impairment of cardiac function (Fig. 1). As noted above, considerable evidence now confirms that both cardiac and renal tissue RAS activities are indeed increased in the compensated stage of heart failure, at a time when plasma renin-angiotensin activity is normal. Such evidence of increased tissue A II peptide biosynthesis (via activated cardiac and renal RAS activities) during stable heart failure may mediate compensatory local cardiac inotropic and lucitropic effects, the redistribution of regional blood flow, and renal sodium retentive effects. Both local and systemic physiological mechanisms contribute to cardiac and renal end-organ function in heart failure. We hypothesize that the activation of local angiotensin biosynthesis may subserve beneficial tissue homeostatic responses without detrimental systemic neurohormonal activation during compensated heart failure. Whether sustained activation of tissue RAS systems during the compensated stage contributes to disease progression in heart failure is not known. However, we have speculated that the transition from the compensated heart-failure state to cardiac decompensation

Table 1
Potential Compensatory and Deleterious Pathophysiological
Effects of Tissue Renin-Angiotensin Systems During Progressive
Heart Failure

Tissue RAS	Compensatory Effects: Adaptive Responses	Deleterious Effects: Maladaptive Responses
Cardiac RAS	positive inotropic effect; cardiac hypertrophy	negative lucitropic effect; left-ventricular dilatation; dysrhythmia induction; subendocardial ischemia
Renal RAS	maintain GFR	sodium and water retention; increased plasma volume
Vascular RAS	regional blood flow redistribution	increased preload; increased afterload

Tissue biosynthesis of A II may be an initially adaptive response to myocardial injury and hemodynamic decompensation. However, prolonged activation of tissue RASs may eventually subserve maladaptive responses and thereby contribute to the progression of heart failure. It is noted that most "compensatory" effects are acute hemodynamic responses. In contrast, many proposed "deleterious" effects are a result of more long-term physiological effects of A II on end-organ structure or function. Abbreviation: GFR: glomerular filtration rate

would be heralded by further activation of both tissue RAS and circulating neurohormonal systems (Fig. 1 and Table 1). This concept of differential temporal contributions of circulating and tissue RASs to the pathophysiology of heart failure may have important pharmacological implications.

Therapeutic Implications of a Tissue RAS Target of Drug Action in Heart Failure

The demonstration of local synthesis of A II in tissues provides a valuable potential therapeutic target for treatment in heart failure. It has been recognized in hypertensive patients that the acute vasodilatory response to an ACE inhibitor is influenced by the activity of the circulating RAS, whereas the long-term hypotensive response to ACE inhibitors may be more dependent on inhibition of tissue ACE activity. Similarly, we have speculated that the short-term hemodynamic improvement elicited by ACE inhibitors may be mediated by inhibition of the circulating RAS, whereas the effect of ACE inhibitors to improve the natural history of heart faiiure in low-renin states may be due to tissue ACE inhibition.[12,14,15,47,48] For example, it has been demonstrated from the SOLVD database that the circulating RAS is normal in patients with left-ventricular dysfunction but without overt heart failure. Despite normal plasma renin activity in these patients, treatment with enalapril blunted the progression of disease and the subsequent development of overt congestive symptoms.[49] The results of the recent SAVE trial have also confirmed the efficacy of captopril treatment in decreasing the frequency of myocardial ischemic events, hospitalization rates, and morality in patients after acute myocardial infarction.[50] Thus, the efficacy of clinical ACE inhibition in low-renin states has been predicted by the results of studies of animal models of heart failure.

If tissue RAS activation may contribute to the pathogenesis of heart failure, then it is attractive to speculate that these RASs may explain differential pharmacological effects of ACE inhibitors. Experimental data demonstrate that plasma pharmacokinetics do not predict the tissue half-life of these agents. For example, captopril administration to spontaneously hypertensive rats (SHR) inhibits blood vessel and renal ACE for days longer than its plasma effects.[51] Captopril, fosinopril, and zofenipril have been reported to produce greater and more prolonged inhibition of SHR cardiac ACE after a single oral dose than ramipril and enalapril.[52] Similar disparities in tissue ACE inhibition by various agents have been demonstrated in brain and renal tissues. The tissue pharmacokinetics of ACE inhibitors in humans are not known. However, the ability of ACE inhibitors to decrease tissue ACE activities in humans has been confirmed by the study of Erman and coworkers; these studies demonstrated significant inhibition of ACE activities in the kidney, heart, aortic, and venous tissues harvested from patients after short-term administration of oral ramipril.[53]

Thus, target tissue penetration or binding of these agents to ACE may underlie clinically important effects. It has been suggested that long-acting ACE inhibitors (e.g., enalapril) may have greater adverse effects on renal function than short-acting agents.[54] These adverse effects were attributed to more prolonged systemic hypotension than occurred with shorter-acting agents. However, as we have shown, true equipotent doses for tissue ACE inhibition are difficult to achieve in these studies. The inability to define tissue-specific ACE-inhibition equipotency in clinical trials may also explain the disparate effects of captopril and lisinopril on the left-ventricular ejection fraction in patients with heart failure[55] and the differing effects of these agents on exercise duration. For example, it has been suggested that the ability of long-term ACE inhibition to improve skeletal muscle blood flow is due to effects on vascular RAS activity.[56] Finally, it is feasible that the ability of these agents to alter disease progression and mortality is due to their relative ability to achieve prolonged binding to tissue ACE. Whereas this possibility is unlikely to be directly assessed in clinical trials, the results of the recent Xamoterol Heart Failure Trial have suggested that background treatment of captopril and enalapril was associated by post-hoc analysis with differing survival benefits in these heart failure patients.[57]

Conclusion

Present experimenal data suggest that tissue RAS contributes to the pathophysiology of heart failure via myocardial RAS effects, effects on afterload (vascular RAS activity), and effects on preload (vascular and renal tissue RAS activity). It is now clear that ACE inhibitors alter the rate of disease progression in both patients and experimental models of heart failure.[10–15,50] The ability of ACE inhibitors to attenuate left-ventricular dilation, decrease morbidity, and improve survival may be due to effects of these agents on these target tissue RASs.

Summary

The circulating RAS plays an important role in the maintenance of cardiovascular homeostasis. Numerous investigations over the past decade have demonstrated the presence of an endogenous RAS in target tissues that is important in cardiovascular regulation. This chapter reviews the evidence that shows that tissue RAS components are regulated in cardiovascular disease states, permitting possible local biosynthesis of A II in target tissues. Recent observations from our laboratory and from other investigators demonstrate that the cardiac and renal RASs are activated in models of hypertension, pressure-overload cardiac hypertrophy, and chronic heart failure in the rat. Data from these experimental models, as well as preliminary clinical data, now suggest that the tissue RAS may modulate the pathophysiology of these cardiac diseases and progression to frank heart failure. Activation of circulating neurohormones is a classic acute homeostatic mechanism, but it has also been shown to predict wors-

ened survival in heart failure. In an analogous manner, activated tissue RAS (and local A II biosynthesis) may initially have beneficial tissue effects when plasma renin-angiotensin activity is normal. These tissue RASs may, however, have deleterious consequences during prolonged activation. The results of recent ACE-inhibitor clinical trials are consistent with the hypothesis that inhibition of the tissue RAS may underlie the ability of these agents to blunt the progression of heart failure from the compensated to the decompensated state.

References

1. Hirsch AT, Pinto YM, Schunkert H, Dzau VJ. Potential role of the tissue renin-angiotensin system in the pathophysiology of congestive heart failure. Am J Cardiol 1990; 66:22D–32D.
2. Lindpaintner K, Ganten D. The cardiac renin-angiotensin system: an appraisal of present experimental and clinical evidence. Circ Res 1991; 68:905–921.
3. Watkins IJ, Burton JA, Haber E, Cant JR, Smith FM, Barger AC. The renin-aldosterone system in congestive heart failure in conscious dogs. J Clin Invest 1976; 57:1606–1617.
4. Hirsch AT, Talsness CE, Schunkert H, Paul M, Dzau VJ. Tissue-specific activation of cardiac angiotensin converting enzyme in experimental heart failure. Circ Res 1991; 69:475–482.
5. Hirsch AT, Cant JR, Dzau VJ, Barger AC. Sequential cardiorenal responses to rapid ventricular pacing in the conscious dog (abstr). FASEB J 1988; 2:A829.
6. Hodsman GP, Kohzuki M, Howes LG, Sumithran E, Tsunoda K, Johnston CI. Neurohormonal responses to chronic myocardial infarction in rats. Circulation 1988; 78:376–381.
7. Dargie HJ, McAlpine HM, Morton JJ. Neuroendocrine activation in acute myocardial infarction. J Cardiovasc Pharmacol 1987; 9(suppl 2): S21–S24.
8. Kubo SH, Clark M, Laragh JH, Borer JS, Cody RJ. Identification of normal neurohormonal activity in mild congestive heart failure and stimulating effect of upright posture and diuretics. Am J Cardiol 1987; 60:1322–1328.
9. Dzau VJ, Colucci WS, Hollenberg NK, Williams GH. Relation of the renin-angiotensin-aldosterone system to clinical state in congestive heart failure. Circulation 1981; 63:645–651.
10. Pfeffer MA, Pfeffer JM, Steinberg C, Finn P. Survival after an experimental myocardial infarction: beneficial effects of long-term therapy with captopril. Circulation 1985; 72:406–412.
11. Sharpe N, Murphy J, Smith H, Hannan S. Treatment of patients with symptomless left ventricular dysfunction after myocardial infarction. Lancet 1988; 1:255–259.
12. The CONSENSUS Trial Study Group. Effects of enalapril on mortality in severe heart failure. N Engl J Med 1987; 316:1429–1431.

13. Pfeffer MA, Lamas GA, Vaughn DE, Parisi AF, Braunwald E. Effect of captopril on progressive ventricular dilatation after anterior myocardial infarction. N Engl J Med 1988; 319:80–86.
14. Cohn JN, Archibald DG, Ziesche S, et al. Effect of vasodilator therapy on mortality in chronic congestive heart failure: results of a Veterans Administration Cooperative Study. N Engl J Med 1986; 314:1547–1552.
15. The SOLVD Investigators. Effect of enalapril on survival in patients with reduced left ventricular ejection fractions and congestive heart failure. N Engl J Med 1991; 325:293–302.
16. Schunkert H, Dzau VJ, Tang SS, Hirsch AT, Abstein CS, Lorell BH, et al. Increased rat cardiac angiotensin converting enzyme activity and mRNA expression in pressure overload hypertrophy. J Clin Invest 1990; 86:1913–1920.
17. Yamada H, Fabris B, Allen AM, Jackson B, Johnston CI, Mendelsohn AO. Localization of angiotensin converting enzyme in rat heart. Circ Res 1991; 68(1):141–149.
18. Finckh M, Hellmann W, Ganten D, Furtwängler A, Allgeier J, Boltz M, et al. Enhanced cardiac angiotensinogen gene expression and angiotensin converting enzyme activity in tachypacing-induced heart failure in rats. Rasic Res Cardiol 1991; 86:303–316.
19. Drexler H, Hanze J, Finch M, Lu W, Just H, Lang RE. Atrial natriuretic peptide in a rat model of cardiac failure. Circulation 1989; 79:620–633.
20. Drexler H, Lindpaintner K, Lu W, Schieffer B, Ganten D. Transient increase in the expression of cardiac angiotensinogen in rat model of myocardial infarction and failure (abstract). Circulation 1989; 80(suppl II):II-459.
21. Urata H, Healy B, Stewart RW, Bumpus FM, Husain A. Angiotensin II receptors in normal and failing human hearts. J Clin Endocrinol Metab 1989; 69:54–66.
22. Rogers TB, Gaa SH, Allen IS. Identification and characterization of functional angiotensin II receptors on cultured heart myocytes. J Pharmacol Exp Ther 1986; 236:438–444.
23. Linz W, Schölkens BA, Han YF. Beneficial effects of the converting enzyme inhibitor, ramipril, in ischemic rat hearts. J Cardiovasc Pharm 1986; 8(suppl 10):S91–S99.
24. van Gilst WH, de Graeff PA, Wessling H, de Langen CDJ. Reduction of reperfusion arrhythmias in the ischemic isolated rat heart by angiotensin converting enzyme inhibitors: a comparison of captopril, enalapril and HOE 498. J Cardiovasc Pharmacol 1987; 9:254–255.
25. Koch-Weser J. Nature of the inotropic action of angiotensin on ventricular myocardium. Circ Res 1965; 16:230–237.
26. Dempsey PJ, McCallum ZT, Kent KM, Cooper T. Direct myocardial effects of angiotensin II. Am J Physiol 1971; 220:477–481.
27. Koch-Weser J. Myocardial actions of angiotensin II. Circ Res 1964; 14:337–344.
28. Ziang J, Linz W, Becker H, Ganten D, Lang RE, Schölkens B, et al. Effects of converting enzyme inhibitors: ramipril and enalapril on peptide action and sympathetic neurotransmission in the isolated rat heart. Eur J Pharmacol 1984; 113:215–223.
29. Ziogas J, Story DF, Rand MJ. Effects of locally generated A II on noradrenergic transmission in guinea pig isolated atria. Eur J Pharmacol 1985; 106:11–18.

30. Foult JM, Tavolaro O, Antony I, Nitenberg A. Direct myocardial and coronary effects of enalaprilat in patients with dilated cardiomyopathy: assessment by a bilateral intracoronary infusion technique. Circulation 1988; 77:337–344.

31. Urata H, Kinoshita A, Misono KS, Bumpus FM, Husain A. Identification of a highly specific chymase as the major angiotensin Il-forming enzyme in the human heart. J Biol Chem 1990; 265:22348–22357.

32. Freidrich SP, Lorell BH, Douglas PS, Gordon S, Grossman W, Benedict C, et al. Intracardiac ACE inhibition improves diastolic distensibility in patients with left ventricular hypertrophydue to aortic stenosis (abstract). Circulation 1992; 86(suppl I):I-119.

33. Naftilan AJ, Pratt RJ, Eldridge CS, Lin HL, Dzau VJ. Angiotensin II induces *c-fos* expression in smooth muscle via transcriptional control. Hypertension 1989; 13:706–711.

34. Katoh Y, Komuro I, Shibasaki Y, Yamaguchi H, Yazaki Y. Angiotensin II induce hypertrophy and oncogene expression in cultured rat heart myocytes (abstract). Circulation 1989; 80 (suppl II):II-450.

35. Wakashima Y, Fouad FM, Tarazi RC. Regression of left ventricular hypertrophy from systemic hypertension by enalapril. Am J Cardiol 1984; 53:1044–1049.

36. Kromer EP, Riegger GA. Effects of long-term angiotensin converting enzyme inhibition on myocardial hypertrophy in experimental aortic stenosis in the rat. Am J Cardiol 1988; 62: 161–163.

37. Tarazi RC, Fouad FM. Reversal of cardiac hypertrophy. Hypertension 1984; 6(suppl III):III-140–III-145.

38. Saito K, Gutkind JS, Saavedva JM. Angiotensin II binding sites in the conduction system of rat hearts. Am J Physiol 1987; 253:H1618–H1622.

39. Cannon PJ. The kidney in heart failure. N Engl J Med 1977; 296:26–32.

40. Ichikawa I, Pfeffer JM, Pfeffer MA, Hostetter TH, Brenner BM. Role of angiotensin II in the altered renal function of congestive heart failure. Circ Res 1984; 55:669–675.

41. Cleland JGF, Dargie HJ. Heart failure, renal function, and angiotensin converting enzyme inhibitors. Kidney Int 1987; 31 (suppl 20): S220–S228.

42. Schunkert H, Ingelfinger JR, Hirsch AT, Tang SS, Litwin SE, Talsness CE, et al. Evidence for tissue-specific activation of renal angiotensinogen mRNA expression in chronic stable experimental heart failure. J Clin Invest 1992; 90:1523–1529.

43. Hirsch AT, Talsness CE, Smith AD, Schunkert H, Ingelfinger JR, Dzau VJ. Differential effects of captopril and enalapril on tissue renin-angiotensin systems in experimental heart failure. Circulation 1992; 86: 1566–1574.

44. Hostetter TH, Pfeffer JM, Pfeffer MA, Dworkin LD, Braunwald E, Brenner BM. Cardiorenal hemodynamics and sodium excretion in rats with myocardial infarction. Am J Physiol 1983; 245:H98–H103.

45. Cohn JN, Levine TB, Olivari MT, Garberg V, Lura D, Francis GS, et al. Plasma norepinephrine as a guide to prognosis in patients with chronic congestive heart failure. N Engl J Med 1984; 311:819–823.

46. Gottlieb SS, Kukin ML, Ahern D, Packer M. Prognostic importance of atrial natriuretic peptide in patients with chronic heart failure. J Am Coll Cardiol 1989; 13:1534–1539.

47. Creager MA, Faxon DP, Halperin SL, Melidossian CD, McCabe CH, Schick EC, et al. Determinants of clinical response and survival in patients with congestive heart failure treated with captopril. Am Heart J 1982; 104:1147–1154.

48. Massie BM, Kramer BL, Topic N. Lack of relationship between the short-term hemodynamic effects of captopril and subsequent clinical responses. Circulation 1984; 69:1135–1141.

49. Francis GS, Benedict C, Johnstone DE, Kirlin PC, Nicklas J, Liang C-S, et al., for the SOLVD investigators. Comparison of neuroendocrine activation in patients with left ventricular dysfunction with and without congestive heart failure. Circulation 1990; 82:1724–1729.

50. Pfeffer MA, Braunwald E, Mové LA, Basta L, Brown EJ, Cuddy TE, et al., on behalf of the SAVE Investigators. Effect of captopril on mortality and morbidity in patients with leftventricular dysfunction after myocardial infarction: results of the survival and ventricular enlargement trial. N Engl J Med 1992; 327:669–677.

51. Cohen L, Kurz KD. Angiotensin converting enzyme inhibition in tissues from spontaneously hypertensive rats after treatment with captopril or MK-421. J Pharmacol Exp Ther 1982; 220:63–69.

52. Cushman DW, Wang FL, Wang WC, Harvey CM, DeForrest JM. Differentiation of angiotensin-converting enzyme (ACE) inhibitors by their selective inhibition of ACE in physiologically important target organs. Am J Hypertens 1989; 2:294–306.

53. Erman A, Winkler J, Batia CG, Rabinov M, Zelykovski A, Tadjer S, et al. Inhibition of angiotensin converting enzyme by ramipril in serum and tissue of man. J Hypertens 1991; 9:1057–1062.

54. Packer M, Lee WH, Yuschak M, Medina N. Comparison of captopril and enalapril in patients with severe chronic heart failure. N Engl J Med 1981; 315:847–853.

55. Giles TG, Katz R, Sullivan JM, Wolfson P, Haugland M, Kirlin P, et al. Short- and long-acting angiotensin converting enzyme inhibitors: a randomized trial of lisinopril versus captopril in the treatment of congestive heart failure. J Am Coll Cardiol 1989; 13:1240–1247.

56. Drexler H, Banhardt U, Meinertz T, Wollschlager H, Lehmann M, Just H. Contrasting peripheral short-term and long-term effects on converting enzyme inhibition in patients with congestive heart failure. Circulation 1989; 9:491–502.

57. Pouleur H, Rousseau MF, Oakley C, Ryden L, for the Xamoterol in Severe Heart Failure Study Group. Difference in mortality between patients treated with captopril or enalapril in the Xamoterol in Severe Heart Failure Study. Am J Cardiol 1991; 68:71–74.

58. Hirsch AT, Dzau VJ. Tissue renin-angiotensin systems in the pathophysiology of heart failure. In: Brachmann J, Dietz R, Kubler W, eds. Heart Failure and Arrhythmias. Heidelberg, Germany: Springer-Verlag, 1990:33–42.

14

The Contribution of Bradykinin to the Cardiovascular Actions of ACE Inhibitors

Wolfgang Linz, Gabriele Wiemer,
Peter Gohlke, Thomas Unger,
and Bernward A. Schölkens

Introduction

New insights into the molecular biology of the renin-angiotensin system (RAS) have led to the understanding that angiotensin is not only synthesized in the circulation but also locally in tissues.[1-5] Thus, the traditional endocrine concept has evolved into the concept of autocrine-paracrine functions of the RAS. Consequently, angiotensin-converting enzyme (ACE) inhibitors may exert part of their pharmacological effects via these autocrine-paracrine mechanisms, including not only the RAS but also the kallikrein-kinin system and prostaglandins.

ACE inhibitors attenuate the biosynthesis of angiotensin II (A II) and, by inhibition of the degradation of bradykinin (BK), accumulate kinins. They interfere with the systemic and local actions of A II and potentiate the cardiovascular and metabolic effects of BK.[6,7] These effects of kinins had been especially underestimated during the last decade.

Bradykinin is a nonapeptide (Arg-Pro-Pro-Gly-Phe-Ser-Pro-Phe-Arg). It is released, along with Lys-bradykinin (kallidin), from precursor kininogens by proteases called kallikreins. Plasma half-lives of the kinins are short, being approximately 15 sec. Bradykinin

Lindpaintner K and Ganten D (editors): *The Cardiac-Renin Angiotensin System,* © Futura Publishing Co., Inc., Armonk, NY, 1994.

is catabolized by at least two enzymes: kininase I and kininase II. The major catabolic enzyme is kininase II, a dipeptidyl carboxypeptidase, which is also well known as ACE. Kininase I removes the carboxyl terminal Arg forming DesArg^9 BK.

Kinins play a role in a variety of biological processes[8-11] via stimulation of the kinin receptors. These are classified as B_1 and B_2, according to the relative potencies of the agonists involved. B_1 kinin receptors are more sensitive to the metabolite DesArg^9 BK, whereas B_2 kinin receptors, which are more abundant, have greater affinity for BK.[8]

In different models, we will demonstrate that, besides the reduction in A II formation, locally increased kinins by ACE inhibition play a central role in the cardiovascular action of ACE inhibitors. For this purpose, we used bovine aortic and human endothelial cell cultures, models of experimental hypertension, rabbits on an atherogenic diet, neointima formation in rats with smooth muscle cell proliferation and migration after endothelial denudation, isolated ischemic rat hearts, myocardial infarction in dogs and rabbits, and left-ventricular hypertrophy in rats.

The Kallikrein-Kinin System

Kinins are the vasoactive factors of the kallikrein-kinin system. They are oligopeptides containing the sequence of BK in their structure and probably act mainly as local hormonal factors by autocrine-paracrine mechanisms. They circulate, if at all, at very low concentrations in the plasma and are rapidly destroyed by a group of peptidases known as kininases. Kininases are found in blood and endothelial cells and other tissues. The main kininases are kininase I, an arginine carboxypeptidase; kininase II, also known as ACE, a peptidyl dipeptidase; and neutral endopeptidase 24.11, also known as enkephalinase. Kininase II or ACE is found in high amounts on the luminal surface of the endothelial cell membrane as an ecto-enzyme. Thus, when kinins are released and enter the circulation, they are rapidly degraded.

Kinins are released from their precursors, the kininogens, by kinin-forming enzymes (kininogenases), the best known of which are plasma and glandular kallikrein. Two subtypes of kinin receptors, B_1 and B_2, have been characterized on the basis of their pharmacological responses to various BK analogues. B_1 kinin receptors, for example, mediate contraction of the isolated rabbit aorta, relaxation of mesenteric arteries, and contraction of the rat duodenum. B_1 kinin receptors are probably not present in normal tissues but are synthesized de novo during tissue injury, stress, or certain pathological conditions. B_2 kinin receptors mediate most of the effects of BK and are the main receptors for the agonist BK. BK receptor antagonists are indispensable tools. Stewart and Vavrek discovered that substitution of D-phenylalanine for proline at position 7 of BK converted it into a specific antagonist for B_1 and B_2 kinin receptors.[12] In our studies, we used mainly HOE 140 as a tool, which at the present time is the most potent, stable, and long-lasting specific B_2 receptor kinin antagonist.[13,14]

Kinins are vasoactive through the release of different autacoids, mainly generated by the endothelium. Activation of the B_2 kinin receptors on endothelial cells led by stimulating phospholipases A_2 and C to the formation of nitric oxide (NO), prostacyclin (PGI_2), and the platelet activating factor (PAF).[15]

Measurements of plasma kinins in patients after ACE inhibitor treatment led to conflicting data on the contribution of kinins to the cardiovascular actions of ACE inhibitors. The heart and vascular tissue contain a local kallikrein-kinin pathway, and blockade of kininase II with ACE inhibitors may stimulate the system by increasing local kinin concentrations. Thus, locally generated kinins in the heart and in the vascular wall may contribute to the cardiovascular actions of ACE inhibitors rather than circulating kinins.[16,17]

Endothelial Cell Function and ACE Inhibition

It has been shown that endothelial cells are able to synthesize and release potent vasoconstrictor peptides such as angiotensins[18] and endothelin.[19] Furthermore, there is some evidence that the potent stimulators of endothelial NO formation, acetylcholine, ATP, and substance P are released from the endothelial cells,[20,21] in this way establishing an effective paracrine system.

Stimulation of endothelial B_2 kinin receptors by BK increases the cytosolic Ca^{2+} concentration, which promotes synthesis of PGI_2, as well as NO, as assessed by 6-keto-prostaglandin $F_{1\alpha}$ (6-keto-$PGF_{1\alpha}$) and cyclic GMP content, respectively, and is associated with relaxation of vascular smooth muscles.[15]

ACE or kininase II is localized on the luminal surface of endothelial cells, where it can interact with ACE inhibitors. Endothelial cells are a target cell population responsible for a large part of the cardiovascular action of ACE inhibitors.

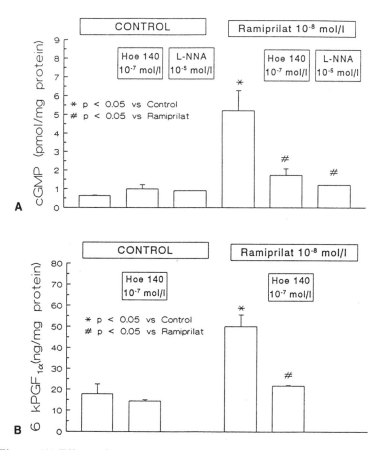

Fig. 1. (A) Effects of ramiprilat (RT) on the accumulation of cyclic GMP in cultured bovine aortic endothelial cells (10 min incubation with RT). HOE 140 (1 × 10⁻⁷ mol/l) was added 5 min before and N^G-nitro-L-arginine (L-NNA; 1 × 10⁻⁵ mol/l) 20 min before the addition of RT. (B) Effects of RT on the accumulation of 6-keto $PGF_{1\alpha}$ in the supernatant of bovine aortic endothelial cells (10 min incubation with RT). Hoe 140 (1 × 10⁻⁷ mol/l) was added to the bovine cells 5 min before the addition of BK. Results are expressed as the mean ± SEM of six to eight experiments performed on four different cell batches. All experiments were performed in the presence of IBMX (10⁻⁴ mol/l) and SOD (3 × 10⁻⁷ mol/l).

We have been interested in whether cultured endothelial cells from different species, including humans, synthesize and release BK and related peptides that may accumulate in the presence of ACE inhibitors, with subsequent stimulation of NO and PGI_2 formation. Inhibition of ACE by ramiprilat, leading to BK accumulation, concentration and time dependently increased the formation of NO and PGI_2. The B_2 kinin receptor antagonist HOE 140 markedly attenuated the cyclic GMP accumulation following the formation of NO and abolished the increase in PGI_2 release (Figure 1). Cultured endothelial cells from different species are capable of producing and releasing BK into the extracellular space in amounts that lead to a sustained stimulation of NO and PGI_2formation, provided that BK degradation is prevented by ACE inhibition.[22] In line with these findings in cultured endothelial cells is the observation in spontaneously hypertensive rats (SHR) that the acute hypotensive effect of ACE inhibitors was attenuated by HOE 140 and a NO synthase inhibitor N^G-monomethyl-L-arginine.[23] The cardiovascular effects of ACE inhibitors may thus be, in part, explained by the local accumulation of endothelium-derived BK[22] that acts in an autocrine and paracrine manner as a potent stimulus for endothelial autacoid formation.

Kinin Contribution to the Antihypertensive Action of ACE Inhibitors

Inactivation of locally produced BK in different vascular beds by the action of BK-degrading vascular enzymes may be an important determinator of BK-related effects on blood pressure and regional blood flow. Therefore, a potentiation of endogenous BK has been implicated in the antihypertensive action of ACE inhibitors since ACE is one of the major BK-degrading enzymes.

In a recent study, the effect of the ACE inhibitor ramiprilat on the metabolism of BK by enzymes localized on endothelial cells and vascular smooth muscle cells (VSMC) of the vascular wall has been investigated in an in vitro model of the isolated rabbit thoracic aorta.[24] The results revealed a marked attenuation of BK breakdown by endothelial enzymes after addition of the ACE inhibitor ramiprilat, most likely by inhibition of endothelial ACE. In addition, in an endothelial-denuded aorta, the ACE inhibitor reduced BK degradation by VSMC enzymes, despite the fact that ACE was absent in this preparation.[24,25] This finding suggests that the ACE inhibitor attenuated BK breakdown by inhibiting BK-degrading enzymes other than ACE in VSMC. In line with this finding, a 50% inhibition of the endopeptidase 24.11 and a 42% inhibition of an amastatin-sensitive aminopeptidase was observed in rat kidney fractions after chronic ACE inhibitor treatment.[26] Furthermore, an inhibition of aminopeptidase P, purified from the pig kidney cortex by several ACE inhibitors, including ramiprilat, was reported.[27] Thus, ACE inhibitors may inhibit BK breakdown by inhibition of ACE, as well as by inhibition of other degrading enzymes.

The development of B_2 kinin receptor antagonists by Vavrek and Stewart in 1985[12] provided tools with which to investigate the contribution of BK to the acute antihypertensive action of ACE inhibitors. Several studies have provided evidence for a contribution of BK in the acute antihypertensive action of ACE inhibitors in different rat models of hypertension. Blockade of B_2 kinin receptors has been shown to attenuate the hypotensive effect following an acute bolus injection of an ACE inhibitor in two-kidney, one-clip (2K1C) hypertensive Wistar rats[28,29] and in rats with hypertension induced by aortic ligation between the renal arteries.[30] In contrast, in kinin-deficient 2K1C hypertensive Brown-Norway (BN) rats, the acute hypotensive effect of an ACE inhibitor was reduced both in magnitude and duration when compared with kinin-replete 2K1C hypertensive control animals. In addition, the ACE inhibitor effect was not affected by the intravenous infusion of a B_2 kinin receptor antagonist.[28] These studies demonstrated that BK contributes to the acute hypotensive action of ACE inhibitors in animal models of renin-dependent hypertension. On the other hand, results from studies in SHR, which are models of genetic hypertension with normal to low plasma renin, were more conflicting. A more recent study in SHR demonstrated an attenuation of the acute antihypertensive action of an ACE inhibitor,[23] whereas other studies did not.[31,32]

All these studies were limited by the fact that the BK receptor antagonists used had a low potency and a very short half-life in vivo and could only be administered intravenously, thus prohibiting chronic studies. The development of the highly potent and long-acting B_2 kinin receptor antagonist HOE 140 has provided a tool to also study the effect of a chronic BK receptor blockade on the antihypertensive action of ACE inhibitors.

In another study, 2K1C hypertensive Wistar rats were pretreated orally with the ACE inhibitor ramipril for 4 weeks.[33] B_2 kinin receptors were then blocked chronically by subcutaneous infusion of HOE 140 via osmotic minipumps for 6 weeks while ramipril treatment was continued. The antihypertensive effect of the ACE inhibitor was partially reversed by the BK receptor antagonist, being significant 2 to 6 weeks after the beginning of the subcutaneous HOE 140 infusion. In another protocol, HOE 140 was coadministered with ramipril in 2K1C hypertensive Wistar rats for 6 weeks.[33] Again, the BK receptor antagonist attenuated the antihypertensive effects of the ACE inhibitor throughout the treatment period. In contrast, chronic B_2 kinin receptor blockade by HOE 140 did not attenuate the depressor effect of coadministered ramipril in SHR and in kinin-deficient 2K1C hypertensive BN rats.[34]

Therefore, BK antagonists seem to be particularly effective in renovascular models of hypertension of kinin-replete animals associated with a stimulated RAS but less effective in genetic hypertension with normal to low plasma renin. The reasons for these rather unexpected findings remain unclear. Possibly, endogenous kinins may gain importance in blood pressure regulation in cases where elevated blood pressure is maintained by circulating pressor agents such as A II. The question of whether the potentiation of endogenous kinins also contributes to the antihypertensive actions of ACE inhibitors in nonrenin-dependent hypertension remains a challenging question to be addressed in future studies.

Experimental Atherosclerosis in Rabbits

Experimental atherosclerosis in rabbits can be induced by a long-term atherogenic diet. To investigate the influence of ACE inhibitor treatment in this pathological situation with marked endothelial dysfunction, rabbits were fed a cholesterol-enriched diet (0.25% cholesterol and 3% coconut oil) for 17 weeks. Concomitantly, they received two dosage regimens of ramipril, a low dose of 0.3 mg/kg/day, which led to an intermittent plasma ACE inhibition, and a tenfold higher dose of 3 mg/kg/day, which induced a persistent plasma ACE inhibition.[35]

Serum cholesterol rose from below 1 mmol/l to between 10 and 20 mmol/l, and ramipril did not change this. At the end of the study, the vascular function of these animals on a long-term atherogenic diet was tested using isolated aortic rings, precontracted with norepinephrine. After reaching a stable plateau, relaxation was induced with acetylcholine. There was a clear difference between the rings from controls and from animals on the long-term atherogenic diet. Rings from animals with atherosclerosis reacted to norepinephrine with a much larger contraction and, following acetylcholine, no relaxation could be observed; by contrast, in many instances, acetylcholine led to an additional contraction of the isolated aortic rings. However, aortic rings from animals on the atherogenic diet, which were concomitantly treated with ramipril, showed a preserved vascular function. The contraction induced by norepinephrine, as well as the relaxation induced by acetylcholine, was identical to the reaction seen with aortic rings from control animals. In rabbits, ramipril treatment was able to protect against the loss of endothelial function caused by the long-term atherogenic diet (Figure 2).

Further evidence came from biochemical measurements that clearly demonstrate that in the atherogenic diet group there is a significant decrease in vascular cyclic GMP content in aortic segments. Following concomitant treatment with ramipril, cyclic GMP content in aortic segments increased significantly.[35] These findings are in line with the observations in cultured endothelial cells showing that ramiprilat enhances the formation and release of NO and PGI_2 by inhibiting the breakdown of endothelium-derived BK.[22]

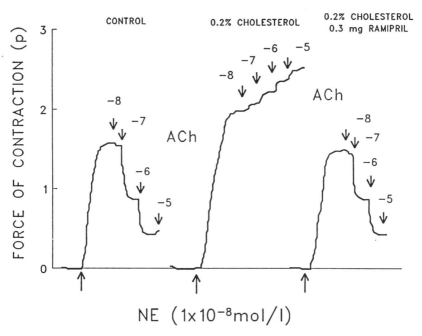

Fig. 2. Response to acetylcholine (ACh) of norepinephrine (NE) precontracted normal and atherosclerotic rabbit aortic rings or athersclerotic- and ramipril-treated rabbit aortic rings.

These pharmacological and biochemical observations on the preservation of endothelial function by ramipril were supported by the morphological observation that aortic surface involvement in rabbits on long-term atherogenic diets was significantly decreased by the treatment with ramipril. In all areas of the aorta investigated, ramipril reduced the surface involvement with respect to atherosclerotic lesions of the aorta. These results clearly show that an ACE inhibitor in a model of experimental atherosclerosis in rabbits is able to preserve endothelial function and vascular reactivity.

In another study of cholesterol-fed rabbits, it was also reported that the ratio of stained area compared with the total intimal surface area significantly decreased with the administration of the ACE inhibitor benazepril. Microscopic examination of the aorta revealed proliferation of the wall and foam cell formation beneath the endothelium in the cholesterol diet group. The formation of foam cells decreased, and the proliferation of the wall was suppressed with benazepril treatment.[36] In another study in cholesterol-fed rabbits, enalapril attenuated atherogenesis; however, the A II antagonist, (subtype AT_1) SC 51316, was without effect on atherosclerosis in this model.[37] During a 9-month treatment period, captopril caused a significant decrease in aortic atherosclerosis in normotensive Watanabe heritable hyperlipidemic rabbits. Total aortic surface involvement by lesions was reduced from 48% in control Watanabe rabbits to 30% with captopril treatment. The cholesterol content of descending thoracic aortas was also reduced by captopril therapy from 25 mg/g wet weight to 10 mg/g.[38] In cholesterol-fed cynomolgus monkeys, captopril treatment for 6 months showed a significantly reduced progression of arterial lesions, most evident in the coronary arteries, which were nearly free from atherosclerosis in captopril-treated animals.[39]

On the basis of these encouraging findings, clinical studies have been designed to prove the antiathersclerotic effects of ACE inhibitors. For example, a study with quinapril (Quinapril Ischemic Event Trial "Quiet Study") and a study with ramipril on the progression of atherosclerosis are underway. The outcome of such clinical studies will show if ACE inhibitors might be used as a kind of substitution therapy in patients with atherosclerosis and a dysfunctional endothelium. Such a correction of endothelial dysfunction in coronary microcirculation of hypercholesterolemic patients by short-term administration of the NO-precursor L-arginine has been reported.[40] In patients with hypercholesterolemia, the increase in coronary blood flow with acetylcholine was significantly attenuated in comparison to control subjects. L-arginine restored the acetylcholine-induced increase in blood flow in patients with hypercholesterolemia but did not affect coronary blood flow in controls.[40]

From the results on the protective effects of ACE inhibitors in animals on a long-term atherogenic diet, evidence accumulates that ACE inhibitors might represent a treatment for endothelial dysfunction in atherosclerosis in man.

Neointima Formation in Rats

Neointimal hyperplasia with smooth muscle cell proliferation is an important feature of the process that occurs after endothelial injury. After injury, smooth muscle cells are activated and begin to proliferate in the media. They migrate across the lamina elastica interna into the intima. Their proliferation continues and reaches its maximum 2 weeks after injury. The mechanisms that produce activation and migration of smooth muscle cells are not fully understood, and several mitogens have been implicated in this process. It was shown that ACE inhibitors reduce myointimal proliferation after endothelial injury in the rat carotid artery and in the rat aorta, suggesting that A II plays a major role in this process.[41,42]

Ramipril decreased the amount of neointima formed 14 days after deendothelialization, as characterized by a significant decrease of intima-media wet weight, however, without any significant effect on intima-media DNA content.[41] These observations suggested that ACE inhibitors may not only act through an inhibition of smooth muscle cell proliferation. Other effects such as inhibition of migration, hypertrophy, and matrix synthesis should also be considered.

These experimental observations, however, did not take into account that one of the effects of ACE inhibitors besides the inhibition of A II formation is the reduction of the breakdown of endogenous kinins. These kinins can release PGI_2 and other factors from endothelial and/or blood cells, such as NO, which may have an antiproliferative effect and may mediate part of the protective effects of ACE inhibitors.

To investigate whether kinins mediate the antiproliferative effect of the ACE inhibitor ramipril, endothelial denudation was achieved in the carotid artery of rats using a balloon catheter.[43] Ramipril markedly reduced neointima formation compared to the control group, as well as to the A II antagonist Losartan-treated group. However, when ramipril was given together with the BK

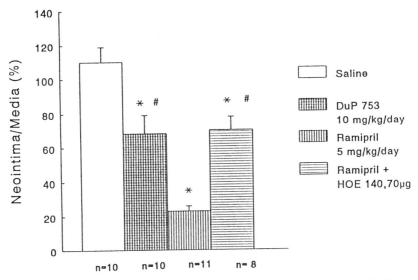

Fig. 3. Changes in neointima formation 2 weeks after carotid artery balloon deendothelialization in rats chronically infused with vehicle (saline), Losartan (10 mg/kg/day), ramipril (5 mg/kg/day), and ramipril plus HOE 140 (70 μg/kg/day). $^*p < 0.05$ compared with vehicle; $^\#p < 0.05$ compared with ramipril (from Scicli AG, et al., modified[16]).

antagonist HOE 140, its effect was significantly blunted (Figure 3). These data provide evidence that endogenous kinins mediate part of the antiproliferative effect of the ACE inhibitor ramipril since administration of the kinin receptor antagonist reversed part but not all of the antiproliferative effect of ramipril. The ACE inhibitor probably affects migration and proliferation by blocking both A II formation and increasing kinin concentrations. These results show that kinins are important mediators in the reduction of neointima formation by ACE inhibitors.

Myocardial Ischemia

Ischemia Reperfusion Injuries in Isolated Working Rat Hearts

The role of BK in the myocardium has received relatively little attention. An early study in dogs showed that locally and systemically administered kinins increased coronary blood flow and improved myocardial metabolism.[44] In 1970, Wilkens et al.[45] reported that the small fall in peripheral blood vessel tissue pH, which follows an ischemic insult, induces an activation of the local kinin system. In 1977, Hashimoto et al.[46] found an increased concentration of BK in the coronary sinus blood after coronary occlusion in the dog. Myocardial ischemia induced by coronary artery stenosis and sympathetic stimulation also caused the heart in the dog to release plasma kinin.[47] In humans, kinin levels in peripheral blood were found to increase soon after myocardial infarction.[48] This led Hashimoto et al. in 1978[48] to the suggestion that kinins released in patients with infarction may have a compensatory cardioprotective effect. On the other hand, it was reported that endothelial dysfunction occurs after ischemia. Reduced NO release and accumulation of neutrophils with

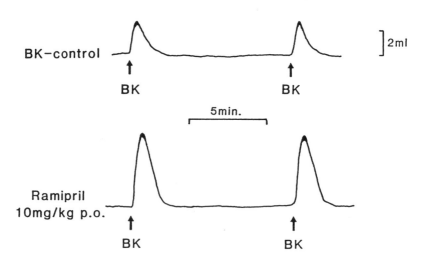

Fig. 4. Effect of bradykinin (BK 10 ng as a bolus) on coronary flow of isolated hearts from ramipril-pretreated guinea pigs (ex vivo).

the generation of superoxide radicals by the reperfused coronary endothelium may play a role in ischemic injuries.[49] In the models of the isolated rat heart with postischemic reperfusion injuries and in dogs with myocardial infarction, we have shown that BK plays a crucial role in these acute ischemic events.[50]

Earlier studies in isolated hearts from different species had shown that hearts from ACE-inhibitor pretreated animals had significantly higher initial values of coronary flow, and that pretreatment with ramipril enhanced the BK-induced increase in coronary flow (Figure 4).[51] Various studies have proven that pretreatment with ACE inhibitors in antihypertensive doses is able to prevent postischemic reperfusion arrhythmias and injuries.[52–54]

In our experimental protocol of ischemia and reperfusion injuries, rat hearts were perfused for an initial 20 minutes (control perfusion or preischemic period). Acute regional myocardial ischemia was produced by clamping the left coronary artery close to its origin for 15 minutes (ischemic period). The occlusion was reopened, and changes during reperfusion were monitored for 30 minutes (reperfusion period).

Using this experimental protocol, the following parameters were measured: cardiodynamics such as left-ventricular pressure, dp/dt_{max}, heart rate, and coronary flow and cytosolic enzymes released into the coronary effluent, such as lactate dehydrogenase, creatine kinase, and lactate. Furthermore, metabolic parameters in the myocardial tissue like lactate, glycogen, the energy-rich phosphates ATP and creatine phosphate, and, lastly, the ECG to record reperfusion arrhythmias were determined.

Cardiac Effects of Angiotensin I, Angiotensin II, and Bradykinin

In this isolated working rat heart model, perfusion of the heart with either A I or A II resulted in a deterioration of function characterized by a decrease in left-ventricular pressure, coronary flow, high energy-rich phosphate levels, and an increase of cytosolic enzymes in the coronary sinus. The incidence and duration of ventricular fibrillation were enhanced by perfusion with A I or A II, indicating that a conversion to A II took place.[54,55] This was reported to be enhanced in hearts impaired by ischemia,[56] thus favoring coronary constriction during myocardial ischemia.[57]

In comparison to the action of A II, BK perfusion (1×10^{-12} to 1×10^{-8} mol/l) of isolated working rat hearts with postischemic reperfusion arrhythmias induced the reduction of the incidence as well as the duration of ventricular fibrillation and an improvement of cardiodynamics via increased left-ventricular pressure, contractility, and coronary flow without changes in heart rate. These effects were accompanied by the reduced activities of the cytosolic enzymes lactate dehydrogenase and creatine kinase, as well as lactate output. In the myocardial tissue, lactate content was reduced, and the energy-rich phosphates increased compared to the saline-perfused control hearts. Glycogen stores were also preserved.[58] In line with these findings in isolated rat hearts, BK profoundly reduced the severity of ischemia-induced arrhythmias in anesthetized dogs.[59] Thus, A II and BK exert opposite effects in the isolated rat heart preparation: A II deteriorates but BK improves cardiac function and metabolism during ischemia and reperfusion (Figure 5).[60]

When comparing the influence on the coronary flow of agents interfering with the RAS, A II antagonists, renin inhibitors, and ACE inhibitors like ramiprilat, only the ACE inhibitor increased coronary flow in this isolated working rat heart preparation. This also points to a possible participation of BK in the effect of ACE inhibitors on coronary flow.

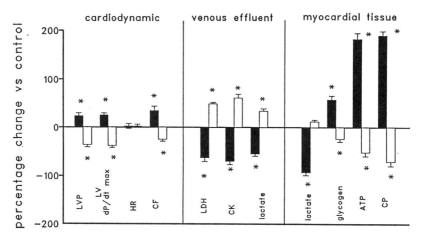

Fig. 5. Cardiodynamic, perfusate, and myocardial tissue values of isolated working ischemic rat hearts perfused with Krebs-Henseleit buffer containing bradykinin (black bars) (1×10^{-9} mol/l; n = 8) or angiotensin II (open bars) (1×10^{-9} mol/l; n = 8). LVP: left-ventricular pressure; LV dp/dt$_{max}$: differentiated left-ventricular pressure; HR: heart rate; CF: coronary flow; LDH: lactate dehydrogenase; CK: creatine kinase; ATP: adenosine triphosphate; CP: creatine phosphate. Values are given as $\pm \delta$ % versus control hearts. $^*p < 0.05$ compared with the vehicle control group.

Cardiac Effects of Bradykinin and ACE Inhibitors

Comparative studies with BK and with ramiprilat in these isolated working rat hearts with postischemic reperfusion arrhythmias surprisingly led to an almost identical fingerprint of changes, even in very low concentrations (1×10^{-10} to 1×10^{-12} mol/l), suggesting that local inhibition of kininase II, most probably synthesized by cardiac endothelial cells and localized on their luminal surface, results in attenuation of BK degradation with subsequent accumulation (Figure 6).[61] These beneficial effects of BK as well as of the ACE inhibitor were abolished in a concentration-dependent manner by perfusion with the B_2 kinin receptor antagonist HOE 140 and a NO synthase inhibitor N^G-nitro-L-arginine (Figures 7 and 8).[62] Additional studies with subchronical pretreatment showed a comparable profile. Ramipril was given orally for 2 weeks in the blood-pressure lowering dose of 1 mg/kg/day and in the non-antihypertensive dose of 10 μg/kg/day.[63] Comparing the changes in ventricular fibrillations, cardiodynamics, and the metabolism of the isolated hearts from rats pretreated with high and low doses of ramipril, it becomes obvious that both regimens result in comparable cardioprotective effects.[63]

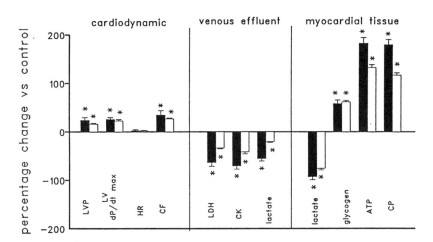

Fig. 6. Cardiodynamic, perfusate, and myocardial tissue values of isolated working ischemic rat hearts perfused with Krebs-Henseleit buffer containing bradykinin (black bars) (1×10^{-9} mol/l; n = 8) or RT (open bars) (1×10^{-8} mol/l); n = 10. For abbreviations and further details see Fig. 5.

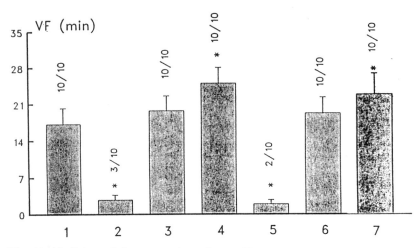

Fig. 7. Abolition of the protective effects of bradykinin and ramiprilat by HOE 140 and L-NNA in isolated working rat hearts with postischemic reperfusion arrhythmias. VF: ventricular fibrillation (in minutes); numbers indicate the incidence of the hearts fibrillating. $^*p < 0.05$ versus control hearts; mean ± SEM. 1 = control; 2 = bradykinin (1×10^{-9} mol/l); 3 = bradykinin (1×10^{-9} mol/l) + HOE 140 (1×10^{-9} mol/l); 4 = bradykinin (1×10^{-9} mol/l) + L-NNA (1×10^{-6} mol/l); 5 = RT (1×10^{-8} mol/l); 6 = RT (1×10^{-6} mol/l) + HOE 140 (1×10^{-9} mol/l); 7 = RT (1×10^{-8} mol/l) + L-NNA (1×10^{-6} mol/l).

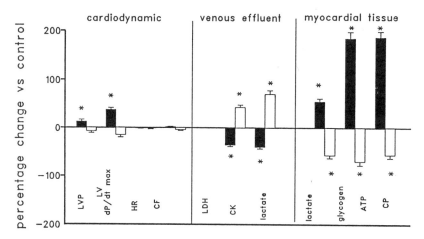

Fig. 8. Cardiodynamic, perfusate, and myocardial tissue values of isolated working ischemic rat hearts perfused with Krebs-Henseleit buffer containing bradykinin (1×10^{-10} mol/l) (black bars) or bradykinin (1×10^{-10} mol/l) + HOE 140 (1×10^{-10} mol/l) (open bars). For abbreviations and further details see Fig. 5.

Prostacyclin (PGI₂) Release From Isolated Rat Hearts

In line with the concept of an enhanced endothelial autacoid formation, by inhibiting the breakdown of endothelium-derived BK by ACE inhibition, is the observation that the perfusion of isolated rat hearts with ramiprilat induced the release of autacoids like PGI_2. This effect required an intact endothelial function since endothelial

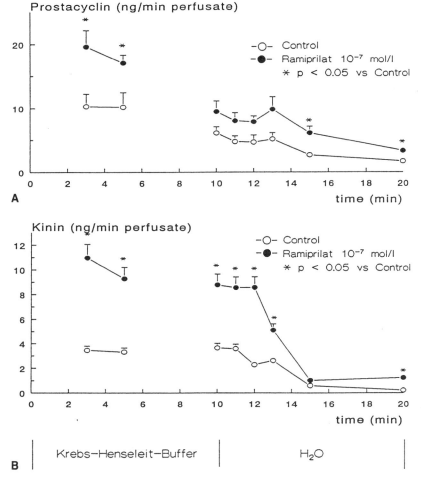

Fig. 9. Prostacyclin and kinin release from isolated rat hearts perfused with the Krebs-Henseleit buffer or the Krebs-Henseleit buffer containing ramiprilat (1×10^{-7} mol/l). Both prostacyclin as well as bradykinin release was abolished when the perfusion medium was switched over distilled water.

impairment by changing perfusion with the Krebs-Henseleit buffer to perfusion with distilled water markedly attenuated PGI_2 release from isolated rat hearts (Figure 9).

Bradykinin may act synergistically with the cyclic AMP-dependent effects of PGI_2 since perfusion of isolated ischemic hearts with PGI_2 reduced the incidence and duration of ventricular fibrillation, increased coronary flow, and decreased cytosolic enzyme release. Inhibition of prostaglandin synthesis with indomethacin, however, prolonged the duration of ventricular fibrillations, reduced coronary flow, increased cytosolic enzyme release, and attenuated the cardioprotective effects of ramiprilat or BK (Figure 10).[64] The stable analogue of PGI_2, iloprost, also induced a cardioprotective effect in a rat model after isoprenaline application.[65] Furthermore, PAF-stimulated neutrophil-mediated myocardial tissue injury was reduced by ramiprilat as well as by BK,[66] and in isolated working rat hearts, ramiprilat inhibited free radical-induced damages mainly by stimulation of PGI_2 synthesis and/or release, whereas captopril exerted additional free radical effects by a mechanism that was probably related to the sulfhydryl group.[67] Other studies with ramiprilat and captopril also suggested that the observed cardiac effects resulted from a reduced BK breakdown and a subsequent increase in PGI_2

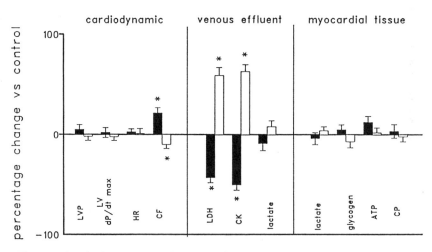

Fig. 10. Cardiodynamic, perfusate, and myocardial tissue values of isolated working ischemic rat hearts perfused with Krebs-Henseleit buffer containing prostacyclin (black bars) (5×10^{-8} mol/l; n = 8) or indomethacin (open bars) (1×10^{-6} mol/l; n = 8). For abbreviations and further details see Fig. 5.

synthesis.[68] In variance with these findings, the cardioprotective effect induced by ramipril with increased synthesis of PGI_2 was still present, whereas captopril did not show any cardioprotective effect.[69] From these data, it can be assumed that the prostacyclin/thromboxane balance seems to be of great importance for the induction or prevention of reperfusion arrhythmias.[70]

Bradykinin Release from Isolated Rat Hearts

Different enzymes in normally perfused and ischemic hearts release a substance with kininlike activity.[71] To prove that BK is formed in the heart, BK was measured with radioimmunoassay (RIA)[72] in the venous effluent from isolated rat hearts perfused with a Krebs-Henseleit buffer. From isolated normoxic rat hearts, a BK outflow of 0.9 ng/ml perfusate per gram of wet weight was measured. Perfusion with ramiprilat increased the BK concentration to 4.4 ng/ml perfusate per gram wet weight. During ischemia of isolated working rat hearts, BK outflow increased more than fivefold and in the ACE-inhibitor perfused hearts to 20 ng/ml perfusate per gram of wet weight. These data allow the conclusion that BK is continously

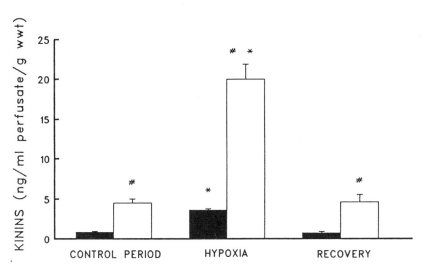

Fig. 11. Kinin release from isolated rat hearts perfused with Krebs-Henseleit buffer closed bars or Krebs-Henseleit buffer containing ramiprilat (1×10^{-7} mol/l) open bars during normoxia (control perfusion period), hypoxia, and reperfusion (recovery). $^{*}p < 0.05$ versus hypoxia; $^{\#}p < 0.05$ versus control.

formed in the isolated rat heart and that ischemia activates BK outflow in the heart. By inhibiting the degradation of kinins, the ACE inhibitor markedly increased BK concentration during normoxia and ischemia (Figure 11).[73] Similar to the PGI_2 experiments, perfusion with distilled water attenuated kinin release from isolated rat hearts (Fig. 9B). Bradykinin released from endothelial cells during ischemia could contribute to the reduction of the sequelae of myocardial ischemia.[46,48,74]

Coronary Ligation in Anesthetized Dogs and Rabbits

In the in vivo situation, the role of BK in the myocardium has received little attention. A fall in blood tissue pH, which follows myocardial ischemia, induced an activation of the local kallikrein-kinin system.[45] After coronary occlusion, an increased concentration of BK in the coronary venous blood was found in the dog.[46] In humans, kinin levels in peripheral blood were found to be increased soon after myocardial infarction.[48] These early observations led to the suggestion that kinin release in myocardial ischemia may have a compensatory cardioprotective effect. Bradykinin infused into the coronary artery of anesthetized dogs during ischemia-reperfusion reduced lactate concentrations in the coronary sinus blood and preserved tissue levels of high energy-rich phosphates in the ischemic area.[75]

In a recent study,[76] the role of local cardiac BK in the infarct-limiting effects of the ACE inhibitor ramiprilat was investigated by use of HOE 140. In anesthetized dogs, the left-descending coronary artery was ligated for 6 hours. Several groups were formed: group 1 received saline into the main stem of the left-coronary artery, starting 30 minutes before the occlusion and lasting for the duration of the experiment. Group 2 received HOE 140 (5 ng/kg per minute). Group 3 received BK in a subhypotensive dose of 1 ng/kg per minute. Group 4 received ramiprilat at the subhypotensive dose of 40 ng/kg per minute. In group 5 ramiprilat was coadministered with HOE 140, and Group 6 received BK together with the BK antagonist. The intracoronary route and very low doses were chosen to obtain a local cardiac effect with no or minimal effects on systemic hemodynamics. During the 6 hours of coronary occlusion, ramiprilat infusion as well as BK had no significant effect on systemic blood pressure.

The size of the infarction of saline-treated dogs averaged 55% of the area at risk. The ACE inhibitor and BK significantly reduced infarct size. This cardioprotective effect of the ACE inhibitor was

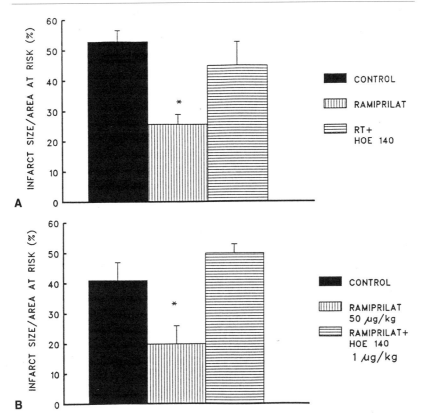

Fig. 12. (A) Reduction in infarct size, as percentage of the area at risk, in control dogs and dogs intracoronarily infused with RT (40 ng/kg/min) and RT plus HOE 140 (0.5 ng/kg/min). Mean ± SEM; $^*p < 0.05$ versus control dogs; n = 8–14 per group. (B) Reduction in infarct size, as percentage of the area at risk, in control rabbits and rabbits treated with RT (50 μg/kg) and RT plus HOE 140 (1 μg/kg). Mean ± SEM; $^*p < 0.05$ versus control rabbits; n = 5 per group. (B: from Hartmann JC, et al. modified[77]).

abolished by the coadministration of the BK antagonist (Figure 12A). Thus, ramiprilat effectively limited infarct size following coronary occlusion in a dose that had no effect on systemic hemodynamics. The observation that the infarct-limiting effect of ramiprilat was reversed by a BK antagonist and that administration of BK also reduced infarct size provided evidence for the involvement of BK in the anti-ischemic effect of the ACE inhibitor. Similar results were found in anesthetized rabbits with myocardial infarction. Ramiprilat pretreatment reduced the infarct size from 40% to 20%, and coadministration of HOE 140 reversed this effect (Figure 12B).[77] Additional evidence for a beneficial role of BK during myocardial ischemia comes from studies in pigs where BK also reduced infarct size[78] and improved electrical stability two weeks after myocardial infarction.[79]

These beneficial effects of BK and ramiprilat in myocardial ischemia were probably mediated by stimulation of endothelial B_2 kinin receptors, resulting in an increase in the cytosolic calcium concentration and followed by an enhanced synthesis and release of PGI_2 and NO.[22]. Both effects were blocked by the B_2 kinin antagonist HOE 140. NO stimulates a soluble guanylyl cyclase to form cyclic GMP, leading to vasodilatation and inhibition of platelet adhesion and aggregation. Additionally, cyclic GMP was found to improve the energy state in the ischemic heart.[80] Finally, BK itself had favorable cardiac metabolic effects by increasing myocardial glucose uptake.[81]

Left-Ventricular Hypertrophy

Rats With Aortic Coarctation (Renal Hypertension)

Left-ventricular hypertrophy (LVH) is an independent risk factor for cardiovascular diseases, such as congestive heart failure, coronary artery disease, and cardiac sudden death.[82]

The RAS has been implicated in the development and maintenance of hypertension and cardiac hypertrophy.[83] In the coarctation model of hypertension, ramipril has been shown to inhibit the development and to induce the regression of cardiac hypertrophy in doses without an effect on blood pressure.[84] In this study, the effects of equipotent antihypertensive doses of ramipril (1 mg/kg/day), the calcium antagonist nifedipine (30 mg/kg/day) and the arterial vasodilator dihydralazine (30 mg/kg/day) on cardiac mass in rats subjected to the banding of the abdominal aorta were compared. Daily treatment over six weeks was started either immediately following acute aortic constriction (prevention experiments) or 6 weeks after aortic banding, when hypertension and cardiac hypertrophy had already developed (regression experiments). Groups of sham-operated animals and untreated animals with aortic banding served as controls. An additional group in the regression experiments received ramipril in the non-antihypertensive lower dose of 10 µg/kg/day.

All three drugs lowered the blood pressure to a similar level, with the exception of the low dose of ramipril, which was without effect on blood pressure. Only the ACE inhibitor induced a significant and complete prevention or regression of cardiac hypertrophy to control values similar to the sham-operated normotensive rats. Surprisingly, animals treated with the low dose of ramipril showed the same complete regression of cardiac hypertrophy as seen in the group receiving the antihypertensive dose of the ACE inhibitor.[84]

A comparable antihypertrophic effect was seen in a recent one-year study in rats with the aim of separating local cardiac effects using a non-antihypertensive dose from those effects on systemic blood pressure when using an antihypertensive dose.[85] Chronic treatment with the ACE inhibitor prevented LVH in the antihypertensive rats, as well as in the low-dose rats, and had no effect on blood pressure. Similar effects were observed on myocardial fibrosis. Plasma ACE activity was inhibited in the ramipril 1 mg group but not in the ramipril 10 μg group, whereas a conversion of A I to A II in isolated aortic strips was suppressed in both treated groups. Plasma catecholamines were increased in the vehicle control group, but treatment with either dose of the ACE inhibitor normalized the values. The myocardial phosphocreatine/ATP ratio as an indicator for the energy state of the heart was reduced in the vehicle control group, whereas the hearts from treated animals showed a normal ratio comparable to hearts from sham-operated animals.

After one year, animals from each group were separated, and treatment was withdrawn. The animals were then housed for an additional 6 months. In the ramipril 1 mg group, blood pressure did not reach the value of the control vehicle group, and surprisingly, LVH and myocardial fibrosis did not recur in animals during withdrawal of treatment (Figure 13).

These experiments showed that long-term ACE inhibition effectively prevented cardiac hypertrophy and myocardial fibrosis, even in the absence of a fall in blood pressure. This protective effect is still present after a six-month treatment withdrawal. Interactions with autocrine-paracrine mechanisms activated by local ACE inhibition involving decreased A II formation, an increased BK accumulation, and an attenuation of sympathetic activities should be considered as contributors to these long-term beneficial cardiac effects of ACE inhibitors.

Some findings indicate that ACE inhibitors may suppress the cardiac hypertrophic response by reducing the formation of A II, which stimulates hypertrophy, matrix protein synthesis, and collagen synthesis.[86,87] However, since inhibition of ACE, besides reducing A II formation, also increases BK levels, BK might also contribute via the generation of NO and PGI_2 to the prevention of the hypertrophic response.

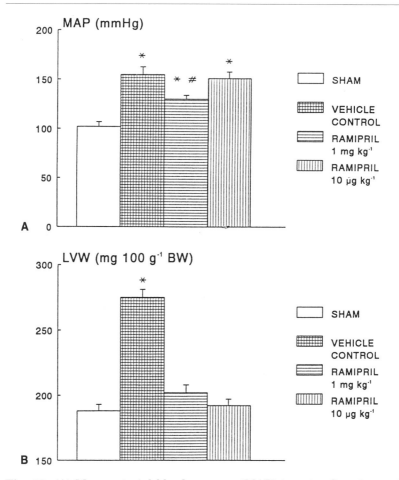

Fig. 13. (A) Mean arterial blood pressure (MAP) in rats after six-month withdrawal of RT treatment. $^*p < 0.05$ versus sham; $^\#p < 0.05$ versus vehicle control. (B) Left-ventricular weight (LVW) in rats after six-month withdrawal of RT treatment; n = 5 per group; $^*p < 0.05$ versus sham.

To evaluate the role of BK in the antihypertrophic effect of ACE inhibitors, the influence of the BK receptor antagonist HOE 140 on the effects of ramipril on LVH in rats with aortic banding was investigated.[88] Ramipril in the antihypertensive dose of 1 mg/kg per day for 6 weeks prevented the increase in blood pressure and the development of LVH. Plasma ACE activity was significantly inhibited. A low non-antihypertensive dose of ramipril 10 µg/kg/day for 6 weeks had no effect on the increase in blood pressure or on plasma

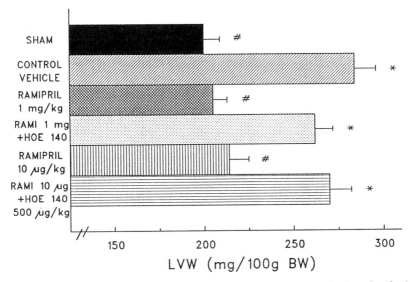

Fig. 14. Effects of orally administered RT (1 mg/kg/day and 10 µg/kg/day) and coadministration of HOE 140 (500 µg/kg/day subcutaneously) on left-ventricular weight (LVW) in rats with aortic banding. $^*p < 0.05$ versus sham; $^\#p < 0.05$ versus control vehicle.

ACE activity but also prevented LVH after aortic banding. The anti-hypertrophic effects of the high dose and the low dose of ramipril, as well as the antihypertensive action of the high dose of ramipril, were abolished by coadministration of the B_2 kinin receptor antago-nist HOE 140 (Figure 14). The specific blockade of A II receptors (subtype AT_1) seems to be less effective than ACE inhibition.[89]

These data demonstrate that ACE inhibitors like ramipril exert beneficial effects on the development of LVH in rats with hyperten-sion caused by aortic banding. The data also demonstrate that these beneficial effects can be prevented by a specific B_2 kinin receptor antagonist, thus delineating the role of BK in the antihypertrophic effects of ACE inhibitors in this experimental model. The results in rats with aortic banding may be explained by the effects of NO and PGI_2 on cell growth. NO-generating vasodilators and cyclic GMP are known to be antimitogenic.[90] Similar effects were found for PGI_2 and cyclic AMP.[91] Therefore, both NO and PGI_2, when increased by BK following ACE inhibition, may contribute to these beneficial effects of ACE inhibitors.[88]

Spontaneously Hypertensive Rats

In spontaneously hypertensive rats (SHR), the preventive effects of chronic treatment with ramipril on myocardial LVH and on capillary length density were investigated. SHR were treated in utero and, subsequently, up to 20 weeks of age with a high dose (1 mg/kg/day) or with a low dose (10 µg/kg/day) of ramipril. Animals on the high dose remained normotensive, whereas those on the low dose developed hypertension in parallel to vehicle-treated controls. At the end of treatment, ACE activity in heart tissue was inhibited dose-dependently in the treated groups. Both groups revealed an increase in myocardial capillary length density (Figure 15), together with increased myocardial glycogen and reduced citric acid concentration. Left-ventricular mass was reduced only in the high-dose-treated, but not in the low-dose-treated, animals.[92]

The underlying mechanism for the ACE-inhibitor-induced myocardial capillary growth is not known. One possible explanation resides in the BK potentiating effect of the ACE inhibitor. BK has been shown to improve myocardial blood flow, even at very low concentrations.[75] An enhanced myocardial blood flow, on the other hand, appears to be the common denominator of all experimental conditions associated with myocardial capillary proliferation.[93] In addition, the increased cardiac glycogen and decreased citric acid

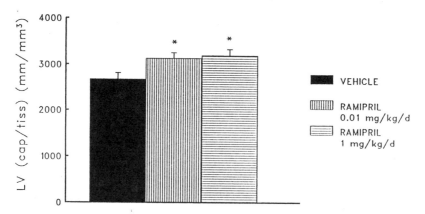

Fig. 15. Cardiac capillaries in hearts from spontaneously hypertensive rats (SHR) treated with ramipril in a non-blood-pressure lowering dose of 10 µg/kg/day and in a blood-pressure-lowering dose of 1 mg/kg/day. SHR were treated in utero and, subsequently, up to 20 weeks of age. $^*p < 0.05$; n = 36 per group.

concentrations, together with a tendency to increased ATP levels in both ramipril-treated groups, are compatible with the known cardiac metabolic effects of BK that enhance myocardial glucose uptake in normoxic isolated rat hearts.[81] Further studies, including specific A II and BK receptor antagonists, will have to address the possible effect of an ACE-inhibitor-induced kinin potentiation on myocardial capillary growth in more detail.

The observation that low-dose ramipril treatment did not affect the development of LVH in the SHR is at variance with the results reported in the coarctation model of hypertension mentioned above. The discrepancy between both studies could be explained by the fact that the coarctation model represents a highly renin-dependent model of experimental hypertension, which may respond to ACE inhibition more drastically than the SHR, a model with normal to low plasma renin.

These results demonstrate that in SHR early-onset treatment with ramipril can induce myocardial capillary growth, even at doses too low to antagonize the development of hypertension or LVH. This ability of ramipril to induce capillary growth might be of great importance for the induction of coronary collateral vessels in humans with coronary artery disease and heart failure.[94]

Conclusion

The cardiovascular actions of ACE inhibitors are not only mediated by the reduction of A II but also by the inhibition of BK degradation. This contribution of BK is evidenced by the comparable effects of ACE inhibitors and BK in different pathophysiological situations. It is also evidenced by the observation that the specific B_2 kinin receptor antagonist HOE 140 blocked the cardiovascular effects of the ACE inhibitors as well as BK in experimental models of atherosclerosis, neointima formation, acute myocardial ischemia, and left-ventricular hypertrophy. The increase in local BK by ACE inhibition exerts protective effects by itself or activates pathways that liberate second messengers such as cyclic GMP via NO increase or cyclic AMP via a PGI_2 increase.

Summary

From pharmacological investigations and clinial studies, it is known that ACE inhibitors exhibit additional local actions, which are not related to hemodynamic changes and which cannot be explained only by interference with the renin-angiotensin system (RAS) with subsequent inhibition of A II formation. Since ACE is identical to kininase II, which inactivates the nonapeptide bradykinin (BK), potentiation of BK might be responsible for these additional effects of ACE inhibitors.

Inhibition of ACE by ramiprilat (RT) concentration and time dependently increased the formation of nitric oxide (NO) and prostacyclin (PGI$_2$) in cultured human and bovine endothelial cells. The new B$_2$ kinin receptor antagonist HOE 140 markedly attenuated the cyclic GMP accumulation following formation of NO and abolished the increase in PGI$_2$ release.

In renovascular models of hypertension associated with a stimulated RAS (2K1C), blood pressure reduction by ramipril was attenuated by HOE 140, whereas in rats with genetic hypertension with normal to low plasma renin, the blood-pressure inhibitory effect of the bradykinin antagonist was less effective. In experimental atherosclerosis in rabbits, ramipril was able to preserve endothelial function and vascular reactivity.

In the balloon deendothelialization model of carotid arteries in rats, it was found that ramipril markedly reduced neointima formation compared to controls and to the A II-antagonist Losartan-treated group. However, when ramipril was given together with HOE 140, its effect was significantly blunted.

To understand the cardioprotective mechanisms of local ACE inhibition by RT in the ischemic heart, HOE 140 and the specific inhibitor of NO synthase N^G-nitro-L-arginine (L-NNA) were tested in isolated working rat hearts subjected to local ischemia by occlusion of the left-coronary artery with reperfusion. Perfusion with RT (1 × 10^{-8} to 1 × 10^{-5} mol/l) induced a reduction of the incidence as well as the duration of ventricular fibrillation and improved cardiodynamics and myocardial metabolism. BK perfusion (1 × 10^{-10} to 1 × 10^{-8} mol/l) induced comparable cardioprotective effects. In addition, perfusion with RT (1 × 10^{-7} mol/l) markedly increased BK outflow in isolated rat hearts measured by RIA. The beneficial effects of RT and BK were abolished by the addition of L-NNA (1 × 10^{-6} mol/l) or HOE 140 (1 × 10^{-9} mol/l). Similar results were found in dogs and rabbits with myocardial infarction.

In rats made hypertensive by aortic banding, the influence of HOE 140 on the antihypertrophic effect of ramipril in left-ventricular hypertrophy (LVH) was investigated. Ramipril in the antihypertensive dose of 1 mg/kg/day for 6 weeks prevented the increase in blood pressure and the development of LVH. The lower non-antihypertensive dose of ramipril (10 μg/kg/day for 6 weeks) had no effect on the increase in blood pressure or on plasma ACE activity but also prevented LVH after aortic banding. The antihypertrophic effect of the higher and lower doses of ramipril, as well as the antihypertensive action of the higher dose of ramipril, was abolished by coadministration of the B₂ kinin antagonist HOE 140.

In spontaneously hypertensive rats (SHR), the preventive effects of chronic treatment with ramipril on myocardial LVH and capillary length density were investigated. SHR were treated in utero and, subsequently, up to 20 weeks of age with a high dose (1 mg/kg/day) or with a low dose (10 μg/kg/day) of ramipril. Animals on a high dose remained normotensive, whereas those on a low dose developed hypertension in parallel to vehicle-treated controls. At the end of the treatment, ACE activity in heart tissue was inhibited dose-dependently in the treated groups. Both groups revealed an increase in myocardial capillary length density. Left-ventricular mass was reduced only in high-dose-treated, but not in low-dose-treated, animals.

On the basis of these experimental findings in different pathophysiological situations, evidence is accumulating that kinins are participating in the cardiovascular actions of ACE inhibitors like ramipril.

References

1. Dzau VJ, Re RN. Evidence for the existence of renin in the heart. Circulation 1987; 75(suppl I):I-134–I-136.
2. Yamada H, Fabris B, Allen AM, Jackson B, Johnston CI, Mendelsohn AO. Localization of angiotensin converting enzyme in rat heart. Circ Res 1991; 68:141–149.
3. Schunkert H, Dzau VJ, Tang SS, Hirsch AT, Apstein CS, Lorell BH. Increased rat cardiac angiotensin converting enzyme activity and mRNA expression in pressure overload left ventricular hypertrophy. J Clin Invest 1990; 36:1913–1920
4. Lindpaintner K, Jin M, Wilhelm MJ, Suzuki F, Linz W, Schölkens BA, et al. Intracardiac generation of angiotensin and its physiologic role. Circulation 1988; 77(suppl I):1–18.
5. Linz W, Schölkens BA, Lindpaintner K, Ganten D. Cardiac renin-angiotensin system. Am J Hypertension 1989; 2:307–310.
6. Kramer HJ, Glänzer K, Meyer-Lehnert H, Mohaupt M, Predel HG. Kinin- and non-kinin-mediated interactions of converting-enzyme inhibitors with vasoactive hormones. J Cardiovasc Pharmacol 1990; 15(suppl 6):S91–S98.
7. Scherf H, Pietsch R, Landsberg G, Kramer HJ, Düsing R. Converting-enzyme inhibitor ramipril stimulates prostacyclin synthesis by isolated

rat aorta: evidence for a kinin-dependent mechanism. Klin Wochenschr 1986; 64:742–745.

8. Regoli D, Barabe J. Pharmacology of bradykinin and related kinins. Pharmacol Rev 1980; 32:1–46.

9. Marceau F, Lussier A, Regoli D, Giroud J. Pharmacology of the kinins: their relevance to tissue injury and inflammation. Gen Pharmacol 1983; 14:209–229.

10. Proud D, Kaplan AP. Kinin formation: mechanisms and role in inflammatory disorders. Ann Rev Immunol 1988; 6:49–83.

11. Wilson DD, de Garavilla L, Kuhn W, Togo J, Burch RM, Steranka L. D-Arg [Hyp3DPhe7] Bradykinin, a bradykinin antagonist, decreases mortality in a rat model of endotoxic shock. Circ Shock 1989; 27:93–101.

12. Vavrek RJ, Stewart JM. Competitive antagonists of bradykinin. Peptides 1985; 6:161–164.

13. Hock FJ, Wirth K, Albus U, et al. HOE 140: a new and long acting bradykinin-antagonist: in vitro studies. Br J Pharmacol 1991; 102: 769–773.

14. Wirth K, Hock FJ, Albus U, et al. HOE 140: a new potent and long acting bradykinin-antagonist: in vivo studies. Br J Pharmacol 1991; 102:774–777.

15. Lückhoff A, Busse R, Winter I, Bassenge E. Characterization of vascular relaxant factor released from cultured endothelial cells. Hypertension 1987; 9:295–303.

16. Scicli AG, Farhy R, Scicli G, Nolly H. The kallikrein-kinin system in heart and vascular tissue. In: Bönner G, Schölkens BA, Scicli AG, eds. The Role of Bradykinin in the Cardiovascular Action of Ramipril. Sussex, United Kingdom: Media Medica, 1992: 17–27.

17. Bönner G, Preis S, Chrosch R. Role of kinins in systemic and pulmonary hemodynamic effects of ramipril in man. In: Bönner G, Schölkens BA, Scicli AG, eds. The Role of Bradykinin in the Cardiovascular Action of Ramipril. Sussex, United Kingdom: Media Medica, 1992: 99–109.

18. Kifor I, Dzau VJ. Endothelial renin-angiotensin pathway: evidence for intracellular synthesis and secretion of angiotensins. Circ Res 1987; 60: 422–428.

19. Yanagishawa M, Kurihara H, Kimura S, Tomboe Y, Kobayashi M, Mitsui Y, et al. A novel potent vasoconstrictor peptide produced by vascular endothelial cells. Nature 1988; 332:411–415.

20. Milner P, Kirkpatrick KA, Ralevic V, Toothill V, Pearson J, Burnstock G. Endothelial cells cultured from human umbilical vein release ATP, substance P, and acetylcholine in response to increased flow. Proc R Soc Lond [Biol] 1990; 241:245–248.

21. Kawashima K, Watanabe N, Oohata H, Fujimoto K, Suzuki T, Ishizaki Y, et al. Synthesis and release of acetylcholine by cultured bovine arterial endothelial cells. Neurosci Lett 1990; 119:156–158.

22. Wiemer G, Schölkens BA, Becker RHA, Busse R. Ramiprilat enhances endothelial autacoid formation by inhibiting breakdown of endothelium-derived bradykinin. Hypertension 1991; 18: 558–563.

23. Cachefeiro V, Sakakibara T, Nasjletti A. Kinins, nitric oxide, and the hypotensive effect of captopril and ramiprilat in hypertension. Hypertension 1992; 19:138–145.

24. Gohlke P, Bünning P, Bönner G, Unger Th. ACE inhibitor effect on

bradykinin metabolism in the vascular wall. Agents and Actions 1992; (suppl.38):III:178–185.

25. Gohlke P, Bünning P, Unger Th. Distribution and metabolism of angiotensin I and II in the blood vessel wall. Hypertension 1992; 20:151–157.

26. Drummer OH, Kourtis S, Johnson H. Effect of chronic enalapril treatment on enzymes responsible for the catabolism of angiotensin I and the formation of angiotensin II. Biochem Pharmacol 1990; 39:513–518.

27. Hooper NM, Hryszko J, Oppong SY, Turner AJ. Inhibition by converting enzyme inhibitors of pig aminopeptidase P. Hypertension 1992; 19: 281–235.

28. Danckwardt L, Shimizu, Bönner G, Rettig R, Unger Th. Converting enzyme inhibition in kinin-deficient Brown Norway rats. Hypertension 1990; 16:429–435.

29. Benetos A, Gavras H, Stewart JM, Vavrek RJ, Hatinoglou S, Gavras I. Vasodepressor role of endogenous bradykinin assessed by a bradykinin antagonist. Hypertension 1986; 8:971–974.

30. Carbonell LF, Carretero OA, Stewart JM, Scicli AG. Effect of a kinin antagonist on the acute antihypertensive activity of enalapril in severe hypertension. Hypertension 1988; 11:239–243.

31. Waeber B, Aubert JF, Vavrek R, Stewart JM, Nussberger J, Brunner HR. Role of bradykinin in the blood pressure response to acute angiotensin converting enzyme inhibition in rats. J Hypertension 1986; 4(suppl 6):S597–S598.

32. Aubert JF, Waeber B, Nussberger J, Vavrek R, Stewart JM, Brunner HR. Lack of a role of circulating bradykinin in the blood pressure response to acute angiotensin converting enzyme inhibition in rats. Agents and Actions 1987; 22:349–354.

33. Bao G, Gohlke P, Qadri F, Unger T. Chronic kinin receptor blockade attenuates the antihypertensive effect of ramipril. Hypertension 1992; 20:74–79.

34. Bao G, Gohlke P, Unger Th. Kinin contribution to chronic antihypertensive actions of ACE inhibitors in hypertensive rats. Agents and Actions 1992; (suppl.38)II:423–430.

35. Becker RHA, Wiemer G, Linz W. Preservation of endothelial function by ramipril in rabbits on a long-term atherogenic diet. J Cardiovasc Pharmacol 1991; 18(suppl 2):S110–S115.

36. Yamamoto S, Takemori E, Hasegawa Y, Kuroda K, Nakao K, Inukai T, et al. General pharmacology of the novel angiotensin converting enzyme inhibitor benazepril hydrochloride. Arzneim Forsch/Drug Res 1991; 41 (II):913–923.

37. Schuh JR, Blehm DJ, Frierdich GE, McMahon EG, Blaine EH. Differential effects of renin-angiotensin system blockade on atherosclerosis in cholesterol-fed rabbits. J Clin Invest 1993; 91:1453–1458.

38. Chobanian AV, Haudenschild CC, Nickerson C, Drago R. Antiatherogenic effect of captopril in the Watanabe heritable hyperlipidemic rabbit. Hypertension 1990; 15:327–331.

39. Aberg G, Ferrer P. Effects of captopril on atherosclerosis in cynomologus monkeys. J Cardiovasc Pharmacol 1990; 15(suppl 5):S65–S72.

40. Drexler H, Zeiher A, Meinzer K, Just H. Correction of endothelial dysfunction in coronary microcirculation of hypercholesterolaemic patients by L-arginine. Lancet 1991; 338:1546–1550.

41. Capron L, Heudes D, Chajara et al. Effect of ramipril, an inhibitor of angiotensin converting enzyme, on the response of rat thoracic aorta to injury with a balloon catheter. J Cardiovasc Pharmacol 1991; 18: 207–211.
42. Powell JS, Clozel JP, Muller RKM, Kuhn H, Hefti F, Hosang M, et al. Inhibitors of angiotensin converting enzyme prevent myointimal proliferation after vascular injury. Science 1989; 245:186–188.
43. Farhy RD, Ho KL, Carretero OA, Scicli AG. Kinins mediate the antiproliferative effect of ramipril in rat carotid artery. Biochem Biophys Res Commun 1992; 182:283–288.
44. Lochner W, Parratt JR. A comparison of the effects of locally and systemically administered kinins on coronary blood flow and myocardial metabolism. Br J Pharmacol 1966; 26:17–26.
45. Wilkens H, Back N, Steger R, Karn J. The influence of blood pH on peripheral vascular tone: possible role of proteases and vaso-active polypeptides. In: Bertelli A, Back N, eds. Shock: Biochemical, Pharmacological and Clinical Aspects. New York: Plenum Press, 1970: 201.
46. Hashimoto K, Hirose M, Furukawa H, Kimura E. Changes in hemodynamics and bradykinin concentration in coronary sinus blood in experimental coronary occlusion. Jpn Heart J 1977; 18:679–689.
47. Matsuki T, Shoji T, Yoshida S, Kudoh Y, Motoe M, Inoue M, et al. Sympathetically induced myocardial ischemia causes the heart to release plasma kinin. Cardiovasc Res 1987; 21:428–432.
48. Hashimoto K, Hamamoto H, Honda Y, Hirose M, Furukawa S, Kimura E. Changes in components of kinin system and hemodynamics in acute myocardial infarction. Am Heart J 1978; 95:619–626.
49. Lefer AM, Tsao PS, Lefer DJ, Ma X-L. Role of endothelial dysfunction in the pathogenesis of reperfusion injury after myocardial ischemia. FASEB J 1991; 5:2029–2034.
50. Martorana PA, Linz W, Schölkens BA. Does bradykinin play a role in the cardiac antiischemic effect of the ACE-inhibitors? Basic Res Cardiol 1991; 86:293–296.
51. Xiang JZ, Linz W, Becker H, Ganten D, Lang RE, Schölkens BA, et al. Effects of converting enzyme inhibitors: ramipril and enalapril on peptide action and sympathetic neurotransmission in the isolated heart. Eur J Pharmacol 1985; 113: 215–223.
52. van Gilst WH, de Graeff PA, Wesseling H, de Langen CDJ. Reduction of reperfusion arrhythmias in the ischemic isolated rat heart by angiotensin converting enzyme inhibitors: a comparison of captopril, enalapril and HOE 498. J Cardiovasc Pharmacol 1986; 8: 722–728.
53. Fleetwood G, Boutinet S, Meier M, Wood JM. Involvement of the renin-angiotensin system in ischemic damage and reperfusion arrhythmias in the isolated perfused rat heart. J Cardiovasc Pharmacol 1991; 17: 351–356.
54. Linz W, Schölkens BA, Han YF. Beneficial effects of the converting enzyme inhibitor, ramipril, in ischemic rat hearts. J Cardiovasc Pharmacol 1986; 8(suppl 10):S91–S99.
55. Linz W, Schölkens BA, Manwen J, Wilhelm M, Ganten D. The heart as a target for converting enzyme inhibitors: studies in ischemic isolated working rat hearts. J Hypertension 1986; 4(suppl.6):S477–S479.
56. Tian R, Neubauer S, Pulzer F, Haas F, Ertl G. Angiotensin I conversion

and coronary constriction by angiotensin II in ischemic and hypoxic isolated rat hearts. Eur J Pharmacol 1991; 203:71–77.

57. Ertl G. Angiotensin converting enzyme inhibitors and ischemic heart disease. Eur Heart J 1988; 9:716–727.
58. Linz W, Schölkens BA. Influence of local converting enzyme inhibition on angiotensin and bradykinin effects in ischemic rat hearts. J Cardiovasc Pharmacol 1987; 10(suppl 7): S75–S82.
59. Vegh A, Szekeres L, Parratt JR. Local intracoronary infusions of bradykinin profoundly reduce the severity of ischemia-induced arrhythmias in anesthetized dogs. Br J Pharmacol 1991; 104:294–295.
60. Schölkens BA, Linz W, Lindpaintner K, Ganten D. Angiotensin deteriorates but bradykinin improves cardiac function following ischemia in isolated rat hearts. J Hypertension 1987; 5 (suppl):S7–S9.
61. Schölkens BA, Linz W, König W. Effects of the angiotensin converting enzyme inhibitor, ramipril, in isolated ischemic rat heart are abolished by a bradykinin antagonist. J Hypertension 1988; (suppl 4):S25–S28.
62. Linz W, Wiemer G, Schölkens BA. ACE inhibition induces NO-formation in cultured bovine endothelial cells and protects isolated ischemic rat hearts. J Mol Cell Cardiol 1992; 24:909–949.
63. Schölkens BA, Linz W, Martorana PA. Experimental cardiovascular benefits of angiotensin converting enzyme inhibitors: beyond blood pressure reduction. J Cardiovasc Pharmacol 1991; 18(suppl 2):S26–S30.
64. Linz W, Schölkens BA, Kaiser J, Just M, Bei-Yin Q, Albus U, et al. Cardiac arrhythmias are ameliorated by local inhibition of angiotensin formation and bradykinin degradation with the converting enzyme inhibitor ramipril. Cardiovasc Drugs and Ther 1989; 3:873–882.
65. Bhargava AS, Preus M, Khater AR, Günzel P. Effect of iloprost on serum creatine kinase and lactate dehydrogenase isoenzymes after isoprenaline-induced cardiac damage in rats. Drug Res 1990; 40(I): 248–252.
66. Felsch A, Schrör K. Platelet activating factor-induced tissue injury in a neutrophil-perfused heart preparation is antagonized by bradykinin and ramiprilat. In: Bönner G, BA Schölkens BA, Scicli AG, eds. The Role of Bradykinin in the Cardiovascular Action of Ramipril. Sussex, United Kingdom: Media Medica, 1992: 69–77.
67. Pi X-J, Chen X. Captopril and ramiprilat protect against free radical injury in isolated working rat hearts. J Mol Cell Cardiol 1989; 21: 1261–1271.
68. van Gilst WH, van Wijngaarden J, Scholtens E, de Graeff PA, de Langen CDJ, Wesseling H. Captopril-induced increase in coronary flow: an SH-dependent effect on arachidonic acid metabolism? J Cardiovasc Pharmacol 1987; 9(suppl 2): S31–S36.
69. Becker BF, Heier M, Gerlach E. Experimental evidence for cardioprotection afforded by ramipril, an inhibitor of angiotensin converting enzyme. In: Schultheib H-P, ed. New Concepts in Viral Heart Disease. Berlin, Germany: Springer-Verlag, 1988: 465–474.
70. Parrat JR, Coker SJ, Wainwright CL. Eicosanoids and susceptibility to ventricular arrhythmias during myocardial ischemia and reperfusion. J Mol Cell Cardiol 1987; 19(suppl V): 55–66.
71. Zeitlin IJ, Fagbemi SO, Parratt JR. Enzymes in normally perfused and ischemic dog hearts which release a substance with kinin like activity. Cardiovasc Res 1989; 23:91–97.

72. Proud D, Togias A, Naclerio RM, Crush SA, Norman PS, Lichtenstein LM. Kinins are generated in vivo following nasal airway challenge of allergic individuals with allergen. J Clin Invest 1983; 72:1678–1685.
73. Baumgarten CR, Linz W, Kunkel G, Schölkens BA, Wiemer G. Ramiprilat increases bradykinin outflow from isolated rat hearts. Br J Pharmacol 1993; 108:293–295.
74. Pitt B, Mason J, Conti CR, Colman RW. Activation of the plasma kallikrein system during myocardial ischemia. Advan Exp Med Biol 1970; 8:403–410.
75. Linz W, Martorana PA, Schölkens BA. Local inhibition of bradykinin degradation in ischemic hearts. J Cardiovasc Pharmacol 1990; 15(suppl 6):S99–S109.
76. Martorana PA, Kettenbach B, Breipohl G, Linz W, Schölkens BA. Reduction of infarct size by local angiotensin-converting enzyme inhibition is abolished by a bradykinin antagonist. Eur J Pharmacol 1990; 182: 395–396.
77. Hartman JC, Wall TM, Hullinger TG, Shebuski RJ. Reduction of myocardial infarct size in rabbits by ramiprilat: reversal by the bradykinin antagonist HOE 140. J Cardiovasc Pharmacol 1993: 21:996–1003.
78. Tio RA, Tobé TJM, Bel KJ, de Langen CDJ, van Gilst WH, Wesseling H. Beneficial effects of bradykinin on porcine ischemic myocardium. Basic Res Cardiol 1991; 86:107–116.
79. Tobé TJM, de Langen CDJ, Tio RA, Bel KJ, Mook PH, Wesseling H. In vivo effect of bradykinin during ischemia and reperfusion: improved electrical stability two weeks after myocardial infarction in the pig. J Cardiovasc Pharmacol 1991; 17:600–607.
80. Vuorinen P, Laustiola K, Metsä-Ketelä T. The effects of cyclic AMP and cyclic GMP on redox state and energy state in hypoxic rat atria. Life Sci 1984; 35:155–161.
81. Rösen P, Eckel J, Reinauer H. Influence of bradykinin on glucose uptake and metabolism studied in isolated cardiac myocytes and isolated perfused rat hearts. Hoppe-Seyler's Z Physiol Chem 1983; 364:431–438.
82. Messerli FH, Ketelhut R. Left ventricular hypertrophy: an independent risk factor. J Cardiovasc Pharmacol 1991; 17 (suppl 4):S59–S67.
83. Schelling P, Fischer H, Ganten D. Angiotensin and cell growth: a link to cardiovascular hypertrophy? J Hypertension 1991; 9:3–15.
84. Linz W, Schölkens BA, Ganten D. Converting enzyme inhibition specifically prevents the development and induces regression of cardiac hypertrophy in rats. Clin Exper Hypertens 1989; A11(7):1325–1350.
85. Linz W, Schaper J, Wiemer G, Albus U, Schölkens BA. Ramipril prevents left ventricular hypertrophy with myocardial fibrosis without blood pressure reduction: a one year study in rats. Br J Pharmacol 1992; 107:970–975.
86. Kato H, Suzuki H, Tajima S, Ogata Y, Tominaga T, Sato A, et al. Angiotensin II stimulates collagen synthesis in cultured vascular smooth muscle cells. J Hypertension 1991; 9:7–22.
87. Giacomelli F, Anversa P, Wiener J. Effect of angiotensin-induced hypertension on rat coronary arteries and myocardium. Am J Pathol 1976; 84:111–125.
88. Linz W, Schölkens BA. A specific B_2 bradykinin receptor antagonist HOE 140 abolishes the antihypertrophic effect of ramipril. Br J Pharmacol 1992; 105:771–772.

89. Linz W, Henning R, Schölkens BA. Role of angiotensin II receptor antagonism and converting enzyme inhibition in the progression and regression of cardiac hypertrophy in rats. J Hypertension 1991; 9(suppl 6):S400–401.
90. Garg UC, Hassid A. Nitric oxide-generating vasodilators and 8-bromocyclic guanosine monophosphate inhibit mitogenesis and proliferation of cultured rat vascular smooth muscle cells. J Clin Invest 1989; 83: 1774–1777.
91. Shirotani P, Yui Y, Hattori R, Kawai C. U-61,431F, a stable prostacyclin analogue, inhibits the proliferation of bovine vascular smooth muscle cells with little antiproliferative effect on endothelial cells. Prostaglandins 1991; 41:97–110.
92. Unger Th, Mattfeld T, Lamberty V, Bock P, Mall G, Linz W, et al. Effect of early onset ACE inhibition on myocardial capillaries in SHR. Hypertension; 1992; 20:478–482.
93. Mall G, Zimmer G, Baden S, Mattfeld T. Capillary neoformation in the rat heart stereological studies on papillary muscles in hypertrophy and physiologic growth. Basic Res Cardiol 1990; 85:531–540.
94. Kass RW, Kotler MN, Yazdanfar S. Stimulation of coronary collateral growth: current developments in angiogenesis and future clinical applications. Am Heart J 1992; 123 (2):486–496.

15

Transgenic Rats Expressing Components of the Renin-Angiotensin System: Focus on Cardiovascular Regulation

Martin Paul, Jürgen Wagner,
Reinhold Kreutz, Maria S. Fernandez-Alfonso,
Yixian Liu, Michael Bader, and Detlev Ganten

Introduction

The renin-angiotensin system (RAS) is one of the best-studied regulatory systems involved in the control of cardiovascular function and volume homeostasis. Its effector peptide, A II, exerts a multiplicity of functions by raising peripheral resistance through vasoconstriction, enhancing renal sodium reabsorption, facilitating catecholamine release from sympathetic nerve endings, or stimulating mineralcorticoid production in the adrenal gland.[1,2] These integrative functions focusing on control of body salt and water homeostasis and blood pressure have led to the hypothesis that malfunction of this system may be related to the pathogenesis of hypertension.[3]

There are also other functions of the RAS that go beyond the understanding of an endocrine system (Figure 1). Angiotensin II, the effector peptide of the RAS, has been implicated as a growth factor or growth modulator in the cardiovascular system, and it has been suggested [4–6] that it plays an important role in the development and maintenance of cardiovascular hypertrophy. This role may have

Lindpaintner K and Ganten D (editors): *The Cardiac-Renin Angiotensin System,* ©
Futura Publishing Co., Inc., Armonk, NY, 1994.

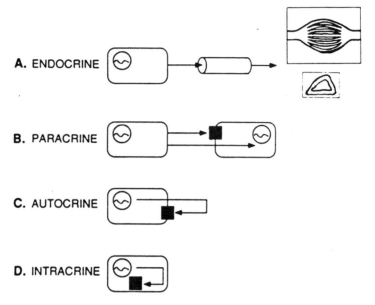

Possible ways of action of tissue angiotensin II.
A The peptide enters the circulation and produces its effects
   at target organs located at distance, e.g. vasculature
   and adrenal gland (endocrine).
B After secretion, the peptide acts on its receptors located
   on adjacent cells (paracrine).
C After release, the peptide acts on its receptors located
   on the same cell (autocrine).
D The peptide acts in the cell of its own synthesis.

Fig. 1. Mechanisms of action of angiotensin II illustrating endocrine, paracrine, autocrine, and intracrine concepts (from Paul M, et al.[51]).

important clinical implications since these findings could provide
the basis for the beneficial effects of converting-enzyme inhibitors
in these situations. Blood pressure-independent, mitogenic, and
growth-promoting effects of A II on endothelial cells, fibroblasts,
and vascular smooth muscle cells (VSMC), possibly via activation
of oncogenes, are well known.[4,7,8] These influences may mediate the
deleterious maladaptations of the cardiovascular system to pathological stimuli.

Due to the predicted major role of the RAS in the pathogenesis
of hypertension and cardiovascular hypertrophy, it has been considered as a candidate gene system for these disorders. Several of its

components have been implicated as genetic factors in the pathogenesis of hypertension such as the renin gene,[9] the angiotensinogen gene, and the gene for the angiotensin-converting enzyme (ACE).[10,11] Since coexpression of the components of the RAS has been demonstrated in the heart or the vasculature, A II formation in the cardiovascular system may not solely be derived from the plasma, but rather be produced by local, tissue-specific RASs and act on the surrounding tissue in a paracrine or autocrine fashion (see [12-14] for a review and Fig. 1). Overexpression of human renin and other components of the RAS in extrarenal tissues in transgenic rats offers one possibility of investigating the impact of tissue-specific human RASs on cardiovascular morphology and function. This review, therefore, will specifically focus on the investigation of the cardiac RAS in transgenic animals overexpressing the components of the RAS.

Methods For Generation of Transgenic Animals

In transgenic experiments, foreign genes have been stably integrated into the genome of a number of species, but mice have been used most extensively in transgenic research. Several factors may account for this: there is a large database of mouse genetics, and transgenic technology can easily be applied in this species. For some areas of research, however, the mouse may not be the most ideal species for transgenic studies (Table 1). Its size puts limitations on

Table 1
Transgenic Rats Versus Mice
in Hypertension Research

Advantages of Mice
Large data base on mouse genetics
Animal size
Costs of maintaining a transgenic colony
Transgenic techniques well established

Advantages of Rats
rat models of hypertension already established
physiological characterization
pharmacological interventions

the methodological arsenal, which can be used for the detailed investigation of phenotypic changes induced by the expression of transgenes. One area of research where this is particularly true is cardiovascular biology. Although investigators have succeeded in applying sophisticated techniques to the measurement of cardiovascular parameters in mice,[15,16] this is still considered an exception.

Other species may be more suited to serve as models for cardiovascular disease. Primary hypertension, for example, is virtually unknown in mice, whereas there are a great number of rat strains that show this disorder and have been extensively used as model systems to study primary hypertension.[17] Experimental hypertension research, therefore, has largely been carried out using rats as models, and there is a great amount of data available to serve as reference points for the measurement of cardiovascular parameters in this species. These considerations made it desirable to establish transgenic rats as experimental models in hypertension research. Transgenic animals are defined by the fact that new genetic material has been integrated in the genome by experimental methods other than breeding. Through incorporation into the germ cells, transgenic founder animals pass the transgene on to their offspring, and a transgenic line can be established.

There are a number of methods available to introduce genetic material into the genome of an animal. Retroviral infection of embryonic cells has been used to generate transgenic mice, but the most widely used method still is microinjection of DNA into the pronucleus of a fertilized oocyte.[18] These cells are obtained from animals that have been mated after their ovulation had been stimulated through gonadotropine treatment. After microinjection, the oocytes are reimplanted into the oviduct or uterus of a pseudopregnant female, which had been mated with a vasectomized or sterile male. The offspring of this animal is then screened for the presence of the transgene by extracting DNA from a small tissue sample, for example, a tail biopsy and by its analysis using established methods such as Southern blotting and/or polymerase chain reaction (PCR) assays.

This general method (Figure 2) can also be applied for the establishment of transgenic rats,[19] but there are several technical details that have to be modified.[20] One is superovulation, which tends to be more difficult to achieve in the rat. This problem can be solved, however, by adapting the procedure of Armstrong and Opavsky[21] using the application of the follicle-stimulating hormone (FSH) via osmotic minipump. By this approach, the first transgenic rat line

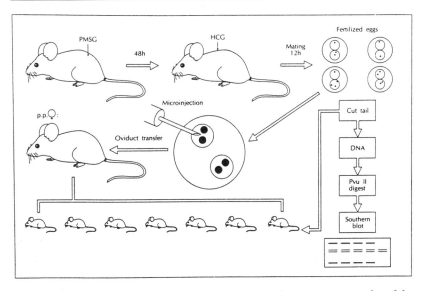

Fig. 2. Generation of transgenic animals. Females are superovulated by gonadotropin treatment and mated with male rats. Fertilized oocytes are microinjected with DNA constructs and reimplanted into the oviduct of a pseudopregnant foster mother. To generate pseudopregnancy, female rats have been mated with vasectomized males. The presence of the transgene in the resulting offspring is tested by analyzing DNA obtained from a tail biopsy by established methods such as Southern blotting (from Wagner J, et al.[19]).

in cardiovascular research was established by Mullins, Peters, and Ganten,[22] who expressed the mouse *Ren-2* gene in rats.

Experimental Approaches in Transgenic Research

Transgenic animals can be used to answer different experimental questions. First, transgenic lines can be established with the purpose of adding an additional gene to develop models for the in vivo study of the transgene's expression and regulation and possible phenotypic changes induced by the transgene. A second widely used application in transgenic research is the establishment of permanent cell lines derived from transgenic animals. For these experiments, a tissue-specific promoter is fused with a gene that has oncogenic potential. An example for such experiments is the work by Sigmund and Gross,[23,24] who linked the regulatory region of the mouse *Ren-2* gene to sequences derived from the SV40 T antigen, which induces tumorigenesis and generated transgenic mice expressing this chimeric construct. The animals showed tumor formation in the kidney, adrenal gland, testis, and subcutaneous tissue. The transformed cells, in addition to their ability to produce renin-mRNA and to secrete renin protein, could be passaged without losing these features specific for juxtaglomerular cells.[25] They may, therefore, provide adequate tissue culture models to study renin biosynthesis, processing, and secretion.

A third application for transgenic animals is their use for the study of gene regulation in vivo. Typically, such a scenario calls for the establishment of transgenics expressing constructs that consist of the regulatory region of a gene under investigation linked to a reporter gene such as the luciferase gene. These constructs can be used for the transient transfection of cells in tissue culture as well as for the generation of transgenic animals. Studies can thus be carried out not only to investigate the tissue-specific responses to stimuli on the level of gene transcription, but also for many other questions such as the identification of cell- and tissue- specific regulatory mechanisms. Experiments investigating these mechanisms for the renin gene are described elsewhere in greater detail.[26–29]

A fourth application of transgenic techniques is the establishment of whole animal models, overexpressing a specific gene in the organism. To achieve this, a heterologous promoter inducing high levels of expression is linked to the gene or cDNA in question. Since extreme overexpression of genes in many cases will prove lethal during fetal life, inducible promoter sequences have proven to be useful. These sequences will show only little activity in the noninduced state, which will allow the prevention of possible deleterious effects of transgene expression during ontogeny. Expression can be induced at a time when the experimental protocol calls for the overexpression. One of the most widely used promoters for such types of experiments is the metallothionein promoter, which can be induced by heavy metals, such as zinc sulphate in the drinking water. This promoter has been used successfully to overexpress rat renin and angiotensinogen genes in transgenic mice.[30]

The Cardiac Renin–Angiotensin System in Transgenic Animals

All components of the RAS are present in the heart (at least on the protein level), and upregulation of the RAS has been described in disorders such as cardiac hypertrophy and failure. Therefore, it has been interesting to investigate the possible pathophysiological changes in the heart induced by an overexpression of components of the RAS. In the following, we will focus our discussion on several transgenic lines: transgenic animals expressing the mouse *Ren-2* gene and transgenic animals expressing the human or rat angiotensinogen gene.

Expression of the Mouse *Ren-2* Gene in Transgenic Animals

The mouse *Ren-2* gene has been used by several investigators for the establishment of transgenic animals. This gene is an additional renin gene present in some mouse strains that has developed most likely from a gene duplication. The protein translated from the *Ren-2* mRNA has been termed renin-2,[31] which is unglycosylated and highly expressed in several extrarenal tissues, most notably the submandibular gland (SMG). Tronik et al.[32] injected a genomic construct containing the entire *Ren-2* gene under control of its authentic 5′ and 3′ sequences into oocytes from mice, which possess only one renin gene (*Ren-1*). Expression analysis in the transgenic offspring obtained from this experiment showed that the transgene was expressed in the SMG and kidney, but not in other tissues such as the heart, liver, and brain.

The same construct was used by Mullins et al.[33,34] to generate transgenic mice. The transgene was expressed in the SMG, kidney, adrenal gland, and testis, but not in other tissues such as the brain, heart, and liver. The studies by Tronik and Mullins do not present any experiments investigating possible pathophysiological effects of the transgene or give details of the effects of transgene expression on RAS proteins in plasma or tissues.

A transgenic rat model expressing the *Ren-2* gene has been introduced by Mullins et al.[20,22] Approximately 100 copies of DNA were injected into pronuclei of rat oocytes. The construct was identical to the one used earlier by Mullins et al. for the establishment of transgenic mice. Five founder animals were identified, and three of them transmitted the transgene to their offspring. The three lines that were derived from these founders have been termed TGR(mREN2)25, 26, and 27. Offspring of lines 26 and 27 developed fulminant hypertension, whereas line 25 showed only slight elevations of blood pressure. The reasons for this are unclear but may be related to the transgene insertion site that is currently under detailed investigation. Lines 25 and 27 have now been bred to homozygosity, but in the case of line 26 this was impossible since all male animals were sterile. The cause for this is most likely an insertional mutation at the integration site of the transgene on the rat genome.

Line 27 develops the highest blood pressure levels (Figure 3) and has been investigated in greater detail. Heterozygous animals of this line develop systolic blood pressures of up to 250 mmHg at 10 weeks of age. Homozygous animals show even higher pressures (up to 300 mmHg) and die from secondary complications of hypertension such as stroke, heart failure, and renal sclerosis if they are not subjected to lifelong antihypertensive treatment. There is a marked sexual dimorphism in these animals, with females having much lower levels than males. This dimorphism may be due to androgen effects, which have been described to upregulate *Ren-2* expression. Indeed, treatment of female transgenic rats with dihydrotestosterone increased blood pressures to male values, whereas castration of males had the opposite effect (J. Bachmann, personal communication).

Since the blood pressure effects must be caused by the "addition" of the mouse *Ren-2* gene, the expression of the transgene, as well

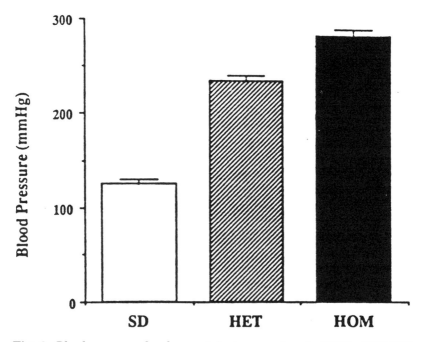

Fig. 3. Blood pressure development in transgenic rats TGR(m*REN2*)27. Blood pressure was measured by the tailcuff method (from Bader M, et al.[38]).

as the parameters of the tissue and plasma RAS, has been determined. As detected by Northern blotting and RNAse protection assay, the transgene is expressed highest in the adrenal gland, followed by organs such as the gastrointestinal tract, lung, and brain and the vasculature. Surprisingly, it was found that plasma active renin was not elevated in transgenic animals, despite a significant rise in prorenin levels. In addition, plasma angiotensinogen, A I, and A II were not changed. These findings were underlined by a depression of renin activity in the kidney, the classical site of renin biosynthesis. In contrast, a significant elevation of renin activity in several organs, most notably the adrenal gland, was found. Immunohistochemical studies and in situ hybridization indeed showed that kidney renin was greatly suppressed but that high signals of renin immunoreactivity and mRNA were localized in the interzone between the zona glomerulosa and fasciculata of the adrenal gland.[35]

Further studies investigating the role of adrenal renin have now been carried out,[36,37] and results indicate that at least a part of the hypertensive response in these transgenic animals can be explained by the increase in adrenal renin, which may interfere with the synthesis of adrenal steroids. Increased aldosterone biosynthesis as a factor by itself could be ruled out since spironolactone cannot lower the blood pressure in these animals.[38] There is still the possibility, however, that other adrenal steroids are upregulated, and indeed increased concentrations of these steroids have been found in the plasma and urine of the transgenic animals.[36] In addition, preliminary results demonstrate that dexamethasone treatment can lower the blood pressure effectively.[39]

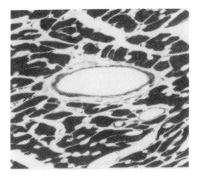 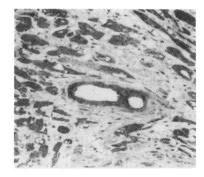

Fig. 4. Morphological analysis of hearts from transgenic rats TGR(mREN2)27. Ultrathin sections x10900 from control (left) and transgenic (right) hearts. The latter show media hypertrophy of coronary vessels and extensive fibrosis (from Bachman S, et al.[35]).

There are indications, however, that other organs also contribute to the blood pressure development in these animals. Measurements of *Ren-2* mRNA, for example, showed its presence in many other organs such as the gastrointestinal tract, the brain, and the blood vessels. The latter may also play an important role in the pathogenesis of blood pressure since recent data using an isolated hindlimb preparation have demonstrated that the conversion of A I to A II is greatly enhanced in transgenic rats, pointing to a contribution of the vascular RAS.[40]

It is interesting to note that transgenic animals develop severe cardiovascular hypertrophy. At later ages this is most likely due to the fulminant hypertension, but the onset of cardiovascular hypertrophy is found at an age when blood pressure is not persistently elevated. Changes seen in the heart include hypertrophy as indicated by the heart weight to body weight ratio and extensive fibrosis (Figure 4). These changes may be influenced by local levels of A II,

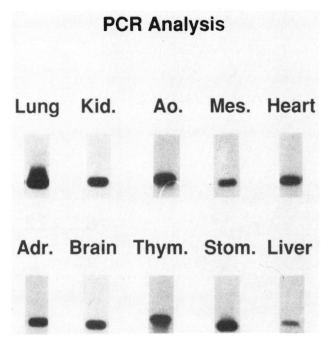

Fig. 5. Expression of ACE in TGR(m*REN2*)27. The gene expression of ACE was measured by reverse transcription (RT) PCR using ACE-specific primers spanning a 380 bp region. The amplified products were blotted onto nylon membranes and hybridized to ACE-specific probes.

which has been postulated to play a role as growth factor or modulator in the cardiovascular system.[4,5,41,42] Since the heart of the transgenic rat itself does not express high levels of renin, it is possible that prorenin is taken up from the circulation and activated so that it contributes to local A II synthesis, which then could stimulate growth mechanisms. This hypothesis is currently under detailed investigation.

In addition, other components of the RAS have been found to be elevated in transgenic animals. Preliminary experiments demonstrate that the gene expression of ACE is stimulated in many tissues of these animals (Figure 5). In addition, the mRNA expression for another potent vasoactive peptide and possible mitogen, endothelin-1, is elevated in the hearts of transgenic animals (Figure 6).

Taken together, the establishment of transgenic rats expressing the mouse *Ren-2* gene has provided an interesting model system to study the regulation and pathophysiological relevance of tissue RASs in vivo. There is increasing evidence that there is enhanced activity of the RAS in the cardiovascular system. In addition, other vasoactive regulatory systems, such as the endothelin system, may be activated.

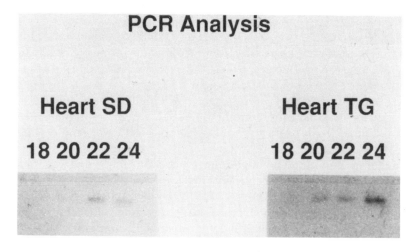

Fig. 6. Expression of endothelin in TGR(m*REN2*). The gene expression of endothelin-1 was investigated by RT-PCR. Endothelin primers span a region of 300 bp of the rat endothelin cDNA. For semiquantitative analysis, samples were taken out after various cycles (18, 20, 22, 24) of the PCR reaction, blotted onto nylon membranes, and hybridized with an endothelin-specific probe.

Expression of Angiotensinogen in Transgenic Animals

Angiotensinogen is the substrate of angiotensin biosynthesis. As an α_2-globulin, it is mainly expressed in the liver, but it is also present in high concentrations in a number of organs, such as the kidney and brain. Angiotensinogen is upregulated in several cardiovascular disorders, such as in cardiac hypertrophy induced by aortic banding.[43,44] It is, therfore, interesting to study the effects of angiotensinogen in transgenic animals on the overall activity of the tissue RAS and to investigate the possible cardiovascular alterations.

Transgenic mice carrying the rat angiotensinogen gene have been first described by Ohkubo et al.[30] These investigators used a mouse metallothionein-I-rat-angiotensinogen fusion gene directing expression predominantly to the liver. Rat angiotensinogen in the mice amounted to 6–8 µg/ml. Transgenic mice in the heterozygous as well as in the homozygous state or after the stimulation of rat angiotensinogen expression by $ZnSO_4$ did not show elevated blood pressure levels. Crossbreeding of these mice with mice transgenic for rat renin under the control of the metallothionein promoter, however, led to elevated blood pressure levels, which could be further enhanced by $ZnSO_4$ treatment or lowered by 1% captopril in the drinking water.

To map the tissue-specific and inducible enhancer elements regulating angiotensinogen gene expression, transgenic mice carrying angiotensinogen minigenes with either 0.75 kb or 4 kb of 5'-flanking region were established. The short fragment was sufficient to mediate induction by glucocorticoids, estrogen, and bacterial endotoxin, as well as tissue-specific expression.[45]

In contrast to the findings of rat renin and angiotensinogen controlled by the metallothionein promoter, where hypertension resulted most likely from the interaction of both transgene products in the plasma of the same animal, transgenic mice expressing only a genomic rat angiotensinogen construct, where the gene was under the control of its own promoter, developed high blood pressure per se.[46] These mouse strains expressed the rat angiotensinogen gene mostly in the liver, kidney, and brain but also in other organs such as the heart. Interestingly, the hypertensive phenotype in these animals is probably not caused by a stimulated plasma RAS since angiotensinogen does not exceed levels of the normotensive, transgenic mice. Transgenic mice carry the same gene under the control of the metallothionein promoter, which directs expression in several organs, but most likely not always in cell types where angiotensinogen is expressed under normal conditions.[30] In contrast, the transgenic mice that express angiotensinogen under control of its native promoter show high angiotensinogen levels in organs such as the liver, brain, and heart, where angiotensinogen is appropriately localized in the same areas as the endogenous angiotensinogen of the mouse.[46] The overexpression of the transgene in these organs is thought to be responsible for the development of hypertension, suggesting a role for the tissue RAS in the pathogenesis of hypertension. In addition, these animals develop cardiac hypertrophy, which is possibly related to a stimulation of the cardiac RAS due to the overexpression of angiotensinogen (S. Kimura, personal communication).

After the use of rat and mouse angiotensinogen, the human angiotensinogen gene has been used to generate transgenic mice.[47] A 14 kb human DNA fragment containing the angiotensinogen gene, including 1.3 kb of the 5'-flanking and 3'-flanking regions, was microinjected into pronuclei from C57Bl/6 mice. Two lines, which showed tissue-specific expression predominantly in the liver and comparably high levels in the kidney and heart, could be obtained. No phenotypic alterations due to the angiotensinogen transgene expression were reported. However, in contrast to rat and mouse angiotensinogen, the interaction of human angiotensinogen with human renin is highly species specific, rendering the interaction with renin from other species difficult.

Human Angiotensinogen in Transgenic Rats

The human angiotensinogen gene comprising five exons, four introns, 1.3 kb of the 5'-flanking and 2.4 kb of the 3'-flanking regions was used to generate transgenic rats. Four lines that transmitted the transgene to their progeny were established.[48] Human angiotensinogen was secreted into the plasma. The different lines exhibited markedly elevated plasma levels ranging from 120 μg/ml up to 5 mg/ml. These angiotensinogen levels surpassed those found in rats of about 40 μg/ml and humans with 60 μg/ml.[49]

Despite the high plasma angiotensinogen concentrations, none of the lines developed hypertension or cardiovascular alterations. As in transgenic mice, the species specificity of human angiotensinogen prevented its interaction with rat renin and thus the production of A II. The human angiotensinogen transgenic protein was functional since infusion of human renin into these animals elicited a hypertensive reponse, which could be blocked by the human renin-specific inhibitor Ro 42–5892.[48]

Human angiotensinogen expression was widespread in a tissue-

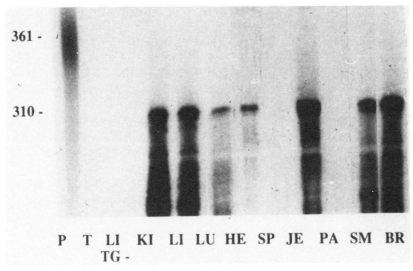

Fig. 7. RNAse protection assay analysis of gene expression of human angiotensinogen in transgenic rats: tissue-specific expression of human angiotensinogen mRNA. Lanes: P: undigested human angiotensinogen antisense RNA probe; T: tRNA; LI: TG- and rat-liver RNA from transgenic negative littermates as negative control; KI: kidney; LI: liver; LU: lung; HE: heart; SP: spleen; PA: pancreas; SM: submandibular gland; BR: brain. In each lane, 50 μg of total RNA were used, except for the liver (5 μg). Specificity was checked by 50 μg of liver transgenic negative RNA as control.

specific distribution. High mRNA levels were found in the liver, kidney, and brain but were also readily demonstrable in the heart by RNAse protection assay (Figure 7).

The angiotensinogen gene from the mouse, rat, and human species has been used to generate transgenic mice and rats. Under the control of the gene's natural promoter, the expression pattern has been stable across species borders, supporting the observed constant gene expression in different animal species.[33] In the case of the heterologous metallothionein promoter, the expression of rat angiotensinogen was directed to the liver and testis, as well as other organs.[30] Transgenic angiotensinogen gene expression could be demonstrated independently of species from the organs involved in cardiovascular regulation. A high expression of the transgene was found in the hearts of mice and rats. In both strains, cardiac expression of the endogenous angiotensinogen gene as well as the angiotensinogen gene from human heart samples has been described.

The exact cellular level of expression has not been defined, but the high amount of human angiotensinogen-mRNA present in the different cardiac compartments may simplify in situ hybridization. Human angiotensinogen expression has been found to be correctly expressed on a cellular level in the liver and proximal tubules of the kidney (S. Bachmann, personal communication) also suggesting appropriate cardiac cell expression.

Most studies so far on angiotensinogen as a transgene have focused on tissue-specific expression in transgenic animals, but the development of hypertension in the presence of angiotensinogen alone or in the presence of rat and human renin[30] suggests a causative role for angiotensinogen in cardiovascular regulation. These findings may prompt investigations depending on if and how the presence of the additional angiotensinogen gene alters cardiac or vascular hypertrophy. Besides a possible effect of the angiotensinogen transgene in the basal state on cardiovascular function, it is tempting to speculate how the angiotensinogen transgene may modify cardiac function and morphology after stimulation in experimental pathophysiological states.

The transgenic rat as animal model for cardiovascular disease may be useful to study the regulation of the human angiotensinogen transgene under conditions such as aortic banding or myocardial infarction. Cardiac-specific regulation of endogenous angiotensinogen gene expression has been demonstrated by aortic banding in the past.[50]In the presence of human renin by the crossbreeding of animals transgenic for this gene to angiotensinogen transgenic rats, the high expression of human angiotensinogen may influence the process of cardiac and vascular hypertrophy and, thereby, provide new insights into these pathophysiological mechanisms.

Conclusions

The general applicability of transgenic animal models for basic research in cardiovascular biology and hypertension has now been established. The study of transgenic rats offers advantages over the use of transgenic mice in particular with respect to the characterization of cardiovascular parameters and pharmacological interventions, which are more readily available in transgenic rat models. On the other hand, transgenic mouse models are still very helpful when investigating the regulation of gene expression in an animal.

One of the predominant candidate systems thought to be involved in the pathogenesis of hypertension has been the RAS. The generation of mice and rats expressing the human genes for renin and angiotensinogen has provided important models not only for the study of regulatory mechanisms of these genes but also for the detailed investigation of possible pathophysiological consequences of their expression. Ultimately, the information obtained from the study of these transgenic animals should provide important insights into the regulation of the RAS in humans. In addition, they also are experimental systems enabling the study of the pharmacological effects of specific substances interfering with the RAS in humans, such as renin inhibitors. Such experiments have the potential of providing important information on the clinical use of these drugs, especially if they influence the specific sequelae of hypertension such as cardiac or vascular hypertrophy. These transgenic animals are particularly useful in investigating the role of tissue-specific RASs such as in the heart and vasculature.

The information that will be derived from future studies of these animals can be used to design experiments, which will further enhance our understanding of tissue-specific gene expression and regulation. This can be achieved through the use of constructs for the generation of transgenic animals, which allow selective expression of components of the RAS in single tissues, for example, through the use of organ- and cell-specific promoters. In addition, future experiments will focus on the investigation of other candidate genes thought to be involved in human hypertension, such as the genes for ACE, the A II receptor, and also other cardiovascular systems.

Summary

Transgenic animals have been introduced as models to study the genetic basis of many diseases. Recently, several candidate genes have been identified for a number of cardiovascular disorders such as hypertension and cardiovascular hypertrophy, which can be further investigated using transgenic techniques. The RAS is a prominent candidate system for some of these diseases. It has been implicated in the pathogenesis of hypertension in humans as well as in the development of cardiac and vascular hypertrophy. The components of this system are expressed in cardiac and vascular tissues, and the existence of local RASs in these tissues has been demonstrated.

Studies on the regulation of the genes of the RAS and their impact on cardiovascular disease in humans, however, are difficult to perform. We and others, therefore, have established transgenic rats and mice expressing components of the system. These animals show an increased expression of the transgenes in the tissues of the cardiovas-

cular system and should become interesting models to study the effects of the RAS in cardiovascular tissues and its regulation in physiological and pathophysiological situations.

References

1. Hackenthal E, Paul M, Ganten D, et al. Morphology, physiology, and molecular biology of renin secretion. Physiol Rev 1990; 70:1076–1116.
2. Dzau VJ, Pratt RE. Renin angiotensin system: biology, physiology, and pharmacology. Heart and Cardiovasc System 2, 1986:1631–1662.
3. Bader M, Kreutz R, Wagner J, et al. Primary hypertension and the renin angiotensin system: from the laboratory experiment to clinical relevance. In: Sassard J, ed. Colloque INSERM, Vol. 218: Genetic Hypertension. London and Paris: John Libbey Eurotext, 1992: 359–370.
4. Schelling P, Fischer H, Ganten D. Angiotensin and cell growth: a link to cardiovascular hypertrophy? J Hypertens 1991; 9:3–15.
5. Paul M, Ganten D. The molecular basis of cardiovascular hypertrophy: the role of the renin angiotensin system. J Cardiovasc Pharmacol 1992; 19(suppl.5):S51–S58.
6. Dzau VJ. Implications of local angiotensin production in cardiovascular physiology and pharmacology. Am J Cardiol 1987; 59:59A–65A.
7. Paquet J-L, Baudouin-Legros M, Brunelle G, Meyer P. Angiotensin II-induced proliferation of aortic myocytes in spontaneously hypertensive rats. J Hypertens 1990; 8:565–572.
8. Taubman MB, Berk BC, Izumo S, Tsuda T, Alexander RW, Nadal-Ginard B. Angiotensin induces c-fos mRNA in aortic smooth muscle: role of Ca2+ mobilization and protein kinase C activation. J Biol Chem 1989; 264:526–530.
9. Dene H, Wang SM, Rapp JP. Restriction fragment length polymorphisms for the renin gene in Dahl rats. J Hypertens 1989; 7:121–126.
10. Hilbert P, Lindpaintner K, Beckmann JS, et al. Chromosomal mapping of two genetic loci associated with blood-pressure regulation in hereditary hypertensive rats. Nature 1991; 353:521–529.
11. Jacob HJ, Lindpaintner K, Lincoln SE, et al. Genetic mapping of a gene causing hypertension in the stroke-prone spontaneously hypertensive rat. Cell 1991; 67:213–224.
12. Unger T, Gohlke P, Paul M, Rettig R. Tissue renin angiotensin systems: fact or fiction. J Cardiovasc Pharmacol 1991; 18 (suppl.2):20–25.
13. Lindpaintner K, Jin M, Wilhelm MJ, et al. Intracardiac generation of angiotensin and its physiological role. Circulation 1988; 77:I-18–I-23.
14. Baker KM, Booz GW, Dostal DE. Cardiac actions of angiotensin II: role of an intracardiac renin-angiotensin system. Ann Rev Physiol 1992; 54:227–241.
15. Mockrin SC, Dzau VJ, Gross KW, Horan MJ. Transgenic animals: new approaches to hypertension research. Hypertension 1991; 17:394–399.
16. Field LJ. Cardiovascular research in transgenic animals. Trends Cardiovasc Med 1991; 1:141–146.
17. Ganten D, Lindpaintner K, Ganten U, et al. Transgenic rats: new animal models in hypertension research. Hypertension 1991; 17:843–855.

18. Palmiter RD, Brinster RL. Germ-line transformation of mice. Ann Rev Genet 1986; 20:465–499.
19. Wagner J, Zeh K, Paul M. Transgenic rats in hypertension research. J Hypertens 1992; 10:601–605.
20. Mullins JJ, Ganten D. Transgenic animals: new approaches to hypertension research. J Hypertens 1990; 8(suppl 7):S35–S37.
21. Armstrong DT, Opavsky MA. Superovulation of immature rats by continuous infusion of FSH. Biol Reprod 1988; 39:511–518.
22. Mullins JJ, Peters J, Ganten D. Fulminant hypertension in transgenic rats harbouring the mouse Ren-2 gene. Nature 1990; 344:541–544.
23. Sigmund CD, Gross KW. Differential expression of the murine and rat renin genes in peripheral subcutaneous tissue. Biochem Biophys Res Commun 1990; 173:218–223.
24. Sigmund CD, Jones CA, Jacob HJ, et al. Pathophysiology of vascular smooth muscle in renin promoter-T-antigen transgenic mice. Am J Physiol 1991; 260:F249–F257.
25. Sigmund CD, Okuyama K, Ingelfinger J, et al. Isolation and characterization of renin-expression cell lines from transgenic mice containing a renin-promoter viral oncogene fusion construct. J Biol Chem 1990; 265: 19916–19922.
26. Paul M, Nakamura N, Pratt RE, Burt DW, Dzau VJ. Cell dependent posttranslational processing and secretion of recombinant mouse renin-2. Am J Physiol 1992; 262:E224–E229.
27. Sigmund CD, Gross KW. Structure, expression, and regulation of the murine renin genes. Hypertension 1991; 18:446–457.
28. Paul M, Burt DW, Krieger JE, Nakamura N, Dzau VJ. Tissue specificity of renin promoter activity and regulation in mice. Am J Physiol 1992; 262:E644–E650.
29. Nakamura N, Burt DW, Paul M, Dzau VJ. Negative control elements and cAMP responsive sequences in the tissue-specific expression of mouse renin genes. Proc Natl Acad Sci USA 1989; 86:56–59.
30. Ohkubo H, Kawakami H, Kakehi Y, et al. Generation of transgenic mice with elevated blood pressure by introduction of the rat renin and angiotensinogen genes. Proc Natl Acad Sci USA 1990; 87:5153–5157.
31. Dzau VJ, Paul M, Nakamura N, Pratt RE, Ingelfinger JR. Role of molecular biology in hypertension research. Hypertension 1989; 13:731–740.
32. Tronik D, Dreyfus M, Babinet C, Rougeon F. Regulated expression of the Ren-2 gene in transgenic mice derived from parental strains carrying only the Ren-1 gene. EMBO J 1987; 6:983–987.
33. Mullins JJ, Sigmund CD, Kane-Haas C, McGowan RA, Gross KW. Expression of the DBA/2J Ren-2 gene in the adrenal gland of transgenic mice. EMBO J 1989; 8:4065–4072.
34. Mullins JJ, Sigmund CD, Kane-Haas C, et al. Studies on the regulation of renin genes using transgenic mice. Clin Exp Hypertens [A] 1988; 10: 1157–1167.
35. Bachmann S., Peters J, Engler E et al. Transgenic rats carrying the mouse renin gene: morphological characterization of a low-renin hypertension model. Kidney Int 1992; 41:24–36.
36. Sander M, Bader M, Djavidani B, et al. The role of the adrenal gland in the hypertensive transgenic rats TGR(mREN2)27. Endocrinology 1992; 131:807–814.

37. Peters J, Sander M, Münter K, et al. The role of adrenal renin in steroid metabolism and development of hypertension in transgenic rats TGR(mREN2)27. In: Sassard J, ed. Colloque INSERM, Vol. 218: Genetic Hypertension. London and Paris: John Libbey Eurotext, 1992:345–347.

38. Bader M, Zhao Y, Sander M, et al. Role of tissue renin in the pathophysiology of hypertension in TGR(mREN2)27 rats. Hypertension 1992; 19: 681–686.

39. Djavidani B, Sander M, Böhm M, et al. Dexamethasone suppresses development of hypertension in TGR(mREN)27. J Hypertens 1992; 10(suppl.4):S10 (abstract).

40. Hilgers KF, Peters J, Veelken R, et al. Increased vascular angiotensin formation in female rats harboring the mouse Ren-2 gene. Hypertension 1992; 19:687–691.

41. Naftilan AJ, Pratt RE, Eldridge CS, Lin HL, Dzau VJ. Angiotensin II induces c-fos expression in smooth muscle via transcriptional control. Hypertension 1989; 13:706–711.

42. Naftilan AJ, Pratt RE, Dzau VJ. Induction of platelet-derived growth factor A-chain and c-myc gene expressions by angiotensin II in cultured rat vascular smooth muscle cells. J Clin Invest 1989; 83:1419–1424.

43. Niedermaier N, Drexler H, Kaling M, Ganten D. Left ventricular hypertrophy and myocardial infarction increase left ventricular angiotensinogen expression. J. Hypertens. 1991; 9(suppl.1):S469 (abstract).

44. Paul M, Wagner J, Liu Y, Niedermaier N. Application of the polymerase chain reaction for the mRNA measurements of the components of the renin-angiotensin system. Naunyn-Schmiedeberg's Arch Pharmacol 1991; 343 (suppl):R70 (abstract).

45. Clouston WM, Lyons IG, Richards RI. Tissue-specific and hormonal regulation of angiotensinogen minigenes in transgenic mice. EMBO J 1989; 8:3337–3343.

46. Kimura S, Mullins JJ, Bunnemann B, et al. High blood pressure in transgenic mice carrying the rat angiotensinogen gene. EMBO J 1992; 11:821–827.

47. Takahashi S, Fukamizu A, Hasegawa T, et al. Expression of the human angiotensinogen gene in transgenic mice and transfected cells. Biochem Biophys Res Commun 1991; 180:1103–1109.

48. Ganten D, Wagner J, Zeh K, et al. Species specificity of renin kinetics in transgenic rats harboring the human renin and angiotensinogen genes. Proc Natl Acad Sci USA 1992; 89:7806–7810.

49. Gardes J, Bouhnik J, Clauser E, Corvol P, Ménard J. Role of angiotensinogen in blood pressure homeostasis. Hypertension 1982; 4:185–189.

50. Baker KM, Chernin MI, Wixson SK, Aceto JF. Renin-angiotensin system involvement in pressure-overload cardiac hypertrophy in rats. Am J Physiol 1990; 259:H324–H332.

51. Paul M, Bachmann, J, Ganten D. The tissue renin-angiotensin systems in cardiovascular disease. Trends Cardiovasc Med 1992; 2: 94–99.

16

Human Heart Chymase

Ahsan Husain, Akio Kinoshita,
Shen-Shu Sung, Hidenori Urata, and
F. Merlin Bumpus

Introduction

The rate-limiting step in the formation of the octapeptide hormone A II is the cleavage of A I from angiotensinogen by the enzyme renin [EC 3.4.23.15].[1] In the blood and several tissues, the further conversion of A I to A II is thought to be effected by A I-converting enzyme (ACE) [EC 3.4.15.1].[2,3] Angiotensin II formed in the blood has multiple diverse physiological effects on the cardiovascular system, including arteriolar vasoconstriction and aldosterone secretion.[1] In the heart, A II produces a positive inotropic and chronotropic effect.[1] Recently, functional high-affinity A II receptors have been identified in the human heart.[4,5]

Specific inhibitors of ACE are used clinically to treat hypertension and congestive heart failure (CHF).[6,7] But, despite an effective inhibition of plasma ACE activity during chronic ACE inhibitor therapy, plasma A II has been reported to return to near-normal levels.[8,9] Evidence that ACE is incompletely blocked in some tissues during treatment has led to the suggestion that residual levels of ACE activity in these tissues may form A II, which is then released into the blood. Still other studies have suggested that A II-forming enzymes other than ACE participate in A II formation.[10,11] While examining human heart tissue in search of another A II-forming enzyme activity besides ACE, we observed that over 75% of the

Lindpaintner K and Ganten D (editors): *The Cardiac-Renin Angiotensin System,* © Futura Publishing Co., Inc., Armonk, NY, 1994.

A II-forming enzyme activity in human left-ventricular membranes was not blocked by ACE inhibitors.[12] In this review, we describe our attempts at understanding the biology of a major A II-forming serine proteinase from the human heart. Structurally, this cardiac proteinase belongs to the chymase family of leukocyte serine proteinases and will subsequently be referred to as human heart chymase.

Purification of Human Heart Chymase

The complete purification of human heart chymase from left-ventricular tissue was accomplished by a five-step procedure.[13] This procedure is summarized in Table 1. Conversion of A I to A II at pH 8.0 was used as the sole means of enzyme assay throughout the purification. The choice of A I as the substrate was dependent on the initial objective, which was to isolate the ACE-inhibitor-resistant enzyme responsible for the major A II-forming activity in human heart tissue. Washed human cardiac membranes contained A II-forming and angiotensinase activities, as well as ACE. The initial preextraction of cardiac membranes with 1% Triton X-100 and 500 mM of KCl effectively removed ACE activity as well as much of the angiotensinase activity. Subsequent purification was effected by gel

Table 1
Purification of Human Heart Chymase (HHC)

Purification Step	Total Protein (mg)	HHC Activity (kU*)	Specific HHC Activity (U*/mg)	Yield of HHC Activity (%)	Purification (fold)
1. Cardiac membrafes†	73,444	129	1.76	100	1
2. 0.5–2 M KCl extract	57,643	458	8.0	355	4.5
3. Gel filtration on 14 × 96 cm Ultrogel AcA54 column	2,203	425	193	329	110
4. Gel filtration on 4.4 × 96 cm Ultrogel AcA54 column	459	411	896	318	509
5. HPLC heparin-affinity column	1.3	268	202,665	207	115,150

* One unit (U) of human heart chymase activity = 1 nmol A II generated per minute.
† Derived from 1.6 kg of human left-ventricle tissue.
‡ From Urata H, et al.[13]

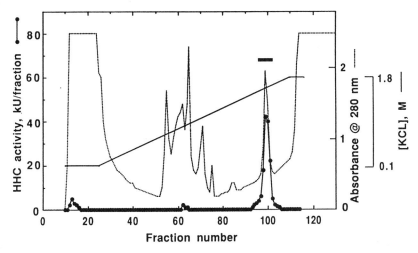

Fig. 1. Final purification of human heart chymase by HPLC heparin-affinity chromatography. Human heart chymase purified by gel filtration was applied to a TSK Heparin-5PW HPLC column. The column was first developed isocratically with 20 mM Tris-HCl buffer, pH 8.0, containing 0.1 M KCl for 12 min at a flow rate of 0.5 ml/min. Human heart chymase was then eluted using a 43-min linear gradient of 20 mM Tris-HCl buffer, pH 8.0, containing 1.8 M KCl and 0.1% Triton X-100. The solid bar represents the human heart chymase containing fractions (from Urata H, et al.[13]).

filtration and HPLC heparin-affinity chromatographies (Figure 1), which, after a 115,000-fold purification, yielded an enzyme preparation with a specific activity of 3.37 μmol A II generated per sec/ mg of protein enzyme. Following heparin-affinity chromatography, SDS-polyacrylamide gel electrophoresis of human heart chymase yielded a broad protein band with an M_r between 29,000 and 31,000 (Figure 2). Upon sequencing, this purified preparation of human heart chymase gave a single amino-terminal sequence, indicating a high degree of enzyme purity. Extensive amino-terminal similarity of this human heart A II-forming enzyme with the chymase (*chymo*tryptic protei*nase*) family of leukocyte serine proteinases suggested that the cardiac enzyme belongs to the chymase family.

Structure of the Human Chymase Gene

Thirty clones were identified by the screening of the γDASH human genomic library under low stringency with the partial rat

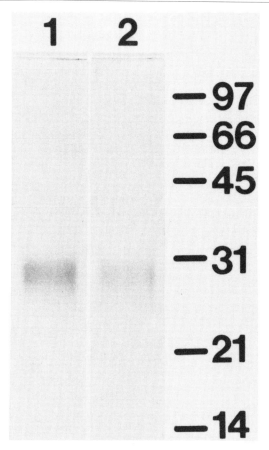

Fig. 2. SDS-polyacrylamide gel electrophoresis analysis of purified human heart chymase. Lanes 1 and 2 were analyzed by SDS-polyacrylamide gel electrophoresis under reducing (10 mM dithiothreitol) and nonreducing conditions, respectively, in 14% acrylamide gels. Proteins were visualized by silver staining. The bars on the right indicate molecular weight standards in kd (from Urata H, et al.[13]).

MCP II (rat mast cell protease II; also rat chymase 2) cDNA probe. An 8 kb Bam HI fragment of the 15 kb insert, isolated from one of these clones, contained the entire human chymase gene.[14] The human chymase gene was also independently cloned by Caughey et al.[15] The nucleotide sequence of the entire human heart chymase gene is shown in Figure 3.[14] The gene is approximately 3 kb in length and has 5 coding blocks and 4 intervening sequences. The 5′ untranslated region contains a CAAT box and a TATA box. A consensus polyadenylation motif, AATAAA, which is followed by a cleavage site motif consisting of a CA sequence located 15 bp downstream along with a GT cluster, is found in the 3' untranslated region (Fig. 3). The first coding block is 58 bp in length; it encodes, in an open reading frame, the first 19 amino acids (-21 to -3) of the preproenzyme. (A similar short first coding block is present in the genes of other serine proteinases, including human cathepsin G,[16] human neutrophil elastase,[17] rat MCP II,[18] and human cytotoxic cell protease.[19]) The second, third, fourth, and fifth coding blocks of the human heart chymase gene encode amino acids -2 to 49, 50 to 94, 95 to 179, and 180 to 226, respectively. A single in-frame stop codon is present at the end of the fifth coding block.

The overall organization of the human heart chymase gene is similar to that of several other serine proteinases.[14] It is, therefore, likely that these genes are derived from a single ancestral gene. These proteinases all have their coding regions located on five coding blocks separated by four intervening sequences, with active-site histidine, aspartic acid, and serine residues located on the second, third, and fifth coding blocks, respectively. The relative positions of these residues within these coding blocks are highly conserved among the chymase subfamily.[14]

Sequences in the 5' untranslated region of the human heart chymase gene contain a TATA box and a CAAT box (Fig. 3). A comparison of the 5' region of the gene with the same location of the rat MCP II gene[184] reveals a homologous sequence (CAGTTCCTGTGGTT) at positions 154 to 166 (Fig.3). This region is homologous to a sequence that confers pancreas-specific gene expression. However, the 5' and 3' untranslated regions of the human heart chymase gene do not contain mast cell specific DNA sequences. Two conserved motifs are also found in the 5' untranslated regions of both human heart chymase[13] and cathepsin G[16] genes. These motifs are CCTTTCTAG (in human heart chymase, 68 to 76); CCTTTCATG (in cathepsin G, -106); and CAGCCTTG (in human heart chymase 170 to 177, cathepsin G, -124). The existence of an enhancer sequence homologous with those in the 5' untranslated regions of the rat MCP II and the cathepsin G genes suggests that a similar enhancer mechanism may participate in the expression of the human heart chymase gene. A sequence (GGGAACT_TC) that is partially homologous to the κB binding site (GGGACTTTC) is found in the 5' untranslated region of the human heart chymase gene.[14] Binding of the nuclear protein factor, NK-κB, by the κB binding site promotes the transcription of the immunoglobulin light chain genes by B lymphocytes.[20] This putative κB-binding site in

```
  1  CTCCAGAAAGTCACCATAGGTTGAGGGTACATCTGAGAAGCCAGCACTTGGAGTTCAGGC   60
 61  TCAAGTTCCTTTCTAGAAAAACACTGGGTGATTCTAGGGGAACTACTGATCAGAAACAGC  120
121  CAATTCAGAGTGAGAGAAGAAAACGTGACCATGCAGTACGTAGGTACGAGCCATGCCC    180
181  CTCTCTTGCCTTCTGGGAGTTTATAAAACCCAAGACTGGAAGGAAAACCAGCATTTGCTCA  240
                                       -21
                 MetLeuLeuLeuProLeuProLeuLeuLeuPheLeuLeuCys
241  GGCAGCCTCTCTGGGAAGATGCTGCTTCTTCCTCTCCCCTGCTGCTCTTTCTCTTGTGC   300
         -3
     SerArgAlaGluAlaG
301  TCCAGAGCTGAAGCTGGTGAGTATCAGGGTTCTTCCCTCTGAAATCTGCTGCAGTATCAG  360
361  CTCCTGAAACAAAGATGTTTAGTCTGAAAATAGCTGACTCCTAAACAGGGTTCCAAGATC  420
421  TCTCTTCAAGAGTCCCAGAGGAAATTTCCACTTGGGATGTGTGCCACCCCACCCCCACCC  480
481  CCACCCACTGCCATTCTCTACAGCCTAGGACAGCCCCCAGGAACAAGGAATTTCACCTCA  540
541  ATTGTAGAAAAGCCCAGAGCAAGTGGAAGGAAAAGGGGTATCCCAGGAAAACAGACATGT  600
601  CCTCTTAATCTTCTGAGCATCAGGGCTACCCATTACTTTGTGACTTCTCACTCTGTGACC  660
661  ATGCTCAAGAGCTATGGAGAAATCTAAAACAGGAACCTGGACAGTGGGTCCTACACAGAG  720
721  ACAGAGGAGGGTGGGCCAGGGCAAGGTGGGAGTGGGAGAAGTCTGAGATGAAAACATCAG  780
781  AATGGAGCAGAGGCAAGAATGAGATTTCACCTGGGAGGTTATGGGTGGGGAAAGATACGA  840
841  AATACAGGAGACAGGAGAGGGAAGATGGGCGGAACACAGGGTGAGAATGAGATTCCAGGG  900
901  AAGTCCTAGCTCAGCTTTAACCCAATTTGTCCATTCATTGGAGAGAGTATCTATGGCCGT  960
                                     -1 +1
                              lyGluIleIleGlyGlyThrGluCysLysPro
961  GTTCAAACCCTGGGGTGCTCTGTTCCAGGGGAGATCATCGGGGGCACAGAATGCAAGCCA 1020

     HisSerArgProTyrMetAlaTyrLeuGluIleValThrSerAsnGlyProSerLysPhe
1021 CATTCCCGCCCCTACATGGCCTACCTGGAAATTGTAACTTCCAACGGTCCCTCAAAATTT 1080

     CysGlyGlyPheLeuIleArgArgAsnPheValLeuThrAlaAlaHisCysAlaGlyAr
1081 TGTGGTGGTTTCCTTATAAGACGGAACTTTGTGCTGACGGCTGCTCATTGTGCAGGAAGG 1140
1141 TGAGACAACAGGGTCTATTTATCTCCAAATGGGAGATGAACAACCAGGTAGCATCCAGGA 1200
1201 TACACCTGCACTGGGGACTGAAGAGGGGGTCCTGGGTCTTGTCAACTTTCAGGAGAGGGA 1260
1261 AGACTTGGGCTGAAAGACTTTAGTCTGTGTTTGAATAGTTCCTTGAGGCTTGGCAGTAG 1320
1321 GAGCTAAGCTCCCTTCGGAGGAAAAGGAGGTCCTGTCCAAGGTCCCTCTTGTTGCAGTAG 1380
1381 CACCCCTCACCCCTACCCAACTCAAGACACAGGCTCACTTTTCAGGGCCCCACCCAGTC 1440
1441 TCAGGGCCACTTCCTCTATGGCCTTTTCAAGAACACTGGCCTCTAGTTCTCAGGGTCCTG 1500
1501 AACCCATCATTTTATGGGAGGCAGAGAACAGGTCTACATGAGACCCCACTTTCCCGTTTA 1560
1561 ACTGATATCTCCTGCTTCAGGGCTGGCCCTCATGCAGGGTTCCCTGAATTAGAAGTGTGA 1620
1621 ACCCTGTCCCCTGAGTCCTCCCTGGCCTGTTCAGTCCCCAGCAATTCCAGGGGTGGTAGA 1680
1681 AATTGTGTCTGTTTCCTGAGAAGCTCTTTCATGAGTTAAGCCTGAGCCCTCAAATCGACA 1740
1741 AGTGGCCCATGAAAAGGGAGATGGGTAGAGTCCGGCGACCCAGTGACAGAGTTTAGTCCT 1800
1801 CTTTTCTCAGAATGAGCTCACCTCAGAAGAAAACCCCAAGCCATCACTGTCGCTCCTTTTC 1860
                                   50
                          gSerIleThrValThrLeuGlyAlaHisAsnIleThrGl
1861 CTTCCTTCTTCCTCACAACAGGTCTATAACAGTCACCCTTGGAGCCCATAACATAACAGA 1920

     uGluGluAspThrTrpGlnLysLeuGluValIleLysGlnPheArgHisProLysTyrAs
1921 GGAAGAAGACACATGGCAGAAGCTTGAGGTTATAAAGCAATTCCGTCATCCAAAATATAA 1980

     nThrSerThrLeuHisHisAspIleMetLeuLeuLys
1981 CACTTCTACTCTTCACCACGGATATCATGTTACTAAAGGTGACAACCACCTCTCTTCTCCCT 2040
2041 TTCCACTTCCCATTCTCCTAAGCTTCTGCTTCAGGTCCTCATTGCCCTGAATTTTTCTTA 2100
2101 AGGACTTGGCTATAACATGAAGCTACTCACCCTTGCCCTCCCTGATCACCTCCAACTGTC 2160
                                 95
                          LeuLysGluLysAlaSe
2161 CAGAGCCCATTTCGAGACTGACGGTCCTTCATTCCCTTCACAGTTGAAGGAGAAAGCCAG 2220

     rLeuThrLeuAlaValGlyThrLeuProPheProSerGlnPheAsnPheValProGlGl
2221 CCTGACCCTGGCTGTGGGGACACTCCCCTTCCCATCACAATTCAACTTTGTCCCACCTGG 2280

     yArgMetCysArgValAlaGlyTrpGlyArgThrGlyValLeuLysProGlySerAspTh
2281 GAGAATGTGCCGGGTGGCTGGCTGGGGAAGAACAGGTGTGTGAAGCGGGGCTCAGCACAC 2340

     rLeuGlnValLysLeuArgLeuMetAspProGlnAlaCysSerHisPheArgAspPh
2341 TCTGCAAGAGGTGAAGCTGAGACTCATGGATCCCCAGGCCTGCAGCCACTTCAGAGACTT 2400

     eAspHisAsnLeuGlnLeuCysValGlyAsnProArgLysThrLysSerAlaPheLys
2401 TGACCACAATCTTCAGCTGTGTGTGGGCAATCCCAGGAAGACAAAATCTGCATTTAAGGT 2460
2461 GATCCTCCAACTAGGTTTCCTCTCCAAAACTCACTGTTCAGGGACCAGAATGCTCTTAGA 2520
2521 AGGAGATGGGGTCAGAAGGTTGTCAGTCAGTGACAGGGTGAGCATCACAGGAATTGCTGT 2580
2581 CCTCCCGTGGTCCAAGACAGCCTCTGACCATCCATTCCAGTCTACTGCACTGGGGGCATG 2640
2641 GGGTGATGTGGAGAATGTGAATGACGGTCCCAAGAAAGGAAGAAGGGGCATCAGAACTAG 2700
2701 ATGTATAAGTGAGGAGCTCCACCTCCTGGGTCTGACTTTAGGTCTCACTGTGACTCCAAG 2760
2761 CTGGCTGGCAGACAGGAGTGGAGGACTTCCCGGGCTCACCTTCTTCTCTCTCTCTGCTCTCT 2820
                180
     GlyAspSerGlyGlyProLeuLeuCysAlaGlyValAlaGlnGlyIleValSer
2821 CTACAGGGAGACTCTGGGGGCCCTCTTCTGTGTGCTGGGGTGGCCCAGGGCATCGTATCC 2880

     TyrGlyArgSerAspAlaLysProProAlaValPheThrArgIleSerHisTyrArgPro
2881 TATGGACGGTCGGATGCAAAGCCCCCTGCTGTCTTCACCCGAATCTCCCATTACACGGCCC 2940

     TrpIleAsnGlnIleLeuGlnAlaAsnEnd
2941 TGGATCAACCAGATCCTGCAGGCAAATTAATCCTGGATCCTGAGCCAGCCTGAAAGGGAA 3000
3001 GCTGGAACTGGACCTGAGCAGCAAAGTGTGTGCCACTCATTCTGGTCTACCCTTGGTCCC 3060
3061 TCAGCCACAACCCTAAGCCTCCAGAAGTATCCTACAGGTCACAGAACTCTCAATAAACCT 3120
3121 CAGTGAAGACACCAGCTTCTAGTCGTGAGTGTGTGTNCCCTCTCTGCTGCTCTCTTCTCCC 3180
3156 TGCACATAGTGACCTGATTCCAGCCCAAGCACCCAAGGATTTGAAGGGGTGTGTGTGTG 3240
3241 TGTGTGTGTGTGTGTGTGTGTGTGTGTAT                              3271
```

Fig. 3. Structure of the human chymase gene. The nucleotide sequence of the five coding blocks, four intervening sequences, and 5′ and 3′ untranslated regions are shown. The deduced encoded amino acids are indicated above the corresponding nucleotides. Numbers at the right and left sides refer to the nucleotides. Overhead numbers refer to the deduced amino acids:

the human heart chymase gene is located immediately 5′ to a sequence that is partially homologous (TGA_TCA) to the phorbol ester reactive element (TGACTCA). Phorbol esters, which activate protein kinase C, induce NK-κB synthesis, not only in B lymphocytes but also in human T cell lines and in HeLa cells. The colocalization of a putative κB-binding site and a phorbol ester reactive element suggests that a protein kinase C mechanism may be involved in the control of human heart chymase gene expression.

Genomic DNA isolated from the leukocytes of normal healthy donors has been examined by Southern blot analysis to investigate whether human chymase is encoded by one or more genes.[14,21] These studies suggest that, unlike rodent chymases, there is a single gene for human heart chymase.

Structure of Human Heart Chymase cDNA

The cDNA for human heart chymase was obtained using polymerase chain reaction (PCR).[14] Based on the DNA sequence of the gene, specific primers were synthesized and used to amplify single-stranded cDNA derived from human heart poly (A)$^+$ mRNA. A PCR product of the correctly predicted length (769 bp) was obtained and isolated after fractionation of the PCR mixture by electrophoresis. The cDNA sequence, as well as the deduced amino acid sequence of human heart chymase, is shown in Figure 4. The nucleotide sequence of the cDNA contains a single ATG codon at the 5′ end, followed in an open reading frame by 741 base pairs encoding 247 amino acids. The amino acid sequences of nine human heart chymase tryptic fragments are found in the cDNA. Residues essential for the catalytic activity of serine proteinases—His[45], Asp[89], and Ser[182]—are conserved in all members and are present in human heart chymase.

−21 to −3, signal peptide; −3 to −1, N-terminal dipeptide of the proenzyme; +1 to 226, mature enzyme. Sequences highlighted in the 5′ untranslated region include a TATA (bp 201 to 206) box and a CAAT (bp 120 to 124) box; two motifs conserved between cathepsin G and human heart chymase (bp 68 to 76 and 170 to 177); and sequences partially homologous to the κB site for the binding of the nuclear protein factor NK-κB (bp 97 to 105) to the phorbol ester reactive element (bp 106 to 111) and to a region of the pancreatic enhancer are indicated by dotted lines (from Urata H, et al.[14]).

```
                                                                 Met    -21
                                          AGCCTCTCTGGGAAG ATG     [18]

Leu Leu Leu Pro Leu Pro Leu Leu Leu Phe Leu Leu Cys Ser Arg Ala Glu Ala Gly Glu   -1
CTG CTT CTT CCT CTC CCC CTG CTG CTC TTT CTC TTG TGC TCC AGA GCT GAA GCT GGG GAG   [78]
«NT

Ile Ile Gly Gly Thr Glu Cys Lys Pro His Ser Arg Pro Tyr Met Ala Tyr Leu Glu Ile   20
ATC ATC GGG GGC ACA GAA TGC AAG CCA CAT TCC CGC CCC TAC ATG GCC TAC CTG GAA ATT   [138]
                  » «T-15                » «T-9

Val Thr Ser Asn Gly Pro Ser Lys Phe Cys Gly Gly Phe Leu Ile Arg Arg Asn Phe Val   40
GTA ACT TCC AAC GGT CCC TCA AAA TTT TGT GGT GGT TTC CTT ATA AGA CGG AAC TTT GTG   [198]
              Δ           » «T-12                                *

Leu Thr Ala Ala His Cys Ala Gly Arg Ser Ile Thr Val Thr Leu Gly Ala His Asn Ile   60
CTG ACG GCT GCT CAT TGT GCA GGA AGG TCT ATA ACA GTC ACC CTT GGA GCC CAT AAC ATA   [258]
              »

Thr Glu Glu Glu Asp Thr Trp Gln Lys Leu Glu Val Ile Lys Gln Phe Arg His Pro Lys   80
ACA GAG GAA GAA GAC ACA TGG CAG AAG CTT GAG GTT ATA AAG CAA TTC CGT CAT CCA AAA   [318]
  *                               Δ                            «T-23

Tyr Asn Thr Ser Thr Leu His His Asp Ile Met Leu Leu Lys Leu Lys Glu Lys Ala Ser   100
TAT AAC ACT TCT ACT CTT CAC CAC GAT ATC ATG TTA CTA AAG TTG AAG GAG AAA GCC AGC   [378]

Leu Thr Leu Ala Val Gly Thr Leu Pro Phe Pro Ser Gln Phe Asn Phe Val Pro Pro Gly   120
CTG ACC CTG GCT GTG GGG ACA CTC CCC TTC CCA TCA CAA TTC AAC TTT GTC CCA CCT GGG   [438]
  »                                  «T-8

Arg Met Cys Arg Val Ala Gly Trp Gly Arg Thr Gly Val Leu Lys Pro Gly Ser Asp Thr   140
AGA ATG TGC CGG GTG GCT GGC TGG GGA AGA ACA GGT GTG TTG AAG CCG GGC TCA GAC ACT   [498]
             »             «T-5                               » «T-11

Leu Gln Glu Val Lys Leu Arg Leu Met Asp Pro Gln Ala Cys Ser His Phe Arg Asp Phe   160
CTG CAA GAG GTG AAG CTG AGA CTC ATG GAT CCC CAG GCC TGC AGC CAC TTC AGA GAC TTT   [558]
                          »                       «T-

Asp His Asn Leu Gln Leu Cys Val Gly Asn Pro Arg Lys Thr Lys Ser Ala Phe Lys Gly   180
GAC CAC AAT CTT CAG CTG TGT GTG GGC AAT CCC AGG AAG ACA AAA TCT GCA TTT AAG GGA   [618]
18  Δ                                                                        »

Asp Ser Gly Gly Pro Leu Leu Cys Ala Gly Val Ala Gln Gly Ile Val Ser Tyr Gly Arg   200
GAC TCT GGG GGC CCT CTT CTG TGT GCT GGG GTG GCC CAG GGC ATC GTA TCC TAT GGA CGG   [678]
«T-6                      »

Ser Asp Ala Lys Pro Pro Ala Val Phe Thr Arg Ile Ser His Tyr Arg Pro Trp Ile Asn   220
TCG GAT GCA AAG CCC CCT GCT GTC TTC ACC CGA ATC TCC CAT TAC CGG CCC TGG ATC AAC   [738]

Gln Ile Leu Gln Ala Asn End                                                  226
CAG ATC CTG CAG GCA AAT TAA TCCTGGATCC                                       [769]
```

Fig. 4. Deduced amino acid sequence of human heart chymase determined from the nucleotide sequence of its cDNA. The positions and amino acid sequences of ten peptides (NT, T-5 to T-23) derived from the purified protein are indicated by the overhead pair of brackets. The dotted lines under certain residues indicate those amino acids that could not be identified by peptide sequencing. The predicted signal peptide, the N-terminal dipeptide of the proenzyme, and the mature enzyme comprise amino acids −21 to −3, −2 to −1, and +1 to 226, respectively. The triad of amino acids, His[45], Asp[89], Ser[182], essential for catalysis by all serine proteinases, are indicated by the open triangles. Two consensus sites for N-linked glycosylation are shown by the asterisks above Asn[59] and Asn[82]. Sequences corresponding to the primers used for PCR in cDNA cloning are indicated by the double lines at the 5′ and 3′ regions of the cDNA. Numbers at the right side refer to amino acids, and the numbers in brackets refer to the nucleotides (from Urata H, et al.[14]).

Selection of the ATG nearest the 5′ end of the open reading frame as the site of the initial methionine predicts that a 21-residue prepropeptide precedes the recognized N-terminus of the mature, active enzyme. The first 19 residues of preprohuman heart chymase are hydrophobic and likely represent a signal peptide. This hydrophobic presequence is similar in size to signal peptides predicted for other mammalian chymases and neutrophil chymotrypsinlike proteinases.[14] It has been proposed that sequence Ala-Xaa-Ala predicts the signal peptidase cleavage site.[22] Since this sequence occurs at the end of the proposed signal peptide in human heart chymase, the human heart chymase signal peptide is likely cleaved at the Ala^{-3}-Gly^{-2} bond. The prosequences of leukocyte chymotrypsinlike proteinases are a pair of acidic residues, usually Glu-Glu.[18,19,23,24] However, human heart chymase[14] and human neutrophil cathepsin G^{25} contain a Gly-Glu sequence at this position. The similarity of the prosequences in these human leukocyte enzymes suggests a common enzymatic activation step.

The calculated mass of the mature human heart chymase is 25,000 daltons.[14] The difference between this calculated mass and the M_r of the purified enzyme[13] ($\approx$30,000) may be due to glycosylation. Human heart chymase contains two consensus N-linked glycosylation sites at Asn^{59} and Asn^{82}. The asparagine at position 59 is likely glycosylated since a blank cycle was obtained in sequencing the tryptic peptide containing this residue (Fig. 4).[14] The further observation that purified human heart chymase binds to concanavalin A-Sepharose and wheat germ agglutinin-Sepharose supports the possibility that human heart chymase is a glycoprotein.[13] The location of these N-linked glycosylation sites is different from those in dog chymase.[24] Only a single consensus N-linked glycosylation site occurs at Asn^{82} in mouse MCP I,[26] whereas rat MCP I[27] and II[18] contain no glycosylation sites.

Human Chymase: Evolutionary Relation to Other Serine Proteinases

Because of the diversity of functions, species origin, and tissue specificity of the trypsin superfamily of enzymes, the precise time-ordered evolutionary tree of human chymase is difficult to derive. However, on the basis of the multiple sequence alignment, we have derived a partial family tree of serine proteinases most closely related to human chymase. A total of 53 enzymes from the trypsin, chymotrypsin, elastase, kallikrein, granzyme, and chymase families were included in the alignment. The resulting family tree, depicted in Figure 5, shows that human chymase belongs to the chymase family of enzymes, which includes mouse, rat, and dog chymases. Structurally, the chymase family is closely related to the granzyme family, and to a lesser extent to the kallikrein family, but is quite

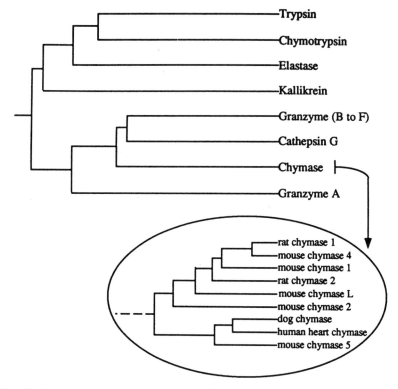

Fig. 5. Evolutionary relation of several mammalian serine proteinases as determined by multiple sequence alignment.

distinct from chymotrypsin and trypsin, the two serine proteinases of the exocrine pancreas. Functionally, chymases show a substrate specificity somewhat similar to that of chymotrypsin, whereas kallikreins and human granzyme A are trypsinlike, and human granzyme B hydrolyzes proteins at Asp-Xaa bonds.[28]

Substrate Specificity of Human Heart Chymase

Human heart chymase rapidly converts A I to A II, and the A I-carboxy-terminal dipeptide His-Leu ($K_m = 60$ μM; $k_{cat} = 160$ sec^{-1});[13,29] A II, however, is not degraded, even after prolonged incubations with human heart chymase.[13] In comparison with other

Table 2
Kinetic Constants for the Conversion of A I to A II
by A II-Forming Enzymes

Species	Enzyme	K_m (μM)	k_{cat} (s^{-1})	k_{cat}/K_m ($\mu M^{-1}s^{-1}$)
Human	heart chymase	60	160	2.7
Rat	tonin	34	39	1.2
Human	ACE	60	8.3	0.14
Human	cathepsin G	290	0.6	0.002

A II-forming enzymes, the hydrolysis of the Phe^8-His^9 bond of A I by human heart chymase has many distinctions. Human heart chymase is an endopeptidase since it converts A I and human tetradecapeptide renin substrate to A II by hydrolyzing the Phe^8-His^9 bond in both these peptides.[13] However, unlike tonin,[30] cathepsin G,[31] and kallikrein,[32] human heart chymase does not form AII from the human protein substrate angiotensinogen (M_r 65,000). When A I is the substrate, the specificity constant (k_{cat}/K_m) for human heart chymase,[13,29] is higher than that for ACE [33] or tonin[30] and much higher than that for cathepsin G[34] (Table 2). These findings indicate that human heart chymase is a highly efficient A II-forming enzyme.

Many similarities and differences exist among mammalian chymases with respect to peptide substrate specificity. For example, human skin[34] and human heart chymases[13,29] readily hydrolyze the Phe^8-His^9 bond in A I to yield A II, but they cannot hydrolyze the Tyr^4-Ile^5 bond in this prohormone or in A II. However, rat MCP I (rat chymase 1) preferentially hydrolyzes the Tyr^4-Ile^5 bond in A I but does not readily convert the prohormone to A II.[35,36] The differences in substrate specificity of human chymase compared to other A II-forming enzymes are summarized in Table 3.

The process of polypeptide catalysis by serine proteinases may be divided into two steps: (1) selection of the scissile bond and (2) catalysis. The mechanism of catalysis per se is common to all serine proteinases and involves the formation and hydrolysis of an acyl enzyme intermediate in which the active-site serine, histidine, and aspartic acid play critical roles. Serine proteinases, however, share many similarities and differences in the way the scissile bond is selected. Trypsin and chymotrypsin place a very high emphasis on the P_1-positioned amino acid of peptide substrates (which for trypsin

Table 3
Comparison of Polypeptide Substrate Specificities of Human Heart Chymase With Other A II-Forming Enzymes

Peptide Hormone Substrate	Enzyme*						
	Human Heart Chymase	Human Skin Chymase	Dog Mastocytoma Chymase	Rat Chymase I	Human Cathepsin G	Human ACE	Rat Tonin
A I	C	C	—	C	C	C	C
A II	N	N/T	—	C	P	N	N
ACTH (1–24)	T	—	—	C	—	—	—
Bradykinin	N	C	—	N	P	C	—
LHRH	N	—	—	—	—	C	—
[Met⁵]enkephalin	T	—	—	—	—	C	—
α-MSH	N	—	—	—	—	—	—
γ-MSH (3–8)	N	—	—	—	—	—	—
Neuromedin C	N	—	—	—	—	—	—
Substance P	T	—	C	C	—	C	C

Extent of peptide bond hydrolysis: C, complete; P, partial; T, trace; N, none.
Abbreviations: LHRH, luteinizing hormone-releasing hormone; MSH, melanocyte-stimulating hormone.
* For references see Urata et al.[13]
† From Urata, H, et al.[13]

is either arginine or lysine and for chymotrypsin is either tyrosine, tryptophan, or phenylalanine). These serine proteinases place considerably less emphasis on the amino acids surrounding the P_1 residue. The primary specificity pocket (S_1) is a major determinant of specificity in nonprimate chymases, as it is in chymotrypsin. Rat chymases show a high preference for phenylalanine, tyrosine, and tryptophan in the P_1 position, but much less emphasis is placed on the extended substrate-binding site[37] (i.e., interactions other than the P_1/S_1 interaction).

We were surprised to find that human chymase has a greater substrate specificity compared to that of rat chymases. We examined the nature of this restricted human chymase specificity using over 40 peptide analogs of A I.[29] We showed that in addition to a P_1 hydrophobic aromatic amino acid, several unique determinants in a peptide substrate, particularly a dipeptide carboxy-terminal leaving group containing no prolines and a P_2 proline, are critical for the selection of the scissile bond (Figure 6). It is significant that all these determinants are present in A I. Thus, variations in the nature of the extended substrate binding site of chymases can make a difference in their physiological role—prohormone activation (as in humans) versus hormone degradation (as in rats).

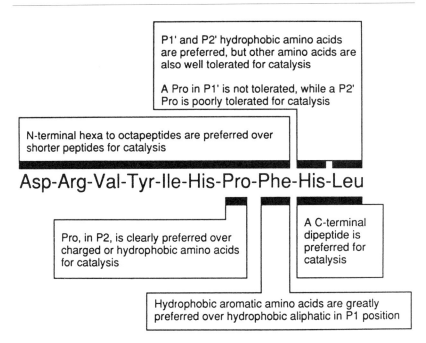

Fig. 6. Summary of determinants of substrate specificity of an A I-converting chymase from the human heart (from Kinoshita A, et al.[29]).

Putative Three-Dimensional Model of Human Chymase

A putative three-dimensional model of human chymase based on the crystal structure of rat MCP II (at 1.9 Å) was constructed.[38] The initial putative tertiary structure of human chymase was obtained by homology modeling, which involves substituting the primary structure of rat MCP II with the human chymase primary structure. About 60% of the residues from human chymase and rat MCP II were identical. Also, it was not necessary to add or delete residues in the rat MCP II structure to model human chymase. This human chymase structure was then energy minimized (5,000 steps) using the program INSIGHT and DISCOVER (Biosym) on a Silicon Graphics workstation. Secondary structure, including the position of β-strands and α-helices as well as water accessibility, was identified using the program DSSP on a Vax 6000–510.[39] Subsequent manipulation of the putative human chymase molecule was performed using the program MIDAS on a Silicon Graphics workstation.[40] The putative three-dimensional model of human chymase is shown in Figure 7 (see color plate, p. A9). This three-dimensional model yields the following tentative conclusions about human chymase. The mature human chymase is comprised of a single 226 residue polypeptide chain. This polypeptide chain is folded into two domains, each of which contains about 110 amino acids. The two domains are both of the antiparallel β-barrel type, each containing six β strands. Two α-helices are present in human chymase, both of which are situated in domain 2: one between β strands two and three of domain 2 and one at the carboxy-terminus of human chymase. Each domain is stabilized, in part, by intradomain disulfides. The domains are linked by a polypeptide hinge. However, no interdomain disulfides are present in human chymase, as they are in trypsinogen and chymotrypsinogen. Domain 1 contributes two of the amino acids of the catalytic triad, His^{45} and Asp^{89}, whereas the active site serine, Ser^{182}, is a part of domain 2. The polypeptide hinge likely contributes to the optimal placement of the active site residues since proteolytic cleavage of the Phe^{114}-Asn^{115} bond in the polypeptide hinge leads to a threefold decrease in catalytic efficiency of human chymase.[13] Docking experiments suggest that the extended substrate binding site lies across the two domains.

To better understand the influence of structure on substrate specificity, we have compared the structure of human heart chymase with that of rat chymases. In contrast to rat MCP I,[36] human heart chymase is a highly specific A II-forming enzyme.[29] Substrate specificity studies indicate that human chymase clearly prefers a dipeptide-leaving group for catalysis, indicating that important differences exist between the S' subsites of various chymases. On the basis of the crystal structure of rat MCP II, Remington et al.[38] have proposed that P_1' to P_3' residues of substrates interact with residues in the loop region formed by residues 35 to 41 (chymotrypsinogen numbering) in chymases. The differences in functional S' subsite preferences between human heart chymase and rat MCP I may not be surprising since residues 35 to 41 (chymotrypsinogen numbering) in rat MCP I are only 30% homologous to those residues in human heart chymase. Of particular interest may be the location of a proline, a rigid kinked amino acid, situated in the middle of the loop region formed by residues 35 to 41 (chymotrypsinogen numbering) between β strand one and two of domain 1 of human heart chymase. Proline is not found in the corresponding loop region of mouse and rat chymases, which could greatly influence the conformation of the S' substrate-binding site region of human heart chymase.

Cellular Localization and Regional Distribution of Chymase in the Heart

EM-immunocytochemical studies using a specific human heart chymase polyclonal antibody indicate the presence of chymaselike immunoreactivity in secretory granules of human cardiac mast cells.[21] Other mammalian chymases studied have also been shown to be stored in an active form in secretory granules of the mast cell.[41] In the human heart, chymaselike immunoreactivity is present in Weibel-Palade bodies of endothelial cells and in cytosolic granules of interstitial mesenchymal cells.[21] These interstitial cells appeared to be actively dividing fibroblasts.

In situ hybridization studies were carried out to clarify whether vesicular chymaselike immunoreactivity in human cardiac cells results from cellular biosynthesis or occurs through protein uptake. Using a highly specific antisense oligonucleotide probe, a chymase mRNA signal was observed in endothelial cells of the intramural venula and in several interstitial cells, including mast cells.[21] These studies are the first to show that human chymase is elaborated in cell types other than the mast cell. This is a unique finding since other known chymases have been described only in mast cells.[41] It is interesting to note that the 5′ and 3′ untranslated regions of the human chymase gene lack important mast-cell specific enhancer sequences found in the mouse and rat chymase genes.[14] Differences in the *cis*-acting elements of the human chymase gene may account for its more widespread cellular distribution than other mammalian chymases.

Using EM-immunocytochemistry, Kaminer et al.[42] have shown that, once chymase in isolated human skin mast cells is released, it attaches to the extracellular matrix. High levels of chymaselike immunoreactivity are localized in the cardiac interstitium and are likely associated with the interstitial extracellular matrix[21] (Figure 8). Human chymase is a highly basic enzyme.[14] Molecular modeling studies on human chymase indicate the presence of several positively charged residues on the surface of this enzyme. It has been suggested that in rat MCP I these positively charged residues play a role in binding to heparin or to other sulfated proteoglycans and glycosaminoglycans found in secretory granules and to the extracellular matrix.[38] The highly basic nature of human chymase is common to all known proteinases found in mast cell granules including tryptase,[43] carboxypeptidase A[44], and cathepsin G.[25] It is also known

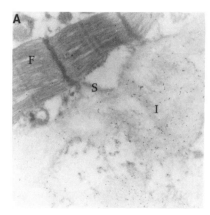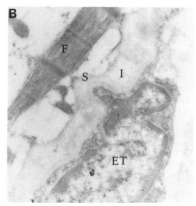

Fig. 8. EM-immunocytochemical localization of inmmunoreactive human chymase in the human cardiac left ventricle. (A) Specific polyclonal antibody to human chymase. (B) Control preimmune serum. Immuno-gold deposits were observed in the interstitial region of the human myocardium but not in myocytes. Abbreviations: F: contractile myofilament; I: interstitial region; S: sarcolemmal membrane; ET: endothelial cell (from Urata H, et al.[21]).

that when these proteinases are bound to heparin or to heparin sulfate, they are relatively resistant to proteolytic degradation and to inactivation by the plasma serine proteinase inhibitor.[45] Chymase in the heart may thus be relatively stable and likely remains active after binding to the extracellular matrix. This latter conclusion is supported by the fact that human chymase is active after binding to heparin immobilized on agarose.[21] Angiotensin II formation occurring from chymase activity associated with the extracellular matrix in the cardiac interstitium may thus be a major site of local A II formation in the human heart.

Evidence for a Functional Chymaselike Angiotensin II–Forming Pathway in Heart Tissue

Extensive studies on the nature of the substrate binding site of human chymase revealed key differences in the way human chymase binds A I prior to catalysis, compared to the interaction between ACE and A I.[29] For example, the N-terminal of A I (i.e., the region constituting the A II primary structure) and the carboxy-terminal His-Leu part of A I are both involved in the binding of A I to human chymase. Only the carboxy-terminal His-Leu part of A I appears to be important in the binding of ACE to A I. On the basis of these important differences, we designed and synthesized the following selective "A II-containing" substrate for human chymase: Asp-Arg-Val-Tyr-Ile-His-Pro-Phe-His-Leu-Pro-DAla, i.e., [Pro^{11},DAla^{12}]A I.

Since a penultimate proline in peptides prevents ACE from cleaving a dipeptide from the carboxy-terminal, [Pro^{11},D Ala^{12}]A I should not be processed by ACE to yield A II. A carboxy-terminal DAla was added to prevent carboxypeptidases from making the penultimate proline into a carboxy-terminal proline. And, as expected,

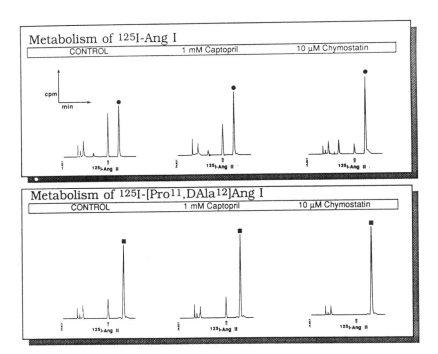

Fig 9. Effects of the ACE inhibitor captopril and the serine proteinase inhibitor chymostatin on the conversion of [^{125}I]A I and [^{125}I]-[Pro^{11},DAla^{12}]A I to [^{125}I]A II by human ventricular membranes. Upper section: [^{125}I]A I conversion to [^{125}I]A II is partially inhibited by captopril as well as by chymostatin. Lower section: [^{125}I]-[Pro^{11},DAla^{12}]A I conversion to [^{125}I]A II is not inhibited by captopril but is completely inhibited by chymostatin. Since human chymase is the major (> 80%) A II-forming serine proteinase in these human cardiac membranes, conversion of [^{125}I]-[Pro^{11},DAla^{12}]A I to [^{125}I]A II appears to be effected by human chymase and not by ACE.

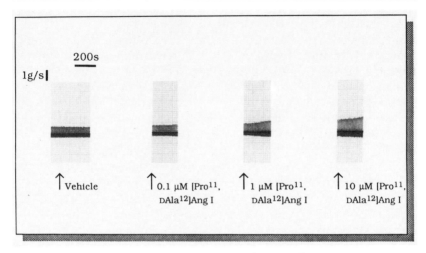

Fig. 10. Positive inotropic responses to [Pro^{11}, DAla^{12}]A I in human atrial trabecular muscle.

ACE did not convert [Pro^{11},DAla^{12}]A I to A II. Since human chymase is an endopeptidase, it should cleave [Pro^{11},DAla^{12}]A I. Pure human chymase converts [Pro^{11},DAla^{12}]A I to A II + His-Leu-Pro-DAla; the k_{cat} for this conversion is 29 sec^{-1}. Comparative k_{cat} for the conversion of A I to A II + His-Leu by human chymase is 160 sec^{-1}. Figure 9 shows differences in specificity between [Pro^{11},DAla^{12}]A I and A I for human chymase. Using human ventricular membranes, the generation of A II from A I is partially inhibited by the ACE inhibitor, captopril, and also by the serine proteinase inhibitor, chymostatin. Conversely, the generation of A II from [Pro^{11},DAla^{12}]A I is not inhibited by captopril and is completely inhibited by chymostatin (Fig. 9). Figure 10 shows positive inotropic responses to [Pro^{11},DAla^{12}]A I in isolated human cardiac trabeculae. Since [Pro^{11},DAla^{12}]A I does not directly interact with the cardiac A II receptor (IC$_{50}$ > 10 µM), these data suggest the presence of a chymaselike A II-forming pathway in the intact human heart tissue other than ACE.

Human Chymase: Clinical Implications

The level of A II in human heart tissue is likely to be regulated by two mechanisms: (1) uptake of circulating A II and (2) local conversion of A I to A II by ACE and potentially by chymase.[46] In blood serum, ACE is the major enzyme that converts A I to A II.[12] By inhibiting ACE, A II formation in the circulation will be markedly reduced. Therefore, the fraction of A II in the heart that is taken up from the circulation also will be reduced. Local A II formation in the heart due to human cardiac ACE will also be decreased during ACE inhibitor therapy.

On the other hand, since chronic ACE inhibitor therapy produces a greater than threefold increase in circulating A I levels,[8] uptake of A I to the heart should be increased. Because chymase levels also are not reduced in cardiac ventricles of patients with idiopathic or ischemic cardiomyopathy[12,21] it is tempting to speculate that chymase-dependent conversion of A I to A II in heart tissue will be increased in patients undergoing ACE inhibitor therapy. We believe that the contribution of ACE and chymase to cardiac A II formation needs to be determined before making conclusions about the role of cardiac A II in congestive heart failure (CHF). Such information may prove valuable in understanding the mechanism of action of ACE inhibitors and A II receptor antagonists in the treatment of hypertension and CHF, particularly if differences in efficacy are apparent.

During chronic ACE inhibitor therapy, levels of circulating A II are only partially decreased. It is conceivable that during chronic ACE inhibitor therapy, A II formed by chymase in the heart, and possibly in other tissues, contributes to blood A II levels. The presence of chymaselike immunoreactivity and activity in the skin, lungs, liver, and coronary arteries would suggest that tissues other than the heart may contribute to levels of circulating A II observed during chronic ACE inhibitor therapy.[21]

As for vascular chymaselike activity, it is interesting to note that A I-mediated contraction of monkey mesenteric and pulmonary arterial strips has been reported to be partially inhibited (by about 55%) by an ACE inhibitor but is completely inhibited by combined ACE inhibitor and chymostatin treatment.[47] Chymostatin, a nonspecific inhibitor of chymotrypsinlike proteinases that inhibit human chymase, could inhibit A I-mediated vascular contraction by inhibiting chymaselike activity in monkey vessels.

Chymase-dependent A II formation may be greater in human cardiac ventricles than in the atria since chymaselike activity is twofold higher in the ventricles than in the atria.[21] ACE activity in the human heart also shows regional variations. Levels of ACE are about threefold higher in the right atrium than in the left ventricle and are twofold higher in the right ventricle than in the left.[12] Under chronic ACE inhibitor therapy, differential changes in cardiac A II concentration may occur. Because of the relative distribution of ACE and chymase in the human heart, atrial A II levels may be reduced more significantly than left-ventricular A II levels during chronic ACE inhibitor therapy. In addition to regional differences in levels of chymase and ACE, differences in the enzymatic properties of chymase and ACE may be important. Chymase and ACE are highly efficient A II-forming enzymes. However, unlike ACE, chymase is more specific and does not cleave bradykinin and substance P.[13] This observation would suggest that chymase-dependent A II formation is not coupled to the simultaneous inactivation of vasodilator peptides as has been shown with ACE—a role perhaps more important in the regulation of myocyte function than in blood pressure regulation.

Summary

We have identified and characterized an A II-forming serine proteinase from the human heart. In human cardiac ventricles, the A II-forming activity of this enzyme is eight times as high as that of the A I-converting enzyme (ACE). This cardiac serine proteinase is the most efficient and specific enzyme described for the conversion of A I to A II. Gene and cDNA cloning studies indicate that this proteinase is a member of the chymase group of enzymes and, based upon structure, should be referred to as human chymase. Southern blot analysis of human genomic DNA indicates that, unlike rodent chymases, human chymase is a single gene product. Northern and Western blot analyses of human heart tissue indicate the existence of chymase mRNA and immunoreactivity in all four cardiac chambers. Lower levels of chymase immunoreactivity are present in the coronary vessels, aorta, and lung. Studies using intact human cardiac trabeculae suggest a functional chymase-mediated conversion of A I to A II. The EM-immunocytochemical studies, which show that a high level of immunoreactive chymase is present in cardiac interstitial spaces between myocytes, also support an A II-forming role for chymase. In the human heart, chymase appears to be stored mainly in cardiac mast cell secretory granules. The identification and characterization of a major A II-forming pathway in the human heart, which is not inhibited by ACE inhibitors, suggests that Ang II formation may continue in heart tissue during chronic ACE inhibitor therapy in patients with CHF.

References

1. Peach MJ. Renin-angiotensin system: biochemistry and mechanisms of action. Physiol Rev 1977; 57:313–370.
2. Soffer RL. Angiotensin-converting enzyme and the regulation of vasoactive peptides. Annu Rev Biochem 1976; 45:73–94.
3. Erdös EG, Skidgel RA. The unusual substrate specificity and the distribution of human angiotensin I converting enzyme. Hypertension 1986; 8(suppl.I):I-34–I-37.
4. Urata H, Healy B, Stewart RW,Bumpus FM,Husain A. Angiotensin II receptors in normal and failing human hearts. J Clin Endocrinol Metab 1989; 69:54–66.
5. Moravec CS, Schluchter MD, Paranandi L, Czerska B, Stewart RW, Rosenkranz E, et al. Inotropic effects of angiotensin II on human cardiac muscle in vitro. Circulation 1990; 82:1973–1984.
6. Waeber B, Gavras I, Brunner HR, Cook CA, Charocopos F, Gravras HP. Prediction of sustained antihypertensive efficacy of chronic captopril therapy: relationships to immediate blood pressure response and control plasma renin activity. Am Heart J 1982; 103:384–390.
7. Cohn JN, Johnson G, Ziesche S, Cobb F, Francis G, Tristani F, et al. A comparison of enalapril with hydralazine-isosorbide dinitrate in the treatment of chronic congestive heart failure. N Engl J Med 1991; 325: 303–310.
8. Nussberger J, Brunner DB, Waeber B, Brunner HR. Specific measurement of angiotensin metabolites and in vivo generated angiotensin II in plasma. Hypertension 1986; 8:476–482.
9. Mento PF, Wilkes BM. Plasma angiotensins and blood pressure during converting enzyme inhibition. Hypertension 1987; 9(suppl. III):III-42–III-48.
10. Campbell DJ. Circulating and tissue angiotensin systems. J Clin Invest 1987; 79:1–6.
11. Smeby RR, Husain A. Angiotensin I and II forming enzymes in the central nervous system. In: Buckley JP, Ferrario CM, eds. Brain Peptides and Catecholamines in Cardiovascular Regulation. New York: Raven Press, 1987: 301–311.
12. Urata H, Healy B, Stewart RW, Bumpus FM, Husain A. Angiotensin II-forming pathways in normal and failing human hearts. Circ Res 1990; 66:883–890.
13. Urata H, Kinoshita A, Misono KS, Bumpus FM, Husain A. Identification of a highly specific chymase as the major angiotensin II-forming enzyme in the human heart. J Biol Chem 1990; 265:22348–22357.
14. Urata H, Kinoshita A, Perez DM, Misono KS, Bumpus FM, Graham RM, et al. Cloning of the gene and cDNA for human heart chymase. J Biol Chem 1991; 266:17173–17179.
15. Caughey GH, Zerweck EH, Vanderslice P. Structure, chromosomal assignment, and deduced amino acid sequence of a human gene for mast cell chymase. J Biol Chem 1991; 266:12956–12963.
16. Hohn PA, Popescu NC, Hanson RD, Salvesen G, Ley TJ. Genomic organization and chromosomal localization of the human cathepsin G gene. J Biol Chem 1989; 264:13412–13419.
17. Takahashi H, Nukiwa T, Basset P, Crystal RG. Myelomonocytic cell

lineage expression of the neutrophil elastase gene. J Biol Chem 1988; 263:2543–2547.

18. Benfey PN, Yin FH, Leder P. Cloning of the mast cell protease, RMCP II: evidence for cell-specific expression and a multi-gene family. J Biol Chem 1987; 262:5377–5384.

19. Meier M, Kwong PC, Fregeau CJ, Atkinson EA, Burrington M, Ehrman N, et al. Cloning of a gene that encodes a new member of the human cytotoxic cell protease family. Biochemistry 1990; 29:4042–4049.

20. Sen R, Baltimore D. Inducibility of κ immunoglobulin enhancer-binding protein NF-κB by a posttranslational mechanism. Cell 1986; 47: 921–928.

21. Urata H, Boehm KD, Phillip A, Kinoshita A, Gabrovsek J, Bumpus FM, et al. Cellular localization and regional distribution of a major angiotensin II-forming chymase in the heart. J Clin Invest 1993; 91: 1269–1281.

22. Carne T, Scheele G. Role of presecretory proteins in the secretory process. In: Cantin M, ed. Cell Biology of the Secretory Process. Basel, Switzerland: S. Karger, 1984: 73–101.

23. Serafin WE, Reynolds DS, Rogelj S, Lane WS, Conder GA, Johnson SS. Identification and molecular cloning of a novel mouse mast cell serine protease. J Biol Chem 1990; 265:423–429.

24. Caughey GH, Raymond WW, Vanderslice P. Dog mast cell chymase: molecular cloning and characterization. Biochemistry 1990; 29: 5166–5171.

25. Salvesen G, Farley D, Shuman J, Przybyla A, Reilly C, Travis J. Molecular cloning of human cathepsin G : structural similarity to mast cell and cytotoxic T lymphocyte proteinases. Biochemistry 1987; 26:2289–2293.

26. Lobe CG, Finlay BB, Paranchych W, Paetkau VH, Bleackley C. Novel serine proteases encoded by two cytotoxic T lymphocyte-specific genes. Science 1986; 232:858–861.

27. Le Trong H, Parmelee DC, Walsh KA, Neurath H, Woodbury RG. Amino acid sequence of rat mast cell protease I (chymase). Biochemistry 1987; 26:6988–6994.

28. Odake S, Kam CM, Narasimhan L, Poe M, Blake JT, Krahenbuhl O, et al. Human and murine cytotoxic T lymphocyte proteases: subsite mapping with peptide thioester substrates and inhibition of enzyme activity and cytolysis by isocoumarins. Biochemistry 1991; 30: 2217–2227.

29. Kinoshita A, Urata H, Bumpus FM, Husain A. Multiple determinants for the high substrate specificity of an angiotensin II-forming chymase from human heart. J Biol Chem 1991; 266:19192–19197.

30. Boucher R, Asselin J, Genest J. A new enzyme leading to the direct formation of angiotensin II. Circ Res 1974; 34 & 35(suppl. I):I-203–I-212.

31. Tonnesen MG, Klempner MS, Austen KF, Wintroub BU. Identification of a human neutrophil angiotensin II-generating protease as cathepsin G. J Clin Invest 1982; 69:25–30.

32. Arakawa K, Maruta H. Ability of kallikrein to generate angiotensin II-like pressor substance and a proposed 'kinin-tensin enzyme system.' Nature 1980; 288:705–706.

33. Erdös EG, Skidgel RA. Structure and functions of human angiotensin I converting enzyme (kininase II). Biochem Soc Trans 1985; 13:42–44.

34. Wintroub BU, Schechter NM, Lazarus GS, Kaempfer CE, Schwartz LB. Angiotensin I conversion by human and rat chymotriptic proteases. J Invest Dermatol 1984; 83:336–339.

35. Reilly CF, Tewksbury DA, Schechter NM, Travis J. Rapid conversion of angiotensin I to angiotensin II by neutrophil and mast cell proteinases. J Biol Chem 1982; 257:8619–8622.

36. Le Trong H, Neurath H, Woodbury RG. Substrate specificity of the chymotrypsin-like protease in secretory granules isolated from rat mast cells. Proc Natl Acad Sci USA 1987; 84:364–367.

37. Powers JC, Tanaka T, Harper JW, Minematsu Y, Barker L, Lincoln D, et al. Mammalian chymotrypsin-like enzymes. Comparative reactivities of rat mast cell proteases, human and dog skin chymases, and human cathepsin G with peptide 4-nitroanilide substrates and with peptide chloromethyl ketone and sulfonyl fluoride inhibitors. Biochemistry 1985; 24:2048–2058.

38. Remington SJ, Woodbury RG, Reynolds RA, Matthews BW, Neurath H. The structure of rat mast cell protease II at 1.9-Å resolution. Biochemistry 1988; 27:8097–8105.

39. Kabsch W, Sander C. Dictionary of protein secondary structure: pattern recognition of hydrogen-bonded and geometrical features. Biopolymers 1983; 22:2577–2637.

40. Ferrin TE, Huang CC, Jarvis LE, Langridge R. The MIDAS display system. J Mol Graphics 1988; 6:13–37.

41. Sayama S, Iozzo RV, Lazarus GS, Schechter NM. Human skin chymotrypsin-like proteinase chymase, subcellular localization to mast cell granules and interaction with heparin and other glycosaminoglycans. J Biol Chem 1987; 262:6808–6815.

42. Kaminer MS, Lavker RM, Walsh LJ, Whitaker D, Zweiman B, Murphy GF. Extracellular localization of human connective tissue mast cell granule contents. J Invest Dermatol 1991; 96:857–863.

43. Schwartz LB, Lewis RA, Austen KF. Tryptase from human pulmonary mast cells: purification and characterization. J Biol Chem 1981; 256: 11939–11943.

44. Goldstein SM, Kaempfer CE, Proud D, Schwartz LB, Irani A, Wintroub BU. Detection and partial characterization of a human mast cell carboxypeptidase. J Immunol 1987; 139:2724–2729.

45. Frommherz KJ, Faller B, Bieth JG. Heparin strongly decreases the rate of inhibition of neutrophil elastase by α_1-proteinase inhibitor. J Biol Chem 1991; 266:15356–15362.

46. Husain A. Formation of angiotensin II in the human heart. ACE Report 1992; 90:1–4.

47. Okunishi H, Miyazaki M, Toda N. Evidence for a putatively new angiotensin II-generating enzyme in the vascular wall. J Hypertens 1984; 2: 277–284.

17

The Cardiac Renin-Angiotensin System and Human Coronary Physiology and Pathology

Karl J. Osterziel and Rainer Dietz

Introduction

In recent years, it has been proved that, in addition to the endocrine renin-angiotensin system (RAS), a local RAS exists in the vessel wall and the heart.[1-3] The discovery of new properties of A II, such as the stimulation of smooth muscle cell hypertrophy and metabolic effects during cardiac ischemia and reperfusion, has stimulated investigations evaluating the importance of the RAS for coronary circulation. Exogenous A II exerts a pronounced vasoconstrictor effect on coronary arteries[4-6] either directly by stimulating A II receptors or indirectly by facilitating noradrenaline release from sympathetic nerve endings.[7] Inhibition of the RAS by captopril increased coronary flow in myocardial ischemia.[8] An increase in coronary flow can also be observed in isolated heart preparations after converting-enzyme inhibition.[9] Moreover, ACE inhibitors may be cardioprotective by reducing myocardial infarct size after coronary ligation in dogs.[10,11]

Angiotensin II may act as a growth factor in the coronary vasculature, leading to hypertrophy of vascular smooth muscle cells (VSMC).[12] The unexpected finding that converting-enzyme inhibi-

Lindpaintner K and Ganten D (editors): *The Cardiac-Renin Angiotensin System,* © Futura Publishing Co., Inc., Armonk, NY, 1994.

tors can attenuate the myointimal hyperplasia after vascular injury has led to the hypothesis that the RAS may be involved in the development of restenosis after coronary balloon angioplasty.[12–15] Further support comes from experiments proving that the RAS is activated in the vessel wall after balloon angioplasty.[16] Dzau et al. have forwarded the hypothesis that the mitogenic effect of A II on VSMC is counterbalanced by an intact endothelium.[12] There is a simultaneous activation of the platelet-derived growth factor (PDGF-AA) and the antiproliferative transforming growth factor —β1 (TGF-β1)—in smooth muscle cells.[12] Removal of the endothelium leads to a loss of endothelium-derived vasodilators, which normally counteract the proliferative action of A II. Consequently, vascular smooth muscle growth occurs by a marked increase of PDGF and the release of the basic fibroblast growth factor (bFGF) from damaged endothelial cells and neointima.[12,17]

On the basis of these experimental data, clinical studies were performed to examine whether inhibition of the RAS may lead to less ischemia, an improvement of exercise tolerance, and a lower rate of restenosis following coronary angioplasty.

Coronary Artery Disease and the Renin–Angiotensin System

An antianginal effect of ACE inhibitors in coronary artery disease could occur through the beneficial systemic effects of an A II blockade, resulting in a decrease of myocardial oxygen demand.[18] The two main determinants of myocardial oxygen consumption, namely, heart rate and systolic blood pressure, remain either unchanged or are reduced by a blockade of the RAS. This may result in a lower oxygen demand at the same level of exercise. At the same time, diastolic blood pressure, the main driving force of coronary flow, remains unchanged or decreases. In addition to the systemic effects of ACE inhibitors, local actions on coronary vessels have to be taken into account in order to examine the antianginal effect of ACE inhibitors.

Acute ACE Inhibition

The circulating RAS is activated in patients with angina pectoris.[19,20] Because coronary blood flow is impaired with activation of the renin system, it should be possible to increase coronary blood flow by ACE inhibitors.[21] Coronary vasodilation by ACE inhibition could occur by blocking A II formation or through a decrease of bradykinin degradation. The local increase of bradykinin leads to an increase of endothelium-derived vasodilating prostaglandins, mainly PGE_2 and PGI_2.[22] Consequently, several studies were performed in patients with coronary artery disease.[19,23-25] In coronary artery disease, however, an altered reaction of the endothelium may also be important when the effects of ACE inhibitors are examined. Even in the absence of hemodynamically significant epicardial stenosis, atherosclerotic coronary arteries show a functionally abnormal endothelium.[26] There was an impaired vasodilator response of the coronary microvasculature after acetylcholine, indicating an impairment of endothelial-dependent vasodilation.[26] Because of a combination of systemic and local effects, it is difficult in clinical studies to separate the effects of the RAS on coronary vessels from systemic effects.[24] But it is likely that acute effects of ACE inhibitors mainly depend on the blockade of circulating renin and not on local renin systems.

First, studies are evaluated in normotensive patients where acute therapy with ACE inhibitors did not decrease blood pressure or heart rate significantly. In patients with stable angina, a significant decrease of maximal ST-segment deviation indicating less ischemia could be observed with different ACE inhibitors.[27-29] This beneficial effect was observed in the majority of patients from the studies mentioned above. However, Rietbrock et al. could not show a significant improvement of exercise-induced ischemia after a single dose of enalapril.[30] When myocardial oxygen demand was increased by atrial pacing, captopril did not reduce myocardial oxygen demand compared to a placebo, and coronary flow did not increase significantly.[28] In patients who showed a decrease of arterial pressure after a single dose of ACE inhibitors, Bussmann et al. observed in 10 out of 14 patients a 30% decrease of ST-segment depression in an open study, whereas Hauf et al. could not demonstrate a significant improvement by ACE inhibition in comparison to a placebo.[31,32]

Several studies even reported an aggravation of angina after ACE inhibition.[33,34] Most likely, this represents an effect of vasodilation in nonstenotic areas, leading to a coronary steal effect in coronary arteries with critical stenosis.

Chronic ACE Inhibition

The effect of chronic treatment with ACE inhibitors on exercise-induced ischemia was investigated in four placebo-controlled studies.[23,25,30,35] Rietbrock found a significant reduction of exercise-induced ischemia not earlier than after 2 weeks of treatment with enalapril.[30]. Gibbs et al. and Thürmann et al. did not find a significant improvement of ST-segment depression during exercise with enalapril or benazepril.[25,35] This was confirmed by another placebo-controlled study comparing the anti-ischemic effects of benazepril with metoprolol.[23] Three weeks of therapy with benazepril did not produce an increase in exercise tolerance, ST-segment changes, blood pressure, and heart rate.[23] In this study, 97% of all ischemic episodes were silent. An unexpected result that seems to be very important is that benazepril reduced the total espisodes of ST-segment depression from 1,549 min/24h to 879 min/24h.[23] It may be hypothesized that coronary vasoconstriction is reduced by ameliorating periods of neurohumoral activation and/or the local effects of low angiotensin and high vasodilatory prostaglandin concentration at the stenotic area. This may finally reduce the incidence and severity of silent ischemia. However, further investigations are necessary to evaluate this potential new effect of ACE inhibitors.

In summary, acute or chronic ACE inhibition in normotensive patients with stable angina pectoris may ameliorate exercise-induced myocardial ischemia. This effect is likely to resume in the blockade of the ischemia-induced activation of the RAS or in the reflectory increase of sympathetic activity.[19,36] However, angina pectoris may not improve in some patients and may worsen in others, so that it is necessary to clearly define the group of patients who benefit from ACE inhibition. In ischemic heart disease, the fall in diastolic aortic pressure and hence the coronary perfusion pressure may result in the aggravation of ischemia.[37,38] The administration of ACE inhibitors may be difficult when several high-grade stenoses of coronary arteries are present. It cannot be excluded at the moment that ACE inhibitors may then lead to a coronary steal phenomenon. This assumption helps in the understanding of why patients with coronary heart disease do not always benefit from ACE inhibition but eventually may even complain about the worsening of angina.[30,33,36–38]

Coronary Blood Flow in Hypertension

In hypertensive patients with angina pectoris, ACE inhibitors may alleviate myocardial ischemia.[36,39] Coronary reserve is diminished, even in the absence of epicardial atherosclerotic lesions.[40]

ACE inhibitors are known to lead to a significant regression of left-ventricular hypertrophy and media hypertrophy of the vascular wall.[40–44] This should lead to less myocardial ischemia in hypertensives treated with ACE inhibitors. In hypertensive patients with a chronically activated circulating RAS, the oral application of 2.5 mg of the ACE inhibitor cilazapril induced an acute sustained increase in coronary blood flow[39] because the decrease of coronary vascular resistance exceeded the decrease of diastolic pressure. However, it was not possible to separate the direct effect of cilazapril on coronary arteries from the indirect decrease of coronary vascular resistance resulting from reduced wall tension.

Coronary Blood Flow in Heart Failure

Coronary blood flow is determined by mechanical, metabolic, and neural factors. The sympathetic nervous system and the RAS are the two major neurohumoral systems modulating coronary vascular resistance and blood flow.[45] ACE inhibitors decrease systemic blood pressure without an increase of heart rate, thereby leading to a lower myocardial oxygen demand.[46] In addition, sympathetic tone is reduced, and reflex increases of sympathetically mediated coronary vasoconstriction are ameliorated.[47] The coronary vascular resistance is reduced by acute ACE inhibition, the magnitude of which depends on the plasma-renin activity.[48] The effect on coronary blood flow is pronounced in patients with heart failure.[33,49] The extravascular and vascular components of coronary resistance are elevated in patients with impaired left-ventricular function. Even when the systemic effects of enalapril are prevented, a selective coronary vasodilation with a decrease of coronary vascular resistance by 18% could be shown.[49] The coronary vasodilation is increased when both components of the increased resistance to coronary flow are reduced by blockade of the RAS. The extraluminal mechanical resistance to flow during diastole is decreased by the reduction of left-ventricular filling pressures. In addition, the increased vasomotor tone due to stimulation of vasoconstrictor forces is reduced,[33] leading to an increase of coronary blood flow by nearly 30%. Usually the discrepancy between the exaggerated energy demand of the failing heart and lowered nutritional flow results in the syndrome of an energy-starving heart in heart failure.[50] This constitutes a negative feedback system since further deterioration of pump function activates those forces that progressively impede the nutritional flow to the heart. Interrupting this negative feedback loop by therapeutic interventions such as the blockade of the RAS, therefore, represents valuable progress in the modern treatment of heart failure. The beneficial effect is obvious from measurements of the arteriovenous difference of lactate release or uptake across the heart in those patients. Following acute ACE inhibition, an improvement in cardiac lactate metabolism, both at rest and during exercise, was observed in 11 of 12 patients with heart failure.[33]

The Renin-Angiotensin System and Coronary Restenosis

Balloon angioplasty has evolved as an alternative treatment for coronary bypass surgery.[51] Despite a high primary success rate of more than 90%, coronary angioplasty is limited by a restenosis rate of about 30%.[51] Research on ways to prevent the development of neointimal proliferation after balloon angioplasty is ongoing. Experimental studies in rats showing that intimal proliferation after vascular injury can be significantly decreased when the RAS was blocked were extremely promising.[13] These experimental results led to a multicenter study (MERCATOR) investigating the effects of ACE inhibition on restenosis after percutaneous transluminal coronary angioplasty (PTCA).[52]

On the basis of the 80% reduction of neointima proliferation in rats after balloon injury by cilazapril, this trial was designed to examine the influences of ACE inhibition on the rate of restenosis after PTCA. In the evening after successful PTCA, 735 patients were randomly assigned to cilazapril (C) or a placebo (P), in addition to standard medical therapy.[52] Five hundred ninety-five patients returned after 6 months for repeat coronary angiography. Changes in minimal coronary lumen diameter were assessed by quantitative angiography immediately after PTCA and again after 6 months. The number of patients who died or had a nonfatal myocardial infarction was evenly distributed between the placebo and cilazapril group. There were also no differences in the requirement for coronary revascularization and in the recurrence rate of angina.

The degree of stenosis, in percentage of diameter, before angioplasty was 61% (P) and 60% (C). PTCA reduced it to 33% in both groups. After 6 months, however, the mean stenosis had increased to 44% in both groups. The cumulative distributions of the severity of stenosis were similar in both groups before and immediately after PTCA and after 6 months. Occurrence of a dissection during PTCA did not influence the long-term results.[53] Consequently, it has to be concluded that, despite convincing data in the rat model, cilazapril does not prevent the myointimal proliferation after coronary balloon angioplasty in humans.

In animal experiments, restenosis could be prevented even when the ACE inhibitor was given within 2 days after wall injury.[13] Therefore, the main question remaining is whether treatment with cilazapril before angioplasty would have yielded different results in the MERCATOR trial.[54] This question could partly be answered by another study on restenosis.[33] The effect of enalapril on restenosis after a repeat PTCA was examined in 24 patients.[33] These patients were at high risk for developing restenosis since they already had had a previous PTCA of the same stenosis.

In a different trial study, 10 mg of enalapril or a placebo were administered 3 days prior to and for 6 months after PTCA. The degree of stenosis before PTCA was similar (89% versus 91%), and the result of the angioplasty was also almost identical in both groups (25% versus 24% stenosis after PTCA). At the time of repeat PTCA, 9 out of 12 patients in the ACE-inhibitor group and 8 out of 12 patients in the placebo group had symptoms of unstable angina. During the stay in the hospital following the angioplasty procedure, none of the patients in either group suffered from angina at rest. All were able to carry out a symptom-limited exercise test. There was no difference in the maximal physical capacity between both groups immediately after PTCA. After a period of 6 months, a high incidence of restenosis was observed in both groups. The luminal narrowing amounted to 72% in the placebo group and 61% in the ACE-inhibitor group, the difference between the groups being not statistically significant. The severity of angina in the control group and in the ACE-inhibitor group was not different during the post-PTCA period. At 6 months following PTCA, maximal symptom-limited physical activity had decreased in both groups compared to the immediate post-PTCA result. Again the difference in exercise capacity between both groups was not statistically significant.

From these data, it has to be concluded that, despite convincing animal experiments, ACE inhibition is not able to prevent or retard restenosis after PTCA in humans.

Summary

The RAS exerts acute as well as chronic effects on the coronary vascular bed. Acute inhibition leads to coronary vasodilation, and chronic inhibition of the renin system reverses coronary artery media hypertrophy and fibrosis. In addition, convincing experimental data show a pronounced inhibition of restenosis after vascular wall injury.

Clinical investigations were based on these findings. They yielded conflicting results in patients with coronary artery disease after acute therapy with inhibitors of ACE. Moreover, some patients experienced an increase of angina pectoris probably due to a coronary steal phenomenon. Chronic ACE inhibition does not improve exercise-induced angina but may ameliorate the severity of silent ischemia.

Because the renin system is likely to be activated in heart failure and hypertension, a blockade by ACE inhibitors may, in addition to other effects, lead to coronary vasodilation and improved nutritional flow and reverse media hypertrophy and fibrosis after chronic treatment. The results of two investigations on the influences of ACE inhibitors on restenosis were disappointing. In both studies there was no significant effect of the blockade of the RAS on the development of restenosis.

References

1. Lindpaintner K, Jin M, Wilhelm MJ, Suzuki F. Intracardiac generation of angiotensin and its physiologic role. Circulation 1988; 77(suppl.I):I-18–I23.
2. Dzau VJ. Circulating versus local renin-angiotensin system in cardiovascular homeostasis. Circulation 1988; 77(suppl. I):I-4–I-13.
3. Naftilan AJ, Ryan TJ, Pratt RE, Dzau VJ. Localization and differential regulation of angiotensinogen mRNA expression in the vessel wall. J Clin Invest 1991; 87:1300–1311.
4. Xiang JZ, Linz W, Becker H, et al. Effects of converting enzyme inhibitors ramipril and enalapril on peptide actions and sympathetic neurotransmission in the isolated heart. Eur J Pharmacol 1984; 113:215–223.
5. Heeg E, Meng K. Die wirkung des bradykinins, angiotensins und vasopressins auf vorhof, papillarmuskel und isoliert durchströmte herzpräparate des meerschweinschens. Naunyn-Schmiedeberg's Arch Pathol 1965; 250:35–40.
6. Tian R, Neubauer S, Pulzer F, Haas U, Ertl G. Angiotensin I conversion and coronary constriction by angiotensin II in ischemic and hypoxic isolated rat hearts. Eur J Pharmacol 1991; 203:71–77.
7. Xiang JZ, Schölkens BA, Han Y. Effects of sympathetic nerve stimulation are attenuated by the converting enzyme inhibitor HOE 498 in isolated rabbit hearts. Clin Exp Hypertens 1993; 6:1853–1859.
8. Ertl G, Alexander RW, Kloner RA. Interaction between coronary occlusion and the renin-angiotensin system in the dog. Basic Res Cardiol 1983; 78:515–518.
9. Linz W, Schölkens BA, Yi-Fan Han. Beneficial effects of the converting enzyme inhibitor ramipril in ischemia hearts. J Hypertens 1986; 8(suppl.10):S91–S99.

10. Re RN, Vizards DL, Brown J, Bryan SE. Angiotensin II receptors in chromatin fragments generated by micrococcal nuclease. Biochem Biophys Res Commun 1984; 119:220–226.
11. Westlin W, Mullane K. Does captopril attenuate reperfusion-induced myocardial dysfunction by scavenging free radicals? Circulation 1988; 77(suppl.I):I-30–I-39.
12. Dzau VJ, Gibbons GH, Pratt RE. Molecular mechanisms of vascular renin-angiotensin system in myointimal hyperplasia. Hypertension 1991; 18(suppl.II):II-100–II-105.
13. Powell JS, Clozel JP, Müller RKM, et al. Inhibitors of angiotensin-converting enzyme prevent myoinitimal injury after vascular injury. Science 1989; 245:186–188.
14. Ross R. The pathogenesis of atherosclerosis: an update. N Engl J Med 1986; 314:448–450.
15. Daemen MJAP, Lombardi DM, Bosma FT, Schwartz SM. Angiotensin II induces smooth muscle cell proliferation in the normal and injured rat arterial wall. Circ Res 1991; 68:450–456.
16. Rakugi H, Jakob HJ, Ingelfinger JR, Krieger JE, Dzau VJ. Angiotensinogen gene expression in the myointima after vascular injury. Hypertension 1990; 16:345 (abstract).
17. Reidy M, Fingerle J, Lindner V. Factors controlling the development of arterial lesions after injury. Circulation 1992; 86:III-43–III-46.
18. Ertl G. Angiotensin converting enzyme inhibitors and ischemic heart disease. Eur Heart J 1988; 9:716–727.
19. Remme WJ, Leeuw PW, Bootsma M, Look MP, Kruijssen D. Systemic neurohumoral activation and vasoconstriction during pacing-induced acute myocardial ischemia in patients with stable angina pectoris. Am J Cardiol 1991; 68:181–186.
20. Dargie HJ, McAlpine HM, Morton JJ. Neuroendocrine activation in acute myocardial infarction. J Cardiovasc Pharmacol 1987; 9 (suppl.2): 21–24.
21. Faxon DP, Craeger MA, Halperin JL, Sussman HA, Bavras H, Ryan TJ. The effect of angiotensin converting enzyme inhibition on coronary blood flow and hemodynamics in patients without coronary artery disease. Int J Cardiol 1982; 2:251–262.
22. Schrör K. Role of prostaglandins in the cardiovascular effects of bradykinin and angiotensin-converting enzyme inhibitors. J Cardiovasc Pharmacol 1992; 20:S68–S73.
23. Klein WW, Khurumi NS, Eber B, Dusleag J. Effects of benazepril and metoprolol OROS alone and in combination on myocardial ischemia in patients with chronic stable angina. J Am Coll Cardiol 1990; 16: 948–956.
24. Thürmann P, Rietbrock N. Current concepts: converting enzyme inhibitors in coronary artery disease. Clin Invest Med 1992; 70:70–76.
25. Thürmann P, Odenthal H-J, Rietbrock N. Converting enzyme inhibition in coronary artery disease: a randomized, placebo-controlled trial with benazepril. J Cardiovasc Pharmacol 1991; 17:718–723.
26. Zeiher AM, Drexler H, Wollschläger H, Just H. Endothelial dysfunction of the coronary microvasculature is associated with impaired coronary blood flow regulation in patients with early atherosclerosis. Circulation 1991; 84:1984–1992.

27. Strozzi C, Cocco G, Portaluppi F, et al. Effects of captopril on the physical work capacity of normotensive patients with stable-effort angina pectoris. Cardiology 1987; 74:226–228.
28. Ikram H, Low CJS, Shirlaw T, Webb CM, Richards AM, Crozier IG. Antianginal, hemodynamic and coronary vascular effects of captopril in stable angina pectoris. Am J Cardiol 1990; 66:164–167.
29. Gasic S, Dudczak R, Korn A, Kleinblösem C. ACE inhibition with cilazapril improves myocardial perfusion to the ischemic regions during exercise. J Cardiovasc Pharmacol 1990; 15:227–232.
30. Rietbrock N, Thürmann P, Kirsten R. Antiischemic effect of enalapril in coronary heart disease: a randomized, placebo-controlled double blind trial on 12 patients. Dtsch Med Wochenschr 1988; 113:300–302.
31. Hauf GF, Buschmann M, Samek L, Roskamm H. Ergibt die ACE inhibition (captopril) einen posaitiven effekt auf deie belastungskoronarinsuffizienz? Z Kardiol 1987; 76(suppl. 2):30.
32. Bussmann WD, Goerke S, Schneider W, Kaltenbach M. Angiotensin-converting-enzym-hemmer bei angian pectoris. Dtsch Med Wochenschr 1988; 14:548–550.
33. Dietz R, Waas W, Süsselbeck T, Willenbrock R, Osterziel KJ. Improvement of cardiac function by angiotensin converting enzyme inhibition: site of action. Circulation 1993; 87(suppl.IV):108–116.
34. Marley E, Pare CMB. Cardiac failure with reserpine. Br Med J 1956; 1:267–269.
35. Gibbs JSR, Crean PA, Wright C, Mockus L, Sutton GC, Fox KM. The variable effects of angiotensin converting enzyme inhibition on myocardial ischemia in chronic stable angina. Br Heart J 1989; 62:112–117.
36. Daly P, Mettauer B, Rouleau JL. Lack of reflex increase in myocardial sympathetic tone after captopril: potential antianginal effect. Circulation 1985; 71:317–325.
37. Gibbs JSR, Crean PA, Mockens L. The variable effects of angiotensin converting enzyme inhibition on myocardial ischemia in chronic stable angina. Br Heart J 1989; 62:112–117.
38. Tardien A, Viret P, Vandroux JC. Effects of captopril on myocardial perfusion in patients with coronary insufficiency: evaluation by the exercise test and quantitative myocardial tonoscintigraphy using thallium-20. Postgrad Med J 1986; 62 (suppl.1):38–41.
39. Magrini F, Reggiani P, Fratianni G, Morganti A, Zanchetti A. Acute effects of cilazapril on coronary hemodynamics in patients with renovascular hypertension. J Cardiovasc Pharmacol 1992; 19 (suppl.5): S128–S133.
40. Strauer BE. Ventricular function and coronary hemodynamics in hypertensive heart disease. Am J Cardiol 1979; 44:999–1006.
41. Grandi AM, Venco A, Barzizza F, Casadei B, Marchesi E, Finardi G. Effect of enalapril on left ventricular mass and performance in essential hypertension. Am J Cardiol 1989; 63:1093–1097.
42. Schwartzkopf B, Motz W, Knauer S, Frenzel H, Strauer BE. Morphometric investigation of intramyocardial arterioles in right septal endomyocardial biopsy of patients with arterial hypertension and left ventricular hypertrophy. J Cardiovasc Pharmacol 1993; 20:S12–S17.
43. Isoyama S, Ito N, Satoh K, Takishima T. Collagen deposition and the reversal of coronary flow reserve in cardiac hypertrophy. Circulation 1992; 20:491–500.

44. Tan L-B, Brilla Ch, Weber KT. Prevention of structural changes in the heart in hypertension by angiotensin converting enzyme inhibition. J Hypertens 1992; 10(suppl 1):S31–S34.
45. Braunwald E, Sobel BE. Coronary blood flow and myocardial ischemia. In: Braunwald E, ed. Heart Disease, 4th ed. Philadelphia: W.B. Saunders Company, 1992: 1161–1199.
46. Vidt DG, Bravo EL, Fouad FM. Captopril. N Engl J Med 1982; 306: 214–219.
47. Mancia G, Giannattasio C, Grassi G, Morganti A, Zanchetti A. Reflex control of circulation and angiotensin converting enzyme inhibition in man. J Hypertens 1988; 6(suppl. 3):S45–S49.
48. Magrini F, Masayoski S, Roberts N, Fouad FM, Tarazi RC, Zanchetti A. Converting enzyme inhibition and coronary blood flow. Circulation 1987; 75:I-168–I-174.
49. Foult JM, Tavolaro O, Antony I, Nitenberg A. Direct myocardial and coronary effects of enalaprilat in patients with dilated cardiomyopathy: assessment by a bilateral intracoronary infusion technique. Circulation 1988; 77:337–344.
50. Katz AM. Cardiomyopathy of overload: a major determinant of prognosis in congestive heart failure. N Engl J Med 1990; 322:100–110.
51. Baim DS. Interventional catheterization techniques: percutaneous transluminal balloon angioplasty, valvuloplasty, and related procedures. In: Braunwald E, ed. Heart Disease, 4th ed. Philadelphia: W. B. Saunders Company, 1992: 1365–1381.
52. MERCATOR Study Group. Does the new angiotensin converting enzyme inhibitor cilazapril prevent restenosis after percutaneous transluminal coronary angioplasty? Results of the MERCATOR study: a multicenter, randomized, double-blind placebo-controlled trial. Multicenter European Research Trial with Cilazapril after Angioplasty to Prevent Transluminal Coronary Obstruction and Restenosis (MERCATOR) Study Group [comment]. Circulation 1992; 86:100–110.
53. Hermans WR, Rensing BJ, Foley DP, et al. Therapeutic dissection after successful coronary balloon angioplasty: no influence on restenosis or on clinical outcome in 693 patients. The MERCATOR Study Group. J Am Coll Cardiol 1992; 20:767–780.
54. Smalling RW. Redoubtable restenosis. Circulation 1992; 86:325–327.

18

Ventricular Remodeling Following Myocardial Infarction: Experimental and Clinical Benefits of ACE Inhibition

Marc A. Pfeffer and Gervasio A. Lamas

Introduction

The development of angiotensin-converting-enzyme (ACE) inhibitor therapy was motivated by the concept that blocking the conversion of A I to the active vasoconstrictor A II would be a useful means for reducing arterial blood pressure. In the 15 years since ACE inhibitors first became available, clinical experience has confirmed their value not only in the treatment of systemic hypertension but also as a cornerstone in the management of symptomatic heart failure.[1] More recently, the clinical utility of ACE inhibitors has broadened to include the treatment of patients during the acute and chronic phases following a myocardial infarction. Experimental evidence demonstrating that a myocardial infarction can initiate a progressive process of global left-ventricular enlargement formed the basis for this new application of ACE inhibitors.[2,3]

Ventricular Remodeling

The enlargement process known as postinfarction ventricular remodeling encompasses both an early phase of infarct expansion

Lindpaintner K and Ganten D (editors): *The Cardiac-Renin Angiotensin System,* © Futura Publishing Co., Inc., Armonk, NY, 1994.

as well as the more insidious hypertrophic responses of the noninfarcted region; together these changes lead to an enlarged and dis-
torted left-ventricular cavity.[4] Hypothesizing that these structural
and geometric changes were, in large part, physiological responses
to abnormal loading conditions, Pfeffer et al.[5] administered ACE
inhibitor therapy to determine whether chronic therapy would favorably influence this enlargement process. Through a series of animal
experiments, Pfeffer et al. demonstrated that long-term therapy
with ACE inhibitors would indeed attenuate this process of global
ventricular enlargement (Figure 1). These investigators found that
rats with experimental myocardial infarction that were chronically
treated with an ACE inhibitor had better-preserved pump function,
smaller ventricular cavities, lower operating pressures and volumes
and, importantly, prolonged survival compared with animals that
had the same degree of histologic damage but did not receive an
ACE inhibitor.[5,6]

The observations made in animal studies provided a rationale

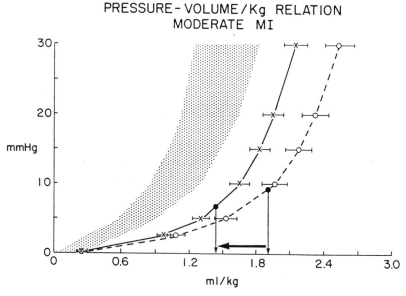

Fig. 1. Left-ventricular passive pressure-volume relation in rats with
chronic infarction. ACE inhibitor therapy (X) demonstrated an attenuation
in the progressive enlargement observed in the placebo-treated (O) group.
The operating volume of the ACE inhibitor (captopril)-treated group was
lower because of both reduced structural changes and distending pressure
(from Pfeffer JM, et al.[5]).

for evaluating the effects of ACE inhibitor therapy in patients experiencing a myocardial infarction.[7-10] The objectives of initial clinical studies were to determine whether ACE inhibitor therapy would favorably influence the process of left-ventricular remodeling that follows infarction. The patients selected were recent survivors of a first anterior Q-wave infarct. Selection criteria included an ejection fraction of ≤ 45% and the absence of overt heart failure. All patients underwent baseline cardiac catheterization (including biplane left ventriculography) at 2 to 4 weeks after the infarct. They were then ramdomly assigned to receive either placebo or captopril therapy in addition to therapy that is conventional during the postinfarction period. Biplane left ventriculography was repeated at 1 year and

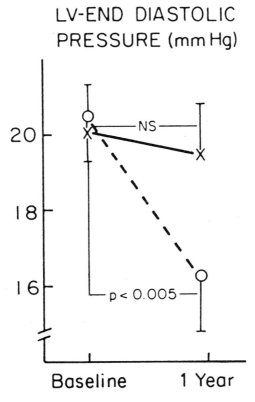

Fig. 2. Left-ventricular end-diastolic pressure in survivors of anterior infarcts at baseline (3 weeks following the acute event) and 1 year thereafter. The open circle represents those randomized to receive captopril therapy. These patients experienced a reduction in filling pressure that was not observed in the conventionally treated group (from Pfeffer MA, et al.[7]).

demonstrated that placebo-treated patients did indeed show further increases in left-ventricular volume over and above their abnormal baseline values.[7] Using each patient as his or her own control, this sensitive evaluation did not detect any enlargement beyond the baseline level in the ACE inhibitor-treated group (Figure 2). Another result in keeping with results from animal studies was the reduced left-ventricular filling pressure observed with active therapy (Figure 3).

In an echocardiography-based study of inferior as well as anterior infarct patients with left-ventricular dysfunction, Sharpe et al.[8] demonstrated ventricular enlargement not only in a placebo-treated

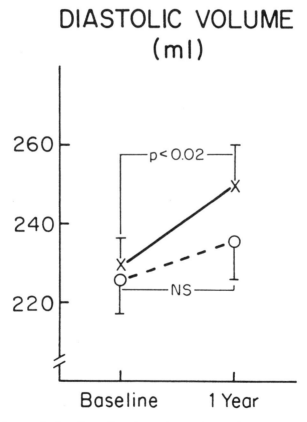

Fig. 3. Left-ventricular diastolic volume in survivors of anterior myocardial infarction. Patients treated with conventional therapy showed an increase in volume over and above their abnormal baseline. In contrast, a significant difference with the paired T test was not observed in the ACE-inhibitor treated group (from Pfeffer MA, et al.[7]).

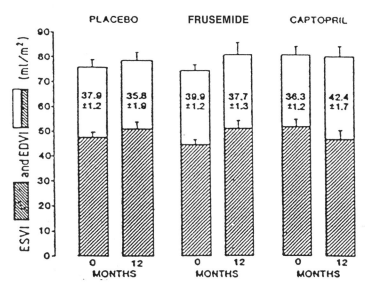

Fig. 4. Quantitative echocardiographic determinations of left-ventricular volumes at baseline and at 1 year, following infarction in patients with LV dysfunction randomized to either placebo, furosemide, or captopril therapy. A time-dependent increase in end-systolic and end-diastolic volumes was observed in the placebo and furosemide groups but not in those groups randomized to captopril therapy (from Sharpe N, et al.[8]).

group but also in a group given furosemide therapy. This randomized trial showed that patients who received captopril therapy did not demonstrate this increase and, at the end of 1 year, had reduced left-ventricular size as compared with placebo- and furosemide-treated patients (Figure 4). More recently, another serial study of survivors of anterior Q-wave infarctions indicated that digoxin therapy was ineffective in preventing progressive enlargement whereas, in contrast, captopril did prevent continued enlargement of the left ventricle.[9] These results provided another independent demonstration of the efficacy of ACE inhibitor therapy.

Acknowledging that the enlargement process (i.e., infarct expansion plus the initiation of global expansion) commences soon (within hours) after myocardial infarction, several groups of investigators have evaluated the safety and effectiveness of early ACE inhibitor therapy in influencing this acute process of ventricular enlargement. Nabel et al.[10] compared the combination of thrombolytic therapy and either a placebo or captopril in changing the ventricular volume during the first week after acute myocardial infarction. The group given thrombolytic therapy plus a placebo had a significant increase in left-ventricular volume that was not seen in the group treated with thrombolytic therapy plus captopril. Oldroyd et al.[11] studied the regional changes in left-ventricular enlargement during the early phase of infarction and demonstrated that administration of captopril within the first 24 hours after a myocardial infarction was associated with less expansion of the infarcted segment than was seen with conventional therapy.

A cautionary note concerning intravenous administration of ACE inhibitors to patients with acute myocardial infarction was raised by Kingma et al.[12] when they reported the occurrence of clinically important hypotension in patients given captopril intravenously shortly after thrombolytic therapy with streptokinase. Similarly, the Data and Safety Monitoring Board of the Cooperative New Scandinavian Enalapril Survival Study II (CONSENSUS II) trial adjusted protocol to reduce the intravenous dose of enalapril and increased the entry blood pressure criterion early in the course of that study when it noted worrisome hypotension.[13] In contrast, oral therapy was found to be safe in the ISIS IV pilot study[14] and in a follow-up study by Sharpe et al.,[15] who administered the ACE inhibitor orally on the first day.

Clinical Outcome Trials

It must be noted that all of the above studies were designed to address the safety and potential efficacy of ACE inhibitor therapy in influencing the process of ventricular enlargement following myocardial infarction. These studies were not designed with sufficient power to address the clinical outcomes. However, the experimental and clinical studies both provided the impetus for an intense international investigative effort to define the role of ACE inhibitors in the management of patients with acute myocardial infarction (Figure 5).

Many of these studies are still in progress. By their design features, these studies may be divided into two groups: those that administer the ACE inhibitor during the acute phase after infarction (within 36 hours) and those that wait to give the initial dose of the ACE inhibitor after clinical stability is achieved (2 to 16 days). Another important distinguishing characteristic of the various trials is whether therapy is administered to the broad population of patients with acute myocardial infarction or whether patients are se-

Chronology: ACE Inhibition, Acute MI, Clinical Endpoint Trials

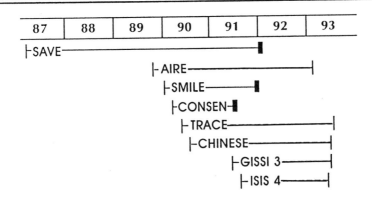

Fig. 5. SAVE, Survival and Ventricular Enlargement; AIRE, Acute Infarction Ramipril Efficacy; SMILE, Survival of Myocardial Infarction Long-term Evaluation; CONSEN, Cooperative New Scandinavian Enalapril Survival Study; TRACE, Study of Trandolapril in patients with reduced left ventricular function after myocardial infarction; CHINESE Chinese Cardiology Society; GISSI 3, Gruppo Italiano per lo Studio della Streptochinasi nell'Infarcto Miocardico III; ISIS 4, Fourth International Study Group of Infarct Survival.

lected on the basis of some measurable assessment of the extent of left-ventricular dysfunction (Table 1).

Results of the Survival And Ventricular Enlargement (SAVE) study[16] provided encouraging information and led the U.S. Food and Drug Administration to issue a new indication for the use of ACE inhibition in survivors of myocardial infarction who have left-ventricular dysfunction. In the SAVE study, patients with left-ventricular dysfunction demonstrated by radionuclide ventriculography (ejection fraction ≤ 40%) were randomly assigned to commence captopril or placebo therapy 3 to 16 days following infarction. The long-term follow-up showed a clear benefit for the group of patients randomized to receive the ACE inhibitor. The 19% reduction in all-cause mortality among patients given an ACE inhibitor as compared with the placebo-treated group was attributable to a lower rate of cardiovascular mortality among the former (Figure 6).[16] This survival benefit was firmly supported by a reduction in the number of patients whose status deteriorated and who developed overt heart failure, as well as by the number of patients who experienced a recurrent myocardial infarction (Figure 7).

Table 1
ACE Inhibition Following MI: Clinic Endpoints

	n	ACE	Patients	Initiation	Follow-up
SAVE	2,231	Cap	EF ≤ 40	3–16 d	3.5 yrs
AIRE	2,000	Ram	CHF	3–10 d	1 yr
TRACE	1,500	Trandol	↓ WMI	1–5 d	1 yr
SMILE	1,500	Zofen	Ant	<24 hrs	1 yr
Chinese Card.	10,000	Cap	All	<36 hrs	5 wk
CONSENSUS II	9,000	Enal	All	<24 hrs	6 mo
ISIS IV	40,000	Cap	All	<24 hrs	5 wk
GISSI III	20,000	Lisin	All	<24 hrs	6 wk

Abbreviations: CONSENSUS II: Cooperative New Scandinavian Enalapril Survival Study II; Cap: Captopril; RAM: Ramipril; Trandol: Trandolapril; Zofen: Zofenopril; Enal: Enalapril; Lisin: Lisinopril; EF: ejection fraction; CHF: congestive heart failure; ↓ WMI: decreased wall motion index—echocardiography; Ant: anterior.

In an important ancillary study,[17] the original hypothesis that ACE inhibitor therapy would attenuate left-ventricular enlargement and improve outcome was directly assessed by echocardiographic measurements. In this large study, it was indeed possible to demonstrate that placebo recipients experienced greater ventricular enlargement and at 1 year had a larger left-ventricular cavity than did the actively treated patients. Moreover, regardless of therapy, patients who experienced an adverse cardiovascular event (i.e., death, development of congestive heart failure (CHF), or recurrent myocardial infarction) had a greater degree of enlargement than those whose course was more benign.[17] Furthermore, although ACE inhibitor therapy effectively reduced the number of patients who demonstrated both enlargement and adverse clinical outcomes, the incidence of ventricular enlargement among ACE inhibitor-treated patients who had an adverse outcome was similar to the incidence among placebo recipients. In other words, poor outcome was associated with enlargement. Thus, these studies supported the investigators' rationale and indicated that a substantial component of the favorable outcome is the reduction in the number of patients who experienced progressive ventricular enlargement.

In the CONSENSUS II study, patients with acute myocardial infarction (within 1 day) were randomized to receive either enalapril (commencing as intravenous enalaprilat) or a placebo; in addition, both groups received conventional therapy.[18] The study was prematurely terminated by the Data Safety Monitoring Committee when

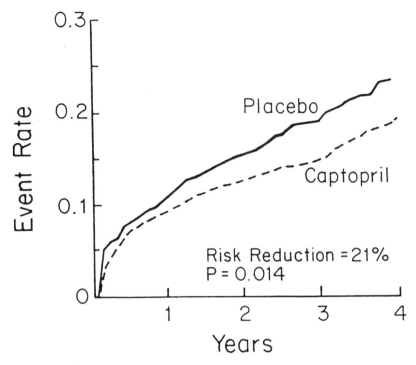

Fig. 6. Cumulative deaths attributed to a cardiovascular etiology in the Survival and Ventricular Enlargement trial (SAVE) (from Pfeffer MA, et al.[16]).

it became apparent that a benefit would not be demonstrated and that there was a trend toward a lower survival rate, especially among elderly patients randomized to active therapy. Although the trial was designed to follow patients for 6 months, the median duration of therapy was only about 4 months.

The preliminary results of the Survival of Myocardial Infarction Long-term Evaluation (SMILE) study were more encouraging regarding the early use of ACE inhibitors in patients with acute myocardial infarction.[19] The SMILE study investigators found that oral administration of the ACE inhibitor zofenopril commencing on the first day and continuing for 6 weeks was associated with a better outcome; the clinical measure used was the combination of death and the development of severe refractory heart failure. It is of interest that this study selected its patients on the basis of having anterior infarction and being viewed as ineligible to receive thrombolytic

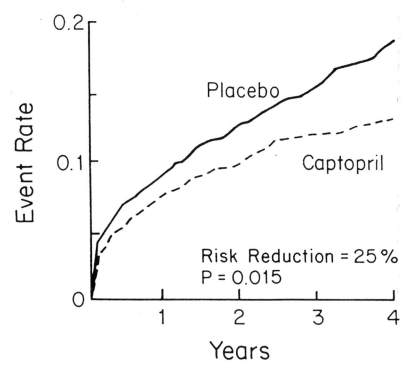

Fig. 7. Recurrent myocardial infarction experience in the Survival and Ventricular Enlargement trial (SAVE) (from Pfeffer MA, et al.[16]).

therapy. In many respects, this is clearly a high-risk group, yet the benefits of ACE inhibitor therapy were apparent in only 6 weeks.

The Fourth International Study of Infarct Survival (ISIS IV), the Gruppo Italiano per lo Studio della Streptochinasi nell'Infarcto Miocardico III (GISSI III) trial, and the Chinese Cooperative Study will undoubtedly provide a great deal of new information regarding the broad use of ACE inhibition during the acute phase of the infarction. The soon-to-be-completed Acute Infarction Ramipril Efficacy (AIRE) study and the Trandolapril in Patients with Reduced Left-Ventricular Function after Myocardial Infarction (TRACE) trial focused their attention on patients selected for dysfunction and will have a longer follow-up period (Table 1). The sum of these intense clinical investigative activities will undoubtedly provide a broad perspective of the overall benefits as well as the risks of ACE inhibition therapy in patients experiencing an acute myocardial infarction. The various studies on the usefulness of ACE inhibition therapy in myocardial infarction have provided a model for experimental and clinical investigative cooperation; the value of this therapy is predicated on a sound fundamental basis that has been borne out first by extensive pilot studies and now by large clinical trials demonstrating efficacy. This new use of ACE inhibitors has not only confirmed the prestudy hypothesis but has led to new mechanistic studies that more fully explain the observed clinical benefits.

Future Directions

It is noteworthy that, in addition to lower rates of death and cardiovascular morbidity, the clinical trials testing the utility of ACE inhibitors for treatment of patients who had a recent myocardial infarction also showed other clinical improvements among ACE inhibitor recipients. These additional indicators of improved status were not directly related to the process of ventricular enlargement. The reduction in rates of recurrent myocardial infarction and the need for invasive revascularization procedures (percutaneous transluminal coronary angioplasty and/or coronary artery bypass surgery) observed in the SAVE study were not related to the left-ventricular ejection fraction as measured at baseline. These observations of a chronic beneficial effect of ACE inhibitors on major coronary events underscore the potential for an even broader application of ACE inhibitors.

Similar observations from the Studies of Left Ventricular Dysfunction (SOLVD), which selected patients with left-ventricular dysfunction who did not necessarily have an acute myocardial infarction, indicated that coronary artery disease was the predominant etiology of the dysfunction. In this large, well-conducted trial, patients randomized to receive the ACE inhibitor enalapril were less likely to experience a myocardial infarction or to be hospitalized for unstable angina during the follow-up period than were patients assigned to placebo therapy[20] (Figure 8). These important anti-ischemic actions of chronic ACE inhibition therapy cannot be fully explained by their documented favorable effects of attenuating ventricular remodeling. The mechanisms by which ACE inhibitors exert a favorable influence on coronary artery disease and its effects remain to be elucidated. The experimental data presented in this volume raise the question whether the inhibition of the local cardiac RAS may play an important role, not shared with other vasodilators, in this process.

Thus, although it was designed as a therapeutic modality to inhibit the conversion of A I to A II, ACE inhibitor therapy is an

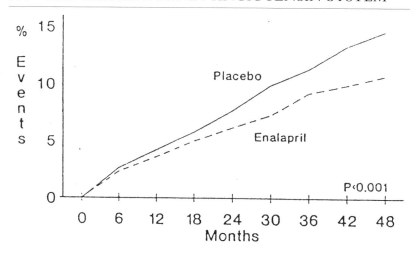

Fig. 8. Development of myocardial infarction in patients with left-ventricular dysfunction from the SOLVD study (from Yusuf S, et al.[20]).

active investigational tool that continues to expand our understanding of the regulation of cardiovascular function and pathophysiology.

Summary

The clinical utility of ACE inhibitors has broadened in recent years from use in systemic hypertension and CHF to provide a new therapy in the management of patients who experience a myocardial infarction. The initial rationale for this new indication stemmed from animal studies that indicated that ACE inhibitor therapy could be used to reduce global systolic and diastolic wall stresses in the infarcted left ventricle and prevent time-dependent deterioration in ventricular function. Clinical studies of quantitative left-ventricular size have supported this concept and indicated that ACE inhibitor therapy can attenuate the progressive ventricular enlargement that may occur following myocardial infarction. Larger trials have now demonstrated that clinical benefits can be achieved with this new use of an ACE inhibitor therapy following myocardial infarction. These benefits include prolonged survival and a reduction in the development of CHF and in the recurrence of further myocardial ischemic events. The diversity of these clinical benefits indicates that mechanisms beyond the original attenuation of ventricular remodeling are operative and points toward an involvement of the local RAS in the complex pathophysiology following myocardial infarction.

References

1. Braunwald E. ACE inhibitors: a cornerstone of the treatment of heart failure. N Engl J Med 1991; 325:351–353.
2. Fletcher PJ, Pfeffer JM, Pfeffer MA, Braunwald E. Left ventricular diastolic pressure-volume relations in rats with healed myocardial infarction: effects on systolic function. Circ Res 1981; 49:618–626.
3. Pfeffer JM, Pfeffer MA, Fletcher PJ, Braunwald E. Progressive ventricular remodeling in rat with myocardial infarction. Am J Physiol 1991; Heart and Circulatory Physiology 29:H1406–H1414.
4. Pfeffer MA, Braunwald E. Ventricular remodeling after myocardial infarction: experimental observations and clinical implications. Circulation 1990; 81:1161–1172.
5. Pfeffer JM, Pfeffer MA, Braunwald E. Influence of chronic captopril therapy on the infarcted left ventricle of the rat. Circ Res 1985; 57:84–95.
6. Pfeffer MA, Pfeffer JM, Steinberg C, Finn P. Survival after an experimental myocardial infarction: beneficial effects of long-term captopril therapy. Circulation 1985; 72:406–412.
7. Pfeffer MA, Lamas GA, Vaughan DE, Parisi AF, Braunwald E. Effect of captopril on progressive ventricular dilatation after anterior myocardial infarction. N Engl J Med 1988; 319:80–86.
8. Sharpe N, Smith H, Murphy J, Hannan S. Treatment of patients with symptomless left ventricular dysfunction after myocardial infarction. Lancet 1988; 1:255–259.
9. Bonaduce D, Petretta M, Arrichiello P, et al. Effects of captopril treatment on left ventricular remodeling and function after anterior myocardial infarction: comparison with digitalis. J Am Coll Cardiol 1992; 19:858–863.
10. Nabel EG, Topol EJ, Galeana A, et al. A randomized placebo-controlled trial of combined early intravenous captopril and recombinant tissue-type plasminogen activator therapy in acute myocardial infarction. J Am Coll Cardiol 1991; 17(2):467–473.
11. Oldroyd KG, Pye MP, Ray SG, et al. Effects of early captopril administration on infarct expansion, left ventricular remodeling and exercise capacity after acute myocardial infarction. Am J Cardiol 1991; 68:713–718.
12. Kingma JH, Louwerenburg JK, van Gilst WH, Six AJ, de Graeff PA, Wesseling H. Concomitant use of captopril during thrombolytic therapy in acute myocardial infarction. In: Sonnenblick EH, Laragh J, Lesch M, eds. New Frontiers in Cardiovascular Therapy: Focus on Angiotensin-Converting Enzyme Inhibition. Princeton, NJ: Excerpta Medica 1989: 277–286.
13. Furberg CD, Campbell RWF, Pitt B. ACE inhibitors after myocardial infarction (letter). N Engl J Med 1993; 328:967–968.
14. ISIS Pilot Study Collaborators' Group. Randomised double-blind trial of oral captopril and of oral nitrates in suspected acute myocardial infarction: safety and practicability. Eur Heart J 1990; 11(abstract suppl).
15. Sharpe N, Smith H, Murphy J, Greaves S, Hart H, Gamble G. Early prevention of left ventricular dysfunction after myocardial infarction

with angiotensin-converting-enzyme inhibition. Lancet 1991; 337: 872–876.

16. Pfeffer MA, Braunwald E, Moyé LA, et al. Effect of captopril on mortality and morbidity in patients with left ventricular dysfunction after myocardial infarction: results of the Survival and Ventricular Enlargement Trial. N Engl J Med 1992; 327:669–677.

17. St. John Sutton M, Pfeffer MA, Plappert T, et al. Quantitative two dimensional echocardiographic measurements are major predictors of adverse cardiovascular events following acute myocardial infarction: the protective effects of captopril. Circulation 1994; 89.

18. Swedberg K, Held P, Kjekshus J, et al. Effects of the early administration of enalapril on mortality in patients with acute myocardial infarction: results of the Cooperative New Scandinavian Enalapril Survival Study II (CONSENSUS II). N Engl J Med 1992; 327:678–684.

19. Ambrosioni E, Borghi C, Boschi S, et al. Early treatment of acute myocardial infarction with ACE inhibition: safety considerations. Am J Cardiol 1991; 68:101D–110D.

20. Yusuf S, Pepine CJ, Garces C, et al. Effect of enalapril on myocardial infarction and unstable angina in patients with low ejection fractions. Lancet 1992; 340:1173–1178.

Index

ACE. *See* Angiotensin-converting enzyme
Adenylate cyclase, angiotensin receptors coupled to, 76, 94
Adrenal adenoma, myocardial fibrosis with, 157
Age
    and angiotensin receptors in heart, 6, 77
    and localization of cardiac renin mRNA, 38–39
    and renin gene expression, 37–38
Aldosteronism, myocardial fibrosis in, 153–162
cAMP, angiotensin II affecting, 114
Angina pectoris, angiotensin-converting enzyme inhibitors in, 220–222, 334–336
Angiotensin I, 1
    activation by cardiac angiotensinogen, 51–55
    concentrations in cardiac areas, 6–7, 48
    and diastolic function in hypertrophied heart, 187, 190
Angiotensin II, 1
    actions on cardiovascular system, 63, 78–79, 102
        cardiac fibroblasts, 108–109
        cardiomyocytes, 103–105
        endothelial cells, 108
        vascular smooth muscle, 106–108
    activation by cardiac angiotensinogen, 51–55
    affecting phosphoinositol metabolism, 76
    and cAMP activity, 114
    and calcium channel activity, 103–104, 113
    cardiac
        concentrations in various areas, 6, 48
        effects in heart failure, 238–239
        localization of receptors for, 5–6, 66–67, 73–75, 184

and ventricular hypertrophy, 239–240
cardiovascular effects of, 289–290
chronotropic effects of, 78, 104, 127–129
and collagen synthesis in rat cardiac fibroblasts, 161
deleterious cardiac effects of, 211
and diastolic function in hypertrophied hearts, 58, 187–188
    in ischemia, 190–193
direct effects of, 1–2
enzymes responsible for formation of, 72
growth effects of, 57–58, 63, 141–148
    on cardiac fibroblasts, 109
    on cardiomyocytes, 105
    on cardiovascular tissue, 143–145
    intracrine action in, 109, 147–148
    on noncardiovascular tissues, 145–149
    role of receptors in, 6
    on vascular smooth muscle, 106–108, 142
    and ventricular hypertrophy, 10–12, 168. *See also* Ventricular hypertrophy
high-affinity binding protein for, 6
increased plasma levels
    after treatment with ACE inhibitors, 169–171
    and myocardial fibrosis, 158–159
indirect effects of, 1
and inositol phosphate activity, 110–111
inotropic effects of, 78, 103–104
and mesangial cell proliferation, 144–145
plasma levels affected by isoproterenol, 171
and prostaglandin production, 114–115
and protein kinase C activity, 111–112

359

receptor subtypes, 102–103, 126. *See also* Receptors for angiotensin II
in cardiac tissue, 74–75, 76, 89–90, 94
and remodeling of ventricles in hypertension, 109
role in cardiovascular pathology, 79–81
  cardiac hypertrophy, 80–81
  congestive heart failure, 80
  ischemic heart disease, 79–80
role in neovascularization, 145
and second messenger regulation, 95
synthesis in heart, 6–8, 71, 202
  chymase affecting, 5, 324–326
  in hypertrophied heart, 189–190
transmembrane signaling by, 109–115
and tyrosine kinase activity, 112–113
and vagus nerve activity, 133–134
vasoconstrictive properties of, 214
Angiotensin-converting enzyme, 1
and activation of angiotensin peptides, 53–54
activity in heart failure, 236–239
activity in pressure-overload cardiac hypertrophy, 185–194
and angiotensin II generation in hypertrophied heart, 189–190
cardiac, 4–5
  characterization of, 69–71
  pathological states affecting, 72–73
  physiological role of, 71–72
  in ventricular hypertrophy, 73, 185–194
and cardiac physiology, 184
concentrations in various areas, 4–5
in coronary vessels, 4–5, 7, 8
distribution in cardiac tissue, 67–69, 91–92
in humans compared to rats, 68–69
inhibitors
  actions in ischemia and reperfusion, 191–193, 206–212
  actions in myocardial infarction affected by bradykinin, 272–274
  affecting bradykinin metabolism, 10, 11
  affecting coronary blood flow, 212–219, 266
  affecting postinfarction ventricular remodeling, 57
  and aggravation of angina, 335, 336
  in angina pectoris, 220–222, 334–336

  cardiac chymase activity affecting, 327–328
  cardiac effects of, 204–206
  in cardiac hypertrophy, 57, 64, 143, 168–171, 221, 236, 274–277
  cardioprotective effects of, 80
  compared to Losartan, 96
  and coronary restenosis after balloon angioplasty, 338–339
  differential pharmacological effects of, 247
  effects in cardiac hypertrophy, 57, 64, 168–171
  effects in isoproterenol-induced cardiac hypertrophy, 174–177
  effects in myocardial ischemia and reperfusion, 267–268
  and endothelial cell function, 255–257
  in heart failure, 11, 246–248, 337–338
  in hypertension, 336–337
  and increased plasma levels of angiotensin II, 169–171
  interaction with organic nitrates, 216
  intravenous, hypotension from, 350
  in myocardial fibrosis, 161
  in myocardial infarction, 219–220
  and postinfarction ventricular remodeling, 57, 80, 220, 345–357
  and regression of cardiac hypertrophy, 168–171
  and release of endothelium-derived relaxing factor, 216
  and renal angiotensinogen levels in heart failure, 241–245
  sulfhydryl-containing, 205, 212, 215, 216, 218
  with thrombolytic therapy, 220, 349–350
localization of receptors in heart, 65–66
Angiotensinogen, 1
cardiac, 47–60
  activation of angiotensin peptides, 51–55
  bimodal pattern of release, 49–51, 64–65
  concentrations in various areas, 3, 48–49
  regulation of expression, 55–59
  mRNA levels, 56–57, 65
  source of, 49–51, 64–65
  human gene expression in transgenic rats, 301–303

intracardiac synthesis of, 3–4, 48–49
in mesangial cells, 144–145
production in spontaneously
hypertensive rats, 143
rat gene expression in transgenic
mice, 300–301
renal levels
in heart failure, 241–245
in myocardial infarction, 240–241
Aorta
angiotensin-converting enzyme in,
67, 71
angiotensin II receptors in, 73
coarctation in rats, ventricular
hypertrophy in, 274–277
Arrhythmias
in ischemia, angiotensin affecting,
240
reperfusion
angiotensin affecting, 211
bradykinin affecting, 265–267
captopril affecting, 208
Atherosclerosis, experimental,
angiotensin-converting enzyme
inhibitors in, 259–262
Atria
angiotensin-converting enzyme in,
68, 71
angiotensin receptors in, 6, 74, 94
renin mRNA in, 27, 38–39
Atrioventricular node. *See* Conduction
system, cardiac
Autonomic nervous system, cardiac,
angiotensin II receptors in, 74,
78–79
Autoradiography in vitro
of angiotensin-converting enzyme
distribution in cardiac tissue,
67–69, 71
of angiotensin II receptors in cardiac
tissue, 73–75

Baroreceptor reflex, angiotensin II
affecting, 131–133
Bartter's syndrome, myocardial fibrosis
in, 157
Blood flow, coronary
angiotensin-converting enzyme
inhibitors affecting, 212–219,
334–338
bradykinin role in, 266
cardiac renin-angiotensin system
affecting, 8–9
Blood pressure
angiotensin affecting, 106
elevated. *See* Hypertension

hypotension from intravenous
administration of ACE
inhibitors, 350
Bradykinin, 253–254
affecting coronary blood flow,
215–219
and effects of sulfhydryl-containing
agents, 218
cardiac effects of, 203, 204–205, 211
cardiac levels affected by ACE
inhibitors, 80
and cardiovascular actions of ACE
inhibitors, 253–281
in experimental atherosclerosis of
rabbits, 259–262
in hypertension, 257–259
in myocardial ischemia, 263–274
and neointima formation in rats,
262–263
in ventricular hypertrophy,
274–279
effects in myocardial ischemia and
reperfusion, 265–267, 272–274
metabolism of
angiotensin-converting enzyme
affecting, 184
angiotensin-converting enzyme
inhibitors affecting, 10, 11
and myocardial capillary growth
induced by ACE inhibitors,
278–279
in production of prostacyclin and
endothelium-derived relaxing
factor, 184, 215, 255
angiotensin-converting enzyme
inhibitors affecting, 257
release from isolated rat hearts,
271–272
vasodilating properties of, 215
Brain cardioregulatory areas,
angiotensin II receptors in,
131–135

Calcium
altered homeostasis in hypertrophied
hearts, 193–194
channels activated by angiotensin II,
103–104, 113
intracellular response to angiotensin,
76, 95, 105, 106
Cancer growth regulation by
angiotensin II, 146
Captopril. *See also* Angiotensin-
converting enzyme, inhibitors
effects during myocardial ischemia
and reperfusion, 207, 209

Cardiomyocytes
  angiotensin II affecting, 103–105
  renin in, 3
Cervical ganglia, angiotensin II
  receptors in, 130
Chymase, cardiac, 5, 309–328
  and angiotensin II generation, 9, 72,
    143–144, 239, 324–326
  clinical implications of, 326–328
  cDNA structure, 315–317
  and effects of ACE inhibitor therapy,
    327–328
  gene structure, 311–315
  localization and distribution of,
    323–324
  purification of, 310–311
  putative three-dimensional model of,
    321–322
  relation to other serine proteinases,
    317–318
  substrate specificity of, 318–321
Circulating renin-angiotensin system,
  233
  role in heart failure, 234–235
Collagen synthesis
  aldosterone affecting, 161
  in hypertensive ventricular
    hypertrophy, 155
Conduction system, cardiac
  angiotensin II receptors in, 6, 74,
    78–79, 94, 126–129, 240
  lack of angiotensin-converting
    enzyme in, 68
Contractility of heart, angiotensin II
  affecting, 9, 78, 79, 193–194
Coronary blood flow
  angiotensin-converting enzyme
    inhibitors affecting, 212–219,
    334–338
    bradykinin role in, 266
  cardiac renin-angiotensin system
    affecting, 8–9
Coronary vessels
  angiotensin-converting enzyme in,
    4–5, 7, 8, 68, 71
  cardiac renin-angiotensin system
    affecting, 333–340
  restenosis after balloon angioplasty
    affected by ACE inhibitors,
    338–339

Deoxycorticosterone levels, elevated,
  myocardial fibrosis in, 155, 157
Diabetes mellitus, angiotensin II
  affecting mesangial cells in,
    144–145

Diacylglycerol production, angiotensin-
  stimulated, 76, 94, 96, 106
Diastolic function in hypertrophied
  hearts, angiotensin II affecting,
    187–188, 239
  in ischemia, 190–193

Enalapril. See also Angiotensin-
  converting enzyme, inhibitors
  effects during myocardial ischemia
    and reperfusion, 207, 209
Endothelial cells
  angiotensin affecting, 108
  interaction with ACE inhibitors,
    255–257
  renin in, 142
Endothelin
  angiotensin affecting, 107, 108
  inotropic effects in ventricular
    myocytes, 112
Endothelium-derived relaxing factor
  actions in ischemic heart disease, 205
  formation from bradykinin, 184, 215,
    255
    angiotensin-converting enzyme
      inhibitors affecting, 257
  release affected by ACE inhibitors,
    216

Fibroblasts, cardiac
  angiotensin affecting, 11, 108–109
  collagen synthesis affected by
    aldosterone and angiotensin, 161
Fibrosis, myocardial
  in mineralocorticoid excess, 153–162
  in animals, 157–161
  in humans, 155–157
  with hypertension, 158–159
  in spontaneously hypertensive rats,
    160
  without hypertension, 159–160
  reactive, 155
  reparative, 155, 159
c-fos expression affected by
  angiotensin, 108
  and cardiac hypertrophy, 12, 80, 105
Fosinoprilat, effects during myocardial
  ischemia and reperfusion, 209

G proteins, angiotensin receptors
  coupled to, 102
Genes for AT_1 receptors, 92–93
Growth effects of angiotensin II, 57–58,
  63, 141–148
  on cardiac fibroblasts, 109
  on cardiomyocytes, 105

on cardiovascular tissue, 143–145
intracrine action in, 109, 147–149
on noncardiovascular tissues,
    145–149
role of receptors in, 6
on vascular smooth muscle, 106–108,
    142
and ventricular hypertrophy, 10–12,
    168. *See also* Ventricular
    hypertrophy

Heart failure
angiotensin-converting enzyme
    activity in, 236–239
angiotensin-converting enzyme
    inhibitors affecting, 11
angiotensin II role in, 80
coronary blood flow affected by ACE
    inhibitors in, 214, 337–338
risk factors in, 153–155
tissue renin-angiotensin systems in,
    233–249
  cardiac, 236–240
  renal, 240–245
  stage-dependent activation of,
      245–246
  therapeutic implications of,
      246–248
Heart rate, angiotensin II affecting,
    9–10, 78, 79, 104, 127–129
Hybridization probing
for cardiac angiotensinogen mRNA,
    49
for cardiac renin mRNA, 25–27
Hypertension
angiotensin-converting enzyme
    inhibitors in
  in angina pectoris, 221
  bradykinin affecting, 257–259
coronary blood flow affected by ACE
    inhibitors in, 214, 336–337
and myocardial fibrosis in
    mineralocorticoid excess,
    158–159
in spontaneously hypertensive rats
  angiotensinogen production in, 143
  and myocardial capillary growth
      induced by ACE inhibitors,
      278–279
  myocardial fibrosis in, 160
and trophic effects of angiotensin on
    vascular smooth muscle, 106–107
ventricular hypertrophy in, 167
  and antihypertrophic effect of ACE
      inhibitors, 274–277

Hypertrophy of heart. *See* Ventricular
    hypertrophy
Hypotension from intravenous
    administration of ACE
    inhibitors, 350

Infarction, myocardial
angiotensin-converting enzyme
    inhibitors in, 80, 219–220
  affecting ventricular remodeling,
      57
bradykinin affecting action of,
    272–274
cardiac angiotensin-converting
    enzyme in, 72–73
renal angiotensinogen levels in,
    240–241
ventricular remodeling after,
    345–357
  angiotensin-converting enzyme
      inhibitors affecting, 57, 80, 220
Inositol triphosphate, angiotensin-
    stimulated production of, 76, 94,
    110–111, 193
Ischemia, myocardial
angiotensin-converting enzyme
    inhibitors in, 335–336
  affecting coronary flow, 212–219
angiotensin II role in, 79–80
  and diastolic function in
      hypertrophied hearts, 190–193
beneficial effects of bradykinin in,
    272–274
and pathophysiological effects of
    cardiac renin-angiotensin
    system, 202–204
and reperfusion injury
  actions of angiotensin-converting
      enzyme inhibitors in, 191–193,
      206–212
  effects of angiotensins and
      bradykinin in, 265–266
  effects of bradykinin and ACE
      inhibitors in, 267–268
  in isolated working rat hearts,
      263–272
Isoproterenol-induced ventricular
    hypertrophy, 171–179

Kallikrein-kinin system, 253–255
Kidneys
mesangial cells affected by
    angiotensin, 144–145
renin-angiotensin system in heart
    failure, 240–245
Kininase I, 254

Kininase II, 254. *See also* Angiotensin-converting enzyme
Kinins, 253–255

Losartan, therapeutic potential of, 96

mas oncogene, and growth sensitivity to angiotensin II, 145–146
Mesangial cells, angiotensin II affecting, 144–145
Mineralocorticoid excess, myocardial fibrosis in, 155–162

Neovascularization, angiotensin II role in, 145
Neuroblastoma cells, growth affected by angiotensin II, 146
Neurohormonal mechanisms in heart failure, 234–235
Nitric acid. *See* Endothelium-derived relaxing factor

Perindopril. *See also* Angiotensin-converting enzyme, inhibitors
effects during myocardial ischemia and reperfusion, 207, 209
Phosphoinositol metabolism stimulated by angiotensin II, 76, 94, 110, 193
Phospholipase C activity affected by angiotensin II, 110
protein kinase C affecting, 111
Platelet activating factor, formation from kinins, 255
Platelet-derived growth factor, angiotensin affecting, 107
Polymerase chain reaction for cardiac renin mRNA detection, 28–34
quantitative studies with, 34–36
Potassium, reduced myocardial stores from mineralocorticoid excess, 155, 159
Pressure-overload hypertrophy
angiotensin role in, 105
cardiac angiotensin-converting enzyme in, 185–194
mRNA for, 71
diastolic function in, angiotensin affecting, 58
Prorenin activity, 39
Prostacyclin
cardioprotective effects of, 211
formation from bradykinin, 184, 215, 255
angiotensin-converting enzyme inhibitors affecting, 215, 257

release from isolated rat hearts, 269–271
Prostaglandin synthesis affected by angiotensin II, 114–115
Protein kinase C
activation by angiotensin II, 11–12, 105, 111–112
and diastolic function in hypertrophied hearts, 194
in mediation of angiotensin effects, 95–96
Pulmonary arteries
angiotensin-converting enzyme in, 67, 71
angiotensin II receptors in, 73

Ramipril. *See also* Angiotensin-converting enzyme, inhibitors
effects during myocardial ischemia and reperfusion, 209
Receptors for angiotensin II
AT_1 receptor, 74–75, 76, 89–90, 102–103, 109–110, 126
on cardiac fibroblasts, 108–109
cloning of, 91–92
genomic analysis of, 92–93
Losartan as antagonist of, 96
regulation of expression, 93
signal transduction by, 94–96
AT_2 receptor, 103, 126
regulation of expression, 93–94
signal transduction by, 96
and baroreceptor reflex, 131–133
in brain cardioregulatory areas, 131–135
in cardiac conduction system, 6, 74, 78–79, 94, 126–129, 240
characteristics of, 75–77
coupled to G-proteins, 102
coupled to second messenger pathways, 76, 94–95, 103
distribution in heart, 5–6, 66–67, 73–75, 184
localization in heart, 66–67
in peripheral sympathetic ganglia, 129–131
regulation of, 77
subtypes of, 74–75, 76, 89–90, 102–103, 126
Remodeling, ventricular
factors affecting fibrosis in, 153–162
in hypertension, angiotensin affecting, 109
postinfarction, angiotensin-converting enzyme inhibitors affecting, 57, 80, 220, 345–357

Renin
  and activation of angiotensin
    peptides, 52–53
  cardiac, 2–3, 65
    early studies of, 21–22
    immunochemical evidence for,
      22–23
    recruitment of cells for synthesis
      of, 36–37
    mRNA studies, 25–39. *See also*
      mRNA of cardiac renin
    role of, 39
    uptake from blood stream, 23
  in cardiovascular tissue, 142
  plasma activity affected by
    isoproterenol, 171–173
  in tumor vessels, 145
Reninlike activity in heart, 21–22
  in cultured cardiac cells, 24
  regulation of levels of, 23–24
Ribonuclease protection assay
  for cardiac angiotensinogen mRNA,
    49
  for cardiac renin mRNA, 27
mRNA of cardiac renin, 25–39
  hybridization probing for, 25–27
    negative findings in, 26–27
  localization of, 27
    in neonatal rats, 38–39
  polymerase chain reaction for, 28–34
    quantitative studies in, 34–36
  regulation of, 34–36
  in transgenic mice, 27–28

Second messengers
  angiotensin receptors coupled to
    pathways for, 76, 94–95, 103
  angiotensin-stimulated production of
    inositol triphosphate in pathways
    for, 76
  regulation by angiotensin, 95,
    101–116
Sinoatrial node. *See* Conduction
    system, cardiac
Sodium levels affecting cardiac renin
    mRNA, 26, 34, 35
Stellate ganglia, angiotensin II
    receptors in, 130
Steroids, anabolic, myocardial fibrosis
    from, 157
Sulfhydryl-containing angiotensin-
    converting enzyme inhibitors
  affecting bradykinin actions on
    coronary flow, 218
  cardiac effects of, 205, 212, 215
  interaction with organic nitrates, 216

Sympathetic ganglia, peripheral,
    angiotensin II receptors in,
    129–131

Thrombolytic therapy, angiotensin-
    converting enzyme inhibitors
    with, 220, 349–350
Tissue renin-angiotensin systems in
    heart failure, 233–249
  cardiac system in, 236–240
  renal system in, 240–245
  stage-dependent activation of,
    245–246
  therapeutic implications of, 246–248
Transforming growth factor-β,
    angiotensin affecting, 107
Transgenic research, 289–305
  experimental approaches in, 293–294
  human angiotensinogen gene
    expression in rats, 301–303
  methods used for animal species in,
    291–293
  mouse *Ren-2* gene expression in,
    295–299
  rat angiotensinogen gene expression
    in mice, 300–301
  renin mRNA in mice, 27–28
Tumor vessels, renin in, 145
Tyrosine kinase activity affected by
    angiotensin II, 113

Vagus nerve activity affected by
    angiotensin II, 133–134
Valves of heart
  angiotensin-converting enzyme in,
    68, 71
  angiotensin II receptors in, 73
Vascular smooth muscle cells
  angiotensin affecting, 106–108, 142
  proliferation affected by ACE
    inhibitors, 262–263
  renin synthesis in, 142
Vena cava, angiotensin-converting
    enzyme in, 67
Ventricles
  angiotensin-converting enzyme in,
    68, 71
  angiotensin II receptors in, 6, 74, 94
  renin mRNA in, 27, 38–39
Ventricular hypertrophy, 167–179
  angiotensin-converting enzyme gene
    expression in, 5
  angiotensin-converting enzyme
    inhibitors in, 57, 64, 143,
    168–171, 221, 236, 274–277
  bradykinin affecting, 276–277

angiotensin II role in, 80–81, 105,
143, 168
cardiac angiotensin-converting
enzyme in, 73, 185–194
cardiac angiotensin in, 239–240
in hypertension, 167
isoproterenol-induced, 171–179
mechanisms of, 167
mediation by renin-angiotensin
system, 10–12
postinfarction
angiotensin-converting enzyme
inhibitors affecting, 57, 80, 220,
345–357

in pressure overload, 167–179. *See
also* Pressure-overload
hypertrophy
in rats with aortic coarctation,
274–277
as risk factor for heart failure,
153–154

Zofenopril. *See also* Angiotensin-
converting enzyme, inhibitors
effects during myocardial ischemia
and reperfusion, 207, 209

Color Appendix

Fig. 1. Computer-generated color autoradiographs showing anatomical distribution of ACE in the rat heart. Coronal sections of the rat heart were obtained from the levels of the great vessels (panels A–D), the atrioventricular junction (panels E–G), and the ventricles (panel H) and incubated with ^{125}I-351A. The density of ACE is indicated by the color calibration bars. Red represents high levels of binding; yellow and green, moderate; and blue, low to undetectable. Abbreviations shown are AO, aorta; AAO, ascending aorta; DAO, descending aorta; AV, aortic valves; PA, pulmonary artery; PV, pulmonary valves; TR, trachea; OES, esophagus; RA and RAP, right atrium and right atrial appendage; LA, left atrium; LV, left ventricle; RV, right ventricle; CA coronary vessels; V, mitral or tricuspid valves; SVC, superior vena cava; MC, myocardium.

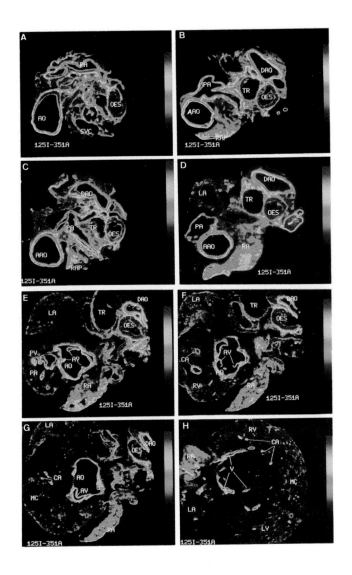

A3

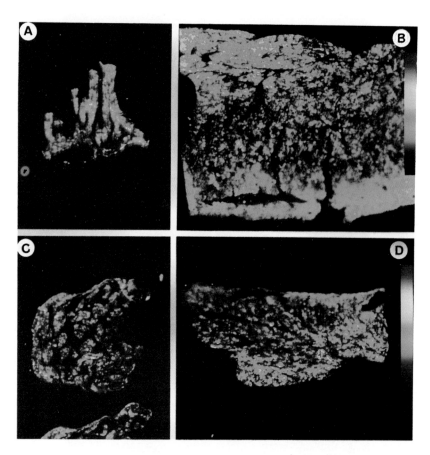

Fig. 4. Computer-generated color autoradiographs showing ACE binding in the human heart. Sections of the left atrium (panel A), left ventricle (panel B), right atrium (panel C), and right ventricle (panel D) of the human heart were processed for localization of ACE using ^{125}I-351A. Nonspecific binding, as determined in parallel incubations containing 1 mM EDTA, is undetectable.

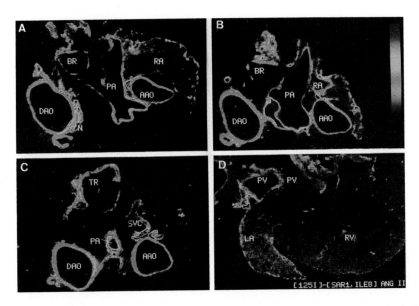

Fig. 5. Computer-generated color autoradiographs showing the anatomical distribution of A II receptors in the rat heart. Coronal sections of the rat heart at the levels of the atrium (panels A and B), great vessels (panel C), and ventricles (panel D) were processed for localization of A II receptor binding using ^{125}I-[Sar^1,Ile^8] A II. Abbreviations not included in Figure 1 are N, nerve trunk; SVC, superior vena cava; BR, bronchus. Interpretation of densities of cardiac A II receptors and other abbreviations are the same as those in Figure 1. (Derived from Allen AM, et al.)[30]

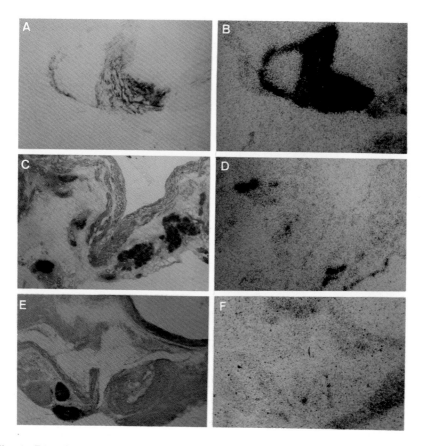

Fig. 6. Distribution of A II receptors in the atrioventricular node (panels A and B) and intracardiac ganglia of the rat heart (panels C–F). Sections in the left-hand panels (A, C, and E) were stained with acetylcholinesterase, and those in the right-hand panels (B, D, and F) are autoradiographs of A II receptor binding, where black regions reflect silver grains and high levels of binding. (Derived from Allen AM, et al.)[30]

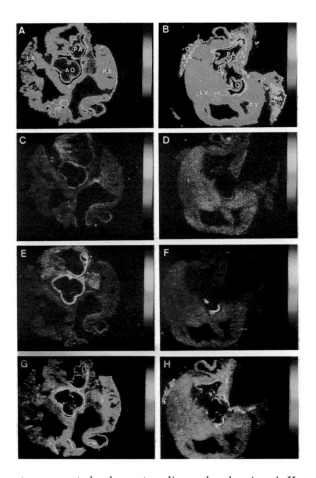

Fig. 8. Computer-generated color autoradiographs showing A II receptor subtypes in the rat heart. Binding is indicated by the color calibration bar, in which red is the highest density, and dark blue background levels. Coronal sections of the rat heart at the levels of the great vessels and atria (panels A, C, E, and G) and the atrioventricular junction (panels B, D, F, and H) were processed for localization of A II receptor binding using ^{125}I-[Sar^1,Ile^8] A II. Panels A and B show total binding; panels C and D show nonspecific binding, which was determined in the presence of an excess (1 μM) of unlabeled A II. Panels E and F indicate that Losartan (10 μM), an AT$_1$-specific antagonist, largely displaced A II receptor binding in the myocardium and the great vessels, whereas PD 123177, an AT^2-specific antagonist, only slightly inhibited binding (panels G and H). This indicates a predominance of AT$_1$ receptors in the rat heart but also some detectable AT$_2$ receptors, especially in the media of the great vessels. For abbreviations shown, see Fig. 1.

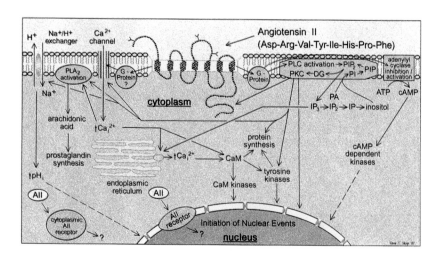

Fig. 1. General scheme by which A II, through the generation of intracellular second messengers, could affect muscle contraction, cell metabolism and growth, and gene expression. Binding of A II to the plasma membrane receptor(s) stimulates, via a G-protein, the lipolytic enzyme PLC, which hydrolyzes phosphatidylinositol 4,5-bisphosphate (PIP_2) to form two intracellular second messengers, diacylglycerol (DG) and inositol 1,4,5-triphosphate (IP_3). In smooth muscle, IP_3 releases Ca^{2+} from intracellular stores, thus increasing intracellular Ca^{2+}, $[Ca^{2+}]_i$, which leads to contraction via phosphorylation and activation of myosin light chain kinase by a Ca^{2+}/calmodulin-dependent (CaM) kinase. The increase in $[Ca^{2+}]_i$ in smooth muscle and other cell types (fibroblasts, etc.) may enhance protein synthesis and gene expression and/or transcription by activation of CaM and tyrosine kinases. Elevation of intracellular Ca^{2+} may also activate phospholipase A_2 (PLA_2), leading to arachidonic acid formation and activation of protein kinase C (PKC) or prostaglandin formation and smooth muscle relaxation. Generation of DG would activate (synergistically with elevated Ca^{2+}, in the case of Ca^{2+}-dependent isoforms) PKC, which in turn could stimulate (a) phospholipase A_2 or (b) gene transcription and protein synthesis via transactivating factors, tyrosine kinases, or the Na^+/H^+ exchanger (undefined pathway). The A II-receptor complex also activates, presumably via a G-protein, the plasma membrane L-type Ca^{2+} channel of cardiomyocytes, increasing $[Ca^{2+}]_i$ and resulting in (a) activation of CaM kinases and (b) the release of Ca^{2+} from the sarcoplasmic reticulum with subsequent contraction. Protein kinase C may directly activate the L-type Ca^{2+} channel and phosphorylate the A II receptor, resulting in desensitization or uncoupling of the A II-receptor complex from second-messenger production.

The A II-receptor complex may couple (positively or negatively) to adenylyl cyclase via a G-protein. The generation of adenosine 3',5'-cyclic monophosphate (cAMP) could affect cellular metabolism, contraction, and gene expression. Prostaglandins could also indirectly stimulate cAMP formation. Angiotensin II (internalized or produced within the cell) could affect gene transcription via interaction with a nuclear A II receptor and/or binding to chromatin.

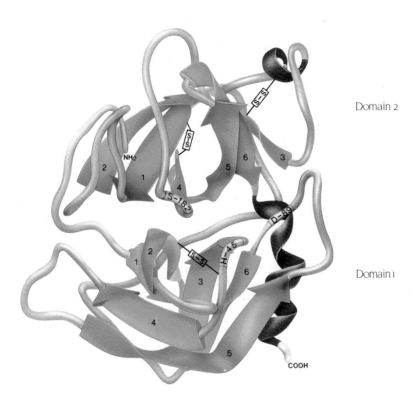

Fig. 7. A schematic model of human chymase. β-strands are shown as green ribbon-arrows. α-helices are shown as red ribbons. Active site serine, histidine, and aspartic acid are indicated as S-182, H-45, and D-89, respectively. Disulfides are shown as—S-S—.